'This beautifully written book has the advantage of coming from the perspective of a highly experienced practitioner-academic. Dr de Valois combines her knowledge of acupuncture in private practice with experience of working in an integrated healthcare team in the NHS – detailing biomedical and acupuncture approaches to managing the consequences of cancer treatments.'

– Dr Christine A. Barry BA BSc PhD, Medical Anthropology Senior Research Fellow, Brunel University (retired)

'This is an important contribution for acupuncture practitioners working in the field of cancer survivorship, bringing together acupuncture theory and available research evidence to provide an invaluable resource to inform practice.'

– Professor Deborah Fenlon PhD RGN, Emeritus Professor of Nursing, Swansea University, Wales

'Integrative medicine at its best!'

– Dr Jill Brook Hervik PhD, physiotherapist/acupuncturist and researcher, Pain Clinic, Vestfold Hospital Trust, Norway

'Meticulously written and researched by an acupuncture pioneer who wants cancer survivors to have the best life possible.'

– Dr Jane Buckle RN BPhil MA PhD, creator of the 'M' Technique, author, former nurse, researcher, and teacher of clinical aromatherapy

'A valuable resource for practitioners; very informative, clear, and written with an intelligent heart.'

– Margré de Vries LicAc BSc (Hons) Acupuncture Dip Shiatsu DO, Acupuncture and Shiatsu practitioner, London UK

ACUPUNCTURE and CANCER SURVIVORSHIP

Recovery, Renewal, and Transformation

Beverley de Valois

Forewords by Jennifer A. Stone MSOM, LAc and
Dr Catherine Zollman MBBS, MRCP, MRCGP

Illustrated by Bruce Hogarth

SINGING DRAGON
LONDON AND PHILADELPHIA

First published in Great Britain in 2023 by Singing Dragon, an imprint of Jessica Kingsley Publishers
Part of John Murray Press

1

A CIP catalogue record for this title is available from the British Library and the Library of Congress

ISBN 978 1 91342 627 9
eISBN 978 1 91342 628 6

Printed and bound in Great Britain by CPI Group

Jessica Kingsley Publishers' policy is to use papers that are natural, renewable and recyclable
products and made from wood grown in sustainable forests. The logging and manufacturing
processes are expected to conform to the environmental regulations of the country of origin.

Jessica Kingsley Publishers
Carmelite House
50 Victoria Embankment
London EC4Y 0DZ

www.singingdragon.com

John Murray Press
Part of Hodder & Stoughton Limited
An Hachette UK Company

For Mom and Jeanne

And for Christy Barry

Contents

Part III: Milestones and Beyond

Part IV: Acupuncture for Transformation and Renewal

Foreword by Jennifer A. Stone

In the mid 1990s, Beverley was living in England and I in the United States.

I was fresh out of Chinese medicine school with an unknown future, and I found myself defending my right to practise in my state of Indiana after receiving a cease-and-desist order for practising medicine (Chinese medicine) without a licence. I was instantly a grass-roots lobbyist.

In England, Beverley read *The Death of a Woman*, the story of a 37-year-old woman dying of cancer, which sparked her passion for helping cancer patients. As a patient of Chinese medicine herself, she understood how acupuncture and Chinese medicine could help the multiple symptoms cancer patients suffer. She altered her trajectory and began to study Chinese medicine and research. She aimed to help validate the medicine and increase the evidence, and ultimately become an activist for acupuncture as an evidence-based adjunct to cancer care.

In 1999, in Indiana in the US, our law finally passed, and acupuncturists were granted licences to practise.

In Reading, England, Beverley completed her programme at the College of Integrated Chinese Medicine and joined the Supportive Oncology Research Team at her new post at Mount Vernon Cancer Centre in Middlesex.

For me, life changed again quickly as doors began to open – I participated in a complementary medicine elective at Indiana University School of Medicine, I was hired to consult and provide acupuncture at Central Indiana Cancer Center, and I joined a research team at Indiana University and performed acupuncture on rats for neuroscience studies. I instantly found a new passion – treating cancer patients and building bridges between the acupuncturists and the researchers with the goal of increasing evidence for the use of acupuncture.

Now both Beverley and I have the shared experience of over 20 years' working at different hospitals and universities in the USA and UK. We spent decades working with incredible mentors, with academic research societies, participating in research working groups, publishing peer-reviewed papers and book chapters, and developing an international network of brilliant like-minded colleagues. Today we are relied on as experts in the field.

In 1995, things were so different. We had different dreams. We could not anticipate how our lives would change and shift and we would end up walking parallel paths on different sides of the Atlantic, eventually coming together through our passion for oncology and acupuncture and increasing the evidence base…and yet, here we are.

This book is valuable not only for clinicians and providers who use acupuncture in oncology, but for all acupuncturists working in hospitals and private practices. Cancer survivors are everywhere, they are patients in all departments and specialties. They often choose acupuncture and other natural therapies as an adjunct to their care.

Beverley has collected empirical evidence treating cancer patients in clinics for over 20 years. Trained in research, her critical mind saw patterns that led to research explorations and ultimately the development of this text.

She includes reports of individual cases in every chapter. The character development in the vignettes and the case studies makes the reader wonder if they're reading a peer-reviewed medical text or more classical literature.

The patients in this book were living their lives, raising their families, working and serving when they got the news 'you have cancer'. Everything changed and their lives were never the same. When you read their stories, you see the kind of people they are, how they felt, what they experienced, and how acupuncture and Chinese medicine helped and changed them.

In addition to providing valuable evidence-based resources for using all styles of acupuncture in cancer survivors, this book is also entertaining. While improving clinical skills, it might also help you have a stronger connection to your patients who are cancer survivors.

I found this book inspiring and believe it will increase your passion for working with these most exceptional patients who have had the shared experience of a cancer diagnosis.

Jennifer A. Stone MSOM, LAc
Assistant Research Faculty
Department of Anesthesia
Department of Pediatric Oncology
Indiana University School of Medicine
Co-Chair Indiana University Integrative Medicine Consortium
Senior Editor, *Medical Acupuncture*, Mary Ann Liebert Publishing

Foreword by Catherine Zollman

As Medical Director of the Integrative Cancer charity, Penny Brohn UK, and an NHS GP with a special interest in cancer medicine, I have regularly seen how helpful, and sometimes life-changing, supportive therapies like acupuncture can be for people after a diagnosis of cancer. However, many acupuncturists lack specific cancer knowledge and training, and are therefore understandably nervous about taking on clients who have had cancer, despite the potential benefits. So when Beverley told me she was writing a practical guide on cancer survivorship for acupuncturists and asked me to write this foreword, I felt very honoured and excited, because this book will fill an important educational gap, and Beverley is one of the few people I know who is truly qualified to write it.

I have known Beverley and admired her unique contribution to the field of integrative oncology since I was a young medical oncology trainee interested in playing my own role in this fascinating and expanding area. She is in the very unusual position of having worked at the 'coal face' as an acupuncturist, seeing patients in a busy NHS cancer centre over decades. At the same time as practising acupuncture, she has contributed to the international understanding of the role of acupuncture in cancer care, by undertaking and publishing a series of well-designed and highly informative research projects. These have demonstrated the far-reaching impacts that acupuncture can have, when integrated with a person's mainstream cancer treatment and management. Beverley's acupuncturist mindset and years of practical experience enable her to see the whole person in front of her, and address their symptoms in relation to their overall health and wellbeing. This holistic approach, combined with her years of cancer experience and the analytic precision and reflective practice she has acquired through her rigorous research, gives Beverley an unusual and multi-faceted perspective, and makes her the perfect guide to examine and explain the full potential of East Asian medicine/acupuncture in the context of cancer survivorship.

After completing active cancer treatment, people often have one or more 'survivorship concerns', which can be physical, emotional, psychological, social, or existential/spiritual, and can vary hugely from individual to individual. Skilled holistic assessment and active intervention are often needed to enable people to live well again. This book explains the cancer survivorship experience, and teaches readers how acupuncture can be used safely, in a way that both directly addresses many common concerns – like menopausal symptoms, fear of recurrence or fatigue – and also takes cancer patients on a journey from 'symptom to self'. It describes approaches which can help acupuncturists support cancer survivors through the many difficulties they may encounter, and into post-traumatic growth. Finally, Beverley looks at long-term resilience and explains how acupuncture, with its ability to both address difficult symptoms and increase people's energy levels, can improve motivation and lead to improved self-care, as well a greater ability to cope with life's continuing challenges.

Beverley appreciates the value of creating a therapeutic alliance, by always listening to and observing the patient (the book is filled with patients' verbatim testimonials and perspectives) and never being surprised by what she sees or hears. Her decades of direct cancer patient contact, and her modest and curious outlook on her work, give her a refreshing humility and an important humanity which she infuses throughout this book. She never mandates; instead she offers examples and suggestions for how practitioners can develop their own practices and techniques. This gives this book a unique combination of wisdom, depth, and the practical utility that ensures readers will refer to it time and time again.

Cancer can create a powerful 'window of opportunity' for change. Some people, with the right support, make profound changes to lifelong habits and patterns that might previously have seemed deeply entrenched, and find themselves living with enhanced general health and wellbeing and a greater appreciation of life. Acupuncturists are in the privileged position of being able to help cancer survivors address their troublesome symptoms while, at the same time, facilitating them to find these personal paths to growth and wellbeing. Increasing numbers of people are living and struggling after a diagnosis of cancer, and I am certain that acupuncturists who read this book, and learn from its many practical and wise observations and suggestions, will gain the knowledge and confidence they need to support more of them into recovery, renewal, and transformation. I wish them every success along the way!

Dr Catherine Zollman MBBS, MRCP, MRCGP
Fellow in Integrative Medicine (University of Arizona)
Medical Director, Penny Brohn UK
NHS GP
Global Ambassador to the UK, International Society of Integrative Oncology
Director, British Society of Integrative Oncology

Acknowledgements

In a career spanning nearly three decades, I have numerous people to thank for their input, insights and inspiration. My immense gratitude to the many mentors, colleagues, teachers, supervisors, patients, academics, researchers, conference and editorial committees, and friends who all contributed to my development as an acupuncturist and researcher, and to the eventual creation of this book.

A special thanks to Val Fear, who inspired me to write this book. And to the many people living with and beyond cancer who chose to have acupuncture, especially those who have generously shared their stories. Thank you also to the chapter reviewers, acknowledged on the next page, who freely gave their time, wisdom, and insight – and especially to those who reviewed multiple drafts of multiple chapters!

I am also grateful to:

- Margaret Kennedy, Erica Yonge, Elaine Clarke, and Pam Thorpe, who opened successive doors in the 1990s, enabling me to become an acupuncturist working with people with cancer.
- Professor Jane Maher, who initiated my research career, for her advice to 'always assess; always collect data'.
- The charitable funders who enabled much of my work, including Dr Richard Ashford, the Milly Apthorp Charitable Trust, the Lynda Jackson Macmillan Centre, and the East and North Hertfordshire Hospitals' Charity.
- The *European Journal of Oriental Medicine*, so instrumental in developing my writing skills.
- The School of Social and Community Medicine, University of Bristol, for my role as Honorary Research Fellow and for ongoing collegial, intellectual, and academic support.
- My publisher, Singing Dragon, and to Handspring before that, especially for granting me Susan Stuart, my Development Editor, whose experience, knowledge, patience, and cheerful support have been invaluable.
- Dr Jane Buckle, Isobel Cosgrove, Angela Hicks, and Jacqui Jensen, the amazing 'doulas' in bringing this book into being.

Special thanks are due to Teresa Young, my research colleague for over 20 years, during which time we have forged a truly creative relationship. Teresa's vision, support, and ingenuity enabled my continuous exploration of acupuncture in the supportive care of people with cancer.

And thank you most especially to my partner, Lee Cotton, whose continuous generosity, support, and love enabled it all.

Reviewers

Dr Richard Ashford MA, MBBChir, FRCP, FRCR, DMRT
Consultant Clinical Oncologist, Mount Vernon Cancer Centre, Northwood, Middlesex, UK

Dr Christine A. Barry BA, BSc, PhD Medical Anthropology
Senior Research Fellow, Brunel University, London, UK (retired)

Maggie Bavington LicAc, MSc Chinese Herbal Medicine
Acupuncturist and Herbalist, London, UK

Dr Eran Ben-Arye MD
Director, Integrative Oncology Program, Lin, Carmel & Zebulun Medical Centers, Clalit Health Service, Haifa, Israel; Primary Researcher, Middle East Research Group in Integrative Oncology (MERGIO), within the Middle East Cancer Consortium (MECC); Society for Integrative Oncology (SIO) Regional Ambassador to Europe and the Middle East; Co-chair of the SIO Online Task Force and SIO Global Task Force

Dr Jane Buckle RN, BPhil, MA, PhD
Creator of the 'M' Technique. Author, former nurse, researcher, teacher of clinical aromatherapy, London, UK

Kim Chan BA (Hons), MA, LicAc, MBAcC
Programme Leader for Acupuncture Skills, Chinese Medicine Lecturer and Clinical Supervisor, College of Integrated Chinese Medicine, Reading, Berkshire, UK

Dr Claudia Citkovitz PhD, MS, LAC
Adjunct Faculty, Massachusetts College of Pharmacy and Health Sciences. Author of *Acupressure and Acupuncture during Birth*

Liz Cook LicAc, MBAcC
Acupuncturist, London, UK

Isobel Cosgrove BA(SS), MA (Oxon), MLitt, FBAcC
Acupuncturist and Founder of UK Supervision Network, London, UK

Louise Derry-Evans BSc TCM (Acupuncture), Dip QiGong Tuina
Acupuncturist, London, UK

Margré de Vries LicAc, BSc (Hons) Acupuncture, Dip Shiatsu DO
Acupuncture and Shiatsu practitioner, London, UK

Dr Shelley Smith DiCecco PT, PhD, CLT-LANA
Assistant Professor, Physical Therapy Department, Philadelphia College of Osteopathic Medicine, Georgia Campus; Owner, LymphEd LLC, a lymphoedema education company; Director, Pelvic Floor and Lymphedema Services, The Sports Rehabilitation Center, Atlanta, Georgia, USA

Amy Din MSc, BSc (Hons), Dip MBAcC
Traditional acupuncturist. Senior Research Assistant, Trial Coordinator, PhD candidate, University of Southampton, UK

Professor Deborah Fenlon PhD, RGN
Emeritus Professor of Nursing, Swansea University, Wales

Dr Rob Glynn-Jones FRCP, FRCR
Consultant Oncologist, Macmillan Lead Clinician in Gastrointestinal and Colorectal Cancer, Mount Vernon Cancer Centre, Northwood, Middlesex, UK. Chief Medical Advisor, Bowel Cancer UK

Dr Ruth A.R. Green MBBS, FRCP, FRCR
Consultant Radiologist, Royal National Orthopaedic Hospital, London, UK

Dr Jill Brook Hervik PhD
Physiotherapist/acupuncturist and researcher. Pain Clinic, Vestfold Hospital Trust, Norway

Angela Hicks BSc, LicAc, FBAcC, MRCHM
Co-founder and President, College of Integrated Chinese Medicine, Reading, Berkshire, UK

Jacqui Jensen BA (Hons), LicAc
Practitioner, Operations Director and Tutor, The Acupuncture Academy Ltd., Leamington, UK

Natalie Kruger BPhty, PgCert Advanced Lymphoedema Management, MPhil candidate
Senior Physiotherapist, Royal Brisbane & Women's Hospital, Australia

Professor Alex Molassiotis RN, PhD
Chair Professor and Head of School of Nursing, The Hong Kong Polytechnic University, Hong Kong

Dr Rhian Noble-Jones PhD, PgD (Advanced Professional Practice in Physiotherapy), PgC (Academic Practice)
Chartered Physiotherapist; Casley-Smith Lymphoedema Method Instructor; National Lymphoedema Researcher, Lymphoedema Network Wales; Associate Lecturer, Swansea University; Senior Honorary Lecturer, University of Glasgow; Chair, British Lymphology Society Scientific Committee; Director, Casley-Smith Lymphoedema Education UK Ltd.

Rachel Peckham MSc, LicAc, FBAcC
Acupuncturist. Trustee and trainer, NADA GB, London, UK

Simon Prideaux LicAc, LicCHM, IBCLC, DO
Osteopath, Lactation Consultant, Acupuncturist, and Medical Herbalist, London, UK

Julia Quick LicAc, MBAcC
Acupuncturist, London, UK

Daniel Schulman BSc, MSc, DiplAc New England School of Acupuncture, DiplAc NCCAOM
Acupuncturist. Writer. Chairperson, Association of Registered Acupuncturists of Prince Edward Island. PEI, Canada

Dr Richard Simcock MBBS, MRCPI, FRCR
Consultant Clinical Oncologist, Sussex Cancer Centre, Brighton, UK

Theresa Sullivan BSN
Senior Staff Nurse, Lynda Jackson Macmillan Centre, Mount Vernon Cancer Centre, Northwood, Middlesex, UK

Raquel Torralba BSc Acupuncture, BSc Physiotherapy, LicAc, MBAcC
Physiotherapist and Acupuncturist, Marlborough, UK

Teresa Young BSc
Supportive Oncology Research Team Lead, Mount Vernon Cancer Centre, Northwood, Middlesex, UK

Preface

This is the first fully peer-reviewed evidence-based book about using acupuncture in the supportive care of cancer survivors post treatment. The reviewers are experts in their own field from Australia, Canada, Hong Kong, Israel, Norway, the UK, and USA, comprising academics, oncology and other healthcare professionals, and acupuncturists. I am grateful for their time and contribution, which have enabled this book to be truly ground-breaking.

This book focuses on the care of people who are in remission and are facing the challenges of adjusting to the 'new normal' after completing primary cancer treatment. Although their cancer has been 'cured', many people experience complex health issues after cancer treatment ends, often requiring the care of professionals from many health-care disciplines. Acupuncture has the potential to be an important contributor in the multidisciplinary care of cancer survivors.

In 1996, David L Sackett wrote that evidence-based medicine 'integrates the best external evidence with individual clinical expertise and patients' choice'.[1] I have sought to embody these three important principles of evidence-based medicine in this book. As well as providing details from research studies to the acupuncture community, I share the discoveries of my clinical practice and research. I am grateful to the patients who chose to have acupuncture and share their stories. Overall, my aim is to make practitioners (and users) of acupuncture aware of the challenges of cancer survivorship and the positive impact acupuncture can have on these.

My journey of working with people with cancer was inspired in 1995, when Margaret Kennedy, my meditation teacher, recommended I read *The Death of a Woman*,[2] a Jungian analyst's account of a 37-year-old woman dying of cancer. On reaching the final page, I knew I had found my vocation. The book opened my eyes to a world of healthcare that, while challenging, also had potential to be rewarding – for both patient and practitioner.

It became my goal to work with people with cancer and I have been privileged to do so for nearly 30 years. In 1996, I began working with inpatients as an aromatherapist with the Macmillan Oncology and Palliative Care Team, led by Elaine Clarke, at London's North Middlesex University Hospital. That same year, acting on advice from my acupuncturist Erica Yonge, I began studying acupuncture at the College of Integrated Chinese Medicine in Reading, UK. On qualifying in 1999, and thanks to Pam Thorpe, I commenced working at the Lynda Jackson Macmillan Centre (LJMC) at Mount Vernon Cancer Centre in Northwood, Middlesex (now part of the East and North Hertfordshire NHS Trust). Following the maxim, 'always assess; always collect data', I quite unexpectedly started on the path to becoming a researcher and joined the Supportive Oncology Research Team (SORT) in 2000. For over 20 years, my role as Research Acupuncturist has enabled me to conduct pioneering research (including a PhD) into using acupuncture and moxibustion in the supportive care of people with cancer.

People diagnosed with cancer are surviving longer after treatment. This is good news. Once considered a terminal illness, cancer is regarded more and more as a *chronic* condition. During the late 1970s, the median survival time for all cancers was just one year from diagnosis.[3] Today, due to improved diagnosis and treatment, expected survival times for many cancers are now longer than ten years. Among my friends, family, and patients are many who mark 20–30 years since their cancer diagnosis.

This change brings new challenges. For many, cancer and its treatments leave a legacy of health problems that may persist long after treatment ends. Healthcare agencies around the world are recognising the long-term consequences of cancer and its treatments, with an increased focus on 'survivorship programmes' to address this growing area of health concern.

As an acupuncturist and researcher, I have observed and systematically assessed the benefits cancer survivors may experience when they have acupuncture treatment. These range from symptom relief to emotional and spiritual support to facilitating improved self-care, as well as the significant shift that comes from being able to accept what has been and what is now. Furthermore, acupuncture offers a drug-free means of healthcare with minimal, if any, side effects – an important feature in meeting the challenges of today's opioid crisis.

At its most powerful, acupuncture treatment can be the catalyst for a process of transformation and profound renewal. Over years of practice and research, I have heard innumerable cancer survivors tell me, 'Acupuncture has given my life back'.

Cancer is one of the most feared diseases in the modern world. It is often daunting to face the complexity of this condition. Yet acupuncture can do so much to increase the wellbeing of cancer survivors. I hope this book can lead to an important cultural shift in the role of acupuncture, making it a vital part of multidisciplinary care in helping people recover after cancer treatment. This is an area of the cancer care continuum which has been underserved by all medical care.

I also hope this book encourages more acupuncturists to use their skills to improve the lives of cancer survivors everywhere. May this book inspire your journey.

Beverley de Valois PhD, LicAc, FBAcC, MBLS
August 2022

References

1. Sackett DL, Rosenberg WM, Gray JA, *et al.* Evidence based medicine: what it is and what it isn't. BMJ Open 1996;312(7023):71–72.
2. Wheelwright JH The death of a woman. New York: St. Martin's Press; 1981.
3. Macmillan Cancer Support Living after diagnosis: median cancer survival times. London: Macmillan Cancer Support; 2012.

Introduction: How to Use this Book

The underlying philosophy of this book is encapsulated in these quotations:

> Evidence based medicine is not 'cookbook' medicine...External clinical evidence can inform, but can never replace, individual clinical expertise... (Sackett *et al.*)[1]

> I personally think that acupuncture is really an 'art' as the choice of points and their combination, besides being determined by the identification of patterns and treatment principle...are also influenced by subtle factors such as the patient's pulse and emotional state at the time of consultation and even factors such as the season, the moon phase and the time of day. (Maciocia, Preface to *The Channels of Acupuncture*)[2]

Sackett and Maciocia, from their very different standpoints, express that both evidence-based medicine and acupuncture are 'arts', relying on individual clinical expertise and judgement.

I offer this book as a bridge between acupuncturists, biomedical healthcare professionals, researchers, and cancer survivors. My purpose in writing is twofold. First, I wish to raise awareness about the challenges of cancer survivorship among the community of acupuncture practitioners, whatever their style of acupuncture. Second, I believe acupuncture is a powerful tool that can improve the wellbeing and quality of life of cancer survivors, and I want to share my experience of working in this field from both evidence- and practice-based perspectives, demonstrating the art involved in each.

Long-term cancer survivorship is a recent phenomenon. It requires all healthcare professionals to develop new methods to meet the needs of survivors. In this book, I present perspectives from biomedicine, East Asian medicine, acupuncture research, clinical experience, as well as case studies to provide a 360-degree perspective of the topics discussed.

Biomedical perspectives

I have assumed that non-medically trained acupuncturists will be supporting survivors who are or have been under the care of oncology healthcare professionals. Thus, I have presented the medical background of cancer treatments and their consequences, to provide insight into what cancer survivors have experienced. I also hope this will facilitate communication between acupuncturists and oncology healthcare professionals.

East Asian medicine perspectives

I have written this book to accommodate practitioners of acupuncture from most, if not all, styles of practice. My own training at the College of Integrated Chinese Medicine integrated Five Element and 'traditional' Chinese medicine theoretical frameworks. In effect, I grew up 'bilingual' in the world of acupuncture, which made me open towards the many styles of acupuncture in practice today. Consequently, I have written this book with a wider focus than on the usual 'TCM'. My purpose is to provide a context within which *any* acupuncturist can bring their own style of practice to improve the quality of life of cancer survivors.

Acupuncture research

Most acupuncturists are not researchers, and accessing research papers often requires costly outlay (although open access publications are becoming more common). My aim is to present the acupuncture point protocols used in research, making them available to the acupuncture community. Sharing these contemporary findings may enlarge our repertoire of approaches.

It has not been my aim to critically evaluate the research studies, and I have relied on summaries from systematic reviews to do this.

Clinical experience

I also present observations and discoveries made in my clinical practice and research in the supportive care of cancer survivors and share tips for clinical practice.

It is not my intention to provide a 'cookbook' of prescriptions or protocols; those that are presented serve as illustrations. My aim is to empower practitioners to find solutions that are relevant to their style of practice, to the context they are working in, and to the characteristics of their patients.

Case studies

Throughout the chapters, I present patient experiences using vignettes and case studies. These provide practical examples to acupuncturists, as well as demonstrating the potential effects of acupuncture to non-acupuncturists and future patients. Acupuncture for people with complex, chronic conditions involves hard work by both practitioner and patient. These illustrate the realities of practice, and I am honest about the challenges and setbacks, as well as celebrating breakthroughs.

All individuals portrayed have given their permission to share their stories, and I have altered certain details to ensure their anonymity. Where possible, I have involved patients in writing their case studies to ensure that they genuinely reflect the experiences of cancer survivors.

Throughout the book, quotations from research participants are presented following the convention used in qualitative research, that is, using the unique code for each participant (e.g. 011 BC, or Participant 45). The abbreviations BC or HNT refer to Breast Cancer and Head Neck Throat respectively.

How to read this book

This book is divided into four parts.

Part I provides the background to cancer survivorship:

- Chapter 1 discusses what cancer survivorship is, and how acupuncture can help. Emily, a breast cancer survivor, eloquently shares her experience of cancer diagnosis, treatment, and acupuncture.
- Chapter 2 details the late and long-term consequences of cancer treatments.
- Chapter 3 explores the emotional impacts of cancer diagnosis and treatment.

Part II presents the specific practical details of acupuncture treatment:

- Chapter 4 discusses how complex conditions can be addressed using simple treatments.
- Chapter 5 presents a 'toolkit' of approaches I have developed for use in my work and serves as an example for other practitioners to develop their own toolkits.
- Chapters 6–10 present the 360-degree perspectives on five common consequences of cancer treatment.

Part III explores wider issues:

- Chapter 11 discusses the milestones of cancer survivorship and the challenges individuals experience at key stages in their lives after cancer treatment.
- Chapter 12 explores how to improve resilience.
- Chapter 13 discusses cancer recurrence and second primary cancers.

Part IV brings this all together in the extended case study of Ann, a breast cancer survivor with lymphoedema, detailing her 13 acupuncture treatments and the (sometimes unexpected) results.

Appendices are available online only and can be downloaded from www.singingdragon. com/catalogue/book/9781913426279:

- Hot Flush and Night Sweats Diary
- Further Information and Resources
- Colour photographs of Figures 8.1, 9.5A, and 9.5B.

Notes on terminology

I have tried primarily to use the term 'East Asian medicine' (EAM) to reflect that acupuncture, moxibustion, and associated practices developed across East Asia – in Japan, Korea, and Vietnam, as well as China.

I have also needed to find terms to distinguish between the styles (or theoretical frameworks) of Five Element acupuncture and that which is often called 'TCM' (Traditional Chinese Medicine). After long discussion with colleagues (many thanks to Dr Felicity Moir and Dr Claudia Citkovitz), I have settled on 'Chinese medicine' to describe the latter. However, when referring to numerous textbooks and research publications that use the term 'TCM', I have followed their terminology.

For acupuncture point names, I have followed the conventions used in *A Manual of Acupuncture*,[3] with one exception, which is that I refer to the Sanjiao (SJ) channel as the Triple Burner (TB).

In endeavouring to keep capitalisation to a minimum, I have again followed the example of *A Manual of Acupuncture*. Thus, I have capitalised the names of the Chinese organs or *zang-fu* (Heart, Spleen, Kidney, etc.) to differentiate them from the biomedical organ names (heart, spleen, kidney). This also applies to differentiate other terms common to both systems (Blood/blood, Conception/conception, etc.).

Finally, I am not conversant in Chinese languages, and my access to the literature emanating from China is limited to that published in English.

Figures

Figures are for illustrative purposes; for details of point location the reader should refer to specialist texts on the subject.

References

1. Sackett DL, Rosenberg WM, Gray JA, *et al.* Evidence based medicine: what it is and what it isn't. BMJ Open 1996;312(7023):71–72.
2. Maciocia G The channels of acupuncture: clinical use of the secondary channels and eight extraordinary vessels. Edinburgh: Churchill Livingstone; 2006.
3. Deadman P, Al-Khafaji M, Baker K A manual of acupuncture. Hove: The Journal of Chinese Medicine; 2007.

Part I

INTRODUCTION TO SURVIVORSHIP

Chapter 1

Cancer Survivorship and the Role of Acupuncture

Introduction

The challenge that cancer survivorship poses to people with a history of cancer, and the potential for acupuncture to address this is encapsulated in the following quotations:

> People with a history of cancer do not rejoin the land of the well when they are deemed cancer free. Rather, they live in the ambiguous space between the well and the sick. (Bell & Ristovski-Slijepcevic, 2013)[1]

> I have been feeling much brighter than I have for some time and have lost the feeling of being sad and depressed. I also have more motivation and interest in things in general … At present I am feeling better than I have felt for the past four years. (Cancer survivor's comments about acupuncture treatment)

This book focuses on using acupuncture and moxibustion for the rehabilitation of people who have completed primary treatment for cancer, and who:

- are in remission
- have ongoing consequences
- are well and require support adapting to having 'had' cancer.

In the words of Bell and Ristovski-Slijepcevic: those people occupying the space between being well and sick. People are living longer after being treated for cancer, thanks to early diagnosis and improved treatments. However, the impact of cancer may continue after treatment ends: people may have problems resulting from the cancer itself or from the treatments used to eradicate it. These 'consequences' may be physical and/or emotional, short-term or chronic, and affect social and working relationships. They may have crucial impacts on quality of life.

Acupuncture can play an important role in helping cancer survivors towards improved wellbeing. It can support recovery after treatment, improve health and wellbeing, and facilitate a return to active living. It can be especially useful in supporting survivors to establish a 'new normal' as they adjust to life with a chronic condition.

This chapter sets the context for this book, discussing the terms *cancer survivor* and *cancer survivorship*. It introduces the concept of the *consequences* of cancer and its treatments and discusses how acupuncture can address these. Feedback from patients and research participants conveys their experience of acupuncture treatment. To conclude this chapter, Emily, a breast cancer survivor, shares a frank account of her journey from diagnosis and treatment through to long-term consequences, and how acupuncture helped her.

TERMINOLOGY

What are 'consequences'?

'Consequences' and 'consequences of cancer and its treatment' are terms used in oncology literature to refer to the wide range of long-term physical and psychosocial changes that appear to be associated with cancer and its treatment, regardless of how long ago the diagnosis and treatment were given. Other terms commonly used in oncology literature include: side effects, late effects, toxicity, adverse effects, long-term effects, chronic effects and consequences of treatment.[2]

Cancer survival

People diagnosed with cancer are surviving longer. In 2018, there were nearly 4.5 million cancer survivors worldwide diagnosed within the previous five years.[3] Today, people live nearly ten times longer after a cancer diagnosis than they did in the 1970s, and half of people diagnosed with cancer are predicted to survive their disease for at least ten years.[4,5]

Table 1.1: Comparison of ten-year survival rates by cancer site 1971–1972 and 2010–2011 (for England and Wales)

Note:
Cancers in **bold** are the 4 most common cancers diagnosed in both the UK and USA.

Cancer type	% 10-year survival 1971–1972	% 10-year survival 2010–2011	% Increase in survival rate
All cancers combined (male)	20	46	26
All cancers combined (female)	28	54	26
Testicular	69	98	29
Malignant melanoma	46	89	43
Prostate	**25**	**84**	**59**
Breast	**40**	**78**	**38**
Non-Hodgkin lymphoma	22	63	41
Bowel	**19**	**57**	**38**
Leukaemia	5	46	39
Brain	6	13	7
Oesophageal	4	12	8
Lung	**4**	**5**	**1**
Pancreas	1	1	0

Source: Cancer Research UK (2014)[5]

Survival times have improved dramatically for many cancers, including breast, colorectal, and testicular cancer, Hodgkin lymphoma, and childhood leukaemia[6] (Table 1.1). Factors facilitating such improved outcomes include screening programmes, early diagnosis, new drugs, and increased understanding of the genetic make-up of some cancers (personalised or precision medicine).

Despite these improvements, many people continue to experience health issues after treatment ends. In the UK, an estimated 25% of cancer survivors are living with long-term consequences of cancer or its treatment.[4] Consequences may continue for many years, and new health problems may emerge – even decades after cancer treatment.[2]

The cancer trajectory

To set the context, an overview of the cancer trajectory is helpful. The Survivorship Pathway (Figure 1.1), developed by the UK's National Cancer Survivorship Initiative (NCSI), provides a model to illustrate the possible states of health or illness a person with cancer may experience.[7]

A simplified diagram, it shows the potential routes a person might take following primary treatment for cancer, examples of which are given in Box 1.1. (The Cancer Control (or Care) Continuum, a similar model developed in the USA, uses the stages aetiology, prevention, early detection, diagnosis, treatment, survivorship, and end of life.)

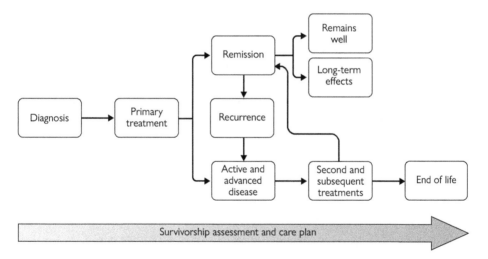

FIGURE 1.1: THE NCSI SURVIVORSHIP PATHWAY[7]

Often, the type of cancer predicts the likely route. For example, most men diagnosed with testicular cancer will have no evidence of disease following primary treatment, nor will they experience any subsequent recurrence. For other cancers (e.g. brain, oesophageal, lung, and pancreatic cancers), few people will be disease-free following primary treatment.

Other factors influence the possible route that any individual might follow. These include the:

- stage of cancer at diagnosis
- rate at which the cancer is likely to grow and spread
- cancer treatments administered (and the decade in which they were administered)
- person's age, gender, and genetic profile
- person's pre-existing health conditions and medications
- social, geographic, and economic factors (personal, regional, national), including the level of healthcare available.

Increasing numbers of people enter remission following primary treatment. While many recover and remain well, others experience health issues that are a legacy of cancer and its treatments. Before discussing the needs of these individuals, it is important to introduce the concepts of *cancer survivor* and *cancer survivorship.*

Box 1.1: Some possible outcomes after primary cancer treatment

- Remission, remains well, no recurrence, e.g. testicular cancer.
- Remission, may experience recurrence some time (months or years) later, e.g. breast, prostate cancer.
- Only a minority of patients will be disease-free, e.g. lung, pancreatic cancer.
- Some patients presenting with active or advanced cancer may die from their cancer within weeks or months, e.g. various cancers.
- Some patients may live with chronic cancer for years; they may die 'with' cancer but 'from' another cause, e.g. elderly prostate cancer patients.
- Cancer responds to treatment for a period and then relapses. The cancer may respond to subsequent treatment, e.g. melanoma patients who receive new treatments repeatedly, each with a short-lived but dramatic improvement.

Who is a cancer survivor?

In biomedicine, 'survivor' refers to individuals who have had a life-threatening disease (cancer or non-cancer) and remained disease-free for at least five years.[1]

The term 'cancer survivor' was used first by the American physician Fitzhugh Mullan in his seminal publication *Seasons of Survival: Reflections of a Physician with Cancer.*[8] Writing from his own cancer experience, he posited that all people diagnosed with cancer were occupied with the process of survival, which he divided into three stages or seasons:

- **Acute survival:** beginning at diagnosis and defined and dominated by cancer treatment.

- **Extended survival:** when treatment ends, and the individual focuses on the consequences of treatment.
- **Permanent survival:** the evolution from the phase of extended survival into a period when the cancer can be considered permanently arrested: 'The patient in this phase is indeed a survivor'.[8]

Mullan co-founded the USA's National Coalition for Cancer Survivorship (NCCS), which shifted the perception of the person with cancer from 'victim' to 'survivor', offering this definition: 'from the time of diagnosis and for the balance of life, an individual diagnosed with cancer is a survivor'.[1,9]

The USA's National Cancer Institute (NCI) extended this definition to acknowledge the wider community of people profoundly affected by the cancer diagnosis of a loved one, adding: 'Family members, friends, and caregivers are also impacted by the survivorship experience and are therefore included in this definition.'[10]

In England, the NCSI developed this definition: 'Someone who is living with or beyond their cancer. This could be someone who has completed their treatment or having ongoing treatment for their cancer.'[7]

Thus, 'cancer survivor' has numerous meanings. In all its forms, it seeks to move away from a 'binary notion of cure versus noncure' to encompass the complexity of having cancer, 'the vagaries, phases and syndromes of survival'.[8]

Many dislike the term 'survivor'. In the UK, focus group participants involved in the NCSI project were divided equally in their preference for the terms 'cancer survivor' and 'people living with and beyond cancer', with both groups feeling strongly about their preferred term (Professor EJ Maher, personal communication, 7 September 2015).

Others prefer 'someone who has had cancer', although this implies that cancer is a past event. As demonstrated throughout this book, the presence of cancer or the threat of cancer may be ongoing for an individual. As a chronic condition, 'cancer is unusual insofar as those successfully treated may be deemed cancer free – although not, for the most part, cured'.[1]

The use of 'cancer survivor' in this book

While respecting that many dislike the term 'cancer survivor', I have chosen to use it in this book. In previous attempts, I found using 'people living with and beyond cancer' awkward and unwieldy, especially when used frequently. Reducing it to an acronym 'PLWABC' is a less attractive option than 'cancer survivor'.

TERMINOLOGY

What does 'cancer survivor' mean in this book?

As discussed, 'cancer survivor' encompasses numerous possibilities. Clarifying the definition has precedents in the medical literature,[11] and in this book it refers to adults who:

- have had cancer diagnosed and treated after the age of 18 years

- completed primary (first-line) treatment for early-stage disease and given with curative intent
- do not currently have evidence of active disease (are in remission)
- have health issues mainly attributed to cancer treatment.

The scope of this definition is illustrated in Figure 1.2. The shaded boxes highlight the aspects of the Survivorship Pathway that are this book's focus.

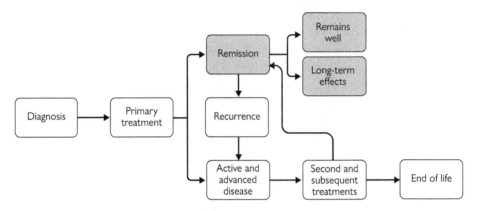

FIGURE I.2: THE SURVIVORSHIP PATHWAY SHOWING THE FOCUS OF THIS BOOK

What is cancer survivorship?

Cancer is viewed increasingly as a chronic, long-term condition, and most cancer survivors will also have at least one other chronic condition.[12] Awareness of the special requirements of this population is increasing. To meet their needs, many countries have developed cancer survivorship programmes or initiatives (Table 1.2) to improve post-treatment care and help people 'embrace their lives beyond illness'.[13] These programmes aim to increase understanding and support for the consequences of cancer treatment.

This marks a shift from the traditional focus on the cancer itself to addressing the broader, individual needs of people living with cancer as a chronic condition. Historically, cancer services have been directed towards:

- primary treatment (the intention to cure cancer)
- palliative and end-of-life care.

Follow-up care typically focused on monitoring the patient for signs of:

- recurrence (the return of cancer in the primary site)
- metastasis (the spread of cancer to another part of the body).

Shading in Figure 1.3 highlights these stages on the Survivorship Pathway. Unlike conditions such as heart attack or stroke, there was no emphasis on post-treatment rehabilitation.[14] Healthcare concentrated on the cancer itself. It did not address the health issues resulting from cancer and its treatments – issues that may last for months or years, may surface many years after treatment ends, and may change over the survivor's lifespan.

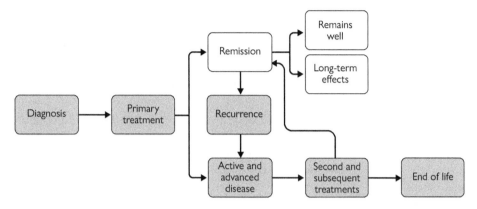

FIGURE I.3: THE SURVIVORSHIP PATHWAY SHOWING THE HISTORICAL FOCUS OF CANCER CARE

Survivorship programmes seek to encompass the physical, psychosocial, spiritual, and existential effects that may be associated with cancer. They aim to enable recovery, health, wellbeing, and return to work after cancer treatment. As well as identifying the continuing healthcare needs of all cancer survivors, programmes endeavour to help people live healthy and active lives for as long as possible.[7]

These programmes also advocate that aftercare should be multidisciplinary, personalised, and take into account the individual's needs and preferences.[14,15] The UK's *Recovery Package*, for example, combines multiple interventions to improve outcomes and care for people living with and beyond cancer, 'supporting them to prepare for the future, identify their individual needs and support rehabilitation to enable them to return to work and/or a near normal lifestyle'.[16]

Table 1.2: Examples of survivorship programmes[14]

Country	Programme name	Website
Australia	Australian Cancer Survivorship Centre	www.petermac.org/cancersurvivorship
	Victorian Cancer Survivorship Programme	www.health.vic.gov.au/health-strategies/victorian-cancer-survivorship-program
Canada	The Canadian Partnership Against Cancer	www.partnershipagainstcancer.ca
Netherlands	Netherlands Cancer Institute	www.nki.nl/research/our-science/survivorship
UK	National Cancer Survivorship Initiative	www.macmillan.org.uk/documents/aboutus/health_professionals/macvoice/sharinggoodpractice_therecoverypackage.pdf
USA	Office of Cancer Survivorship	http://cancercontrol.cancer.gov/ocs

Why focus on these aspects of survivorship?

Just as biomedicine has traditionally focused on cancer treatment and end-of-life care, so has the field of complementary (or integrative) medicine. In general, cancer services offering these therapies have historically supported patients undergoing cancer treatment and nearing the end of life.

Research into these therapies has also focused on these stages of the survivorship pathway. For example, acupuncture for the management of chemotherapy-induced nausea and vomiting (CINV), an acute consequence of active cancer treatment, has been widely researched, with one systematic review identifying over 26 studies of CINV.[17] There is a growing body of investigation into using acupuncture to manage a range of consequences of cancer treatment, including pain, xerostomia (dry mouth), fatigue, and bowel and bladder disorders. Most of these studies focus on patients undergoing active treatment or in late-stage disease. Some address the consequences of long-term adjuvant treatments (such as hot flushes or arthralgia related to adjuvant hormonal treatments); there are few studies investigating the late effects of cancer treatment (such as lymphoedema).

Similarly, English language textbooks about acupuncture or Chinese herbal medicine in cancer care also focus mainly on treatments related to active disease or end-of-life care (see Further Information and Resources in the Appendices, online).

ESSENTIALS

In this book, I make the cultural shift in the approach to care and support for people affected by cancer – away from the predominant focus on cancer as an acute or terminal illness, to a greater focus on recovery and health and wellbeing after cancer treatment.[7] I am concerned mainly with dealing with the aftermath of treatment, and supporting cancer survivors over the long term to deal with cancer as a chronic condition.

While I discuss the management of common symptoms experienced by cancer survivors post treatment, my aims for using acupuncture correspond with those of survivorship programmes – to enhance recovery, improve health and wellbeing, and facilitate a return to active living.

How does this book support integration into cancer survivorship programmes?

Awareness of possible consequences, an important aspect of supporting cancer survivors, is low among the public, healthcare professionals, and cancer survivors. Research identified that only 40% of UK cancer survivors were aware of the long-term consequences of cancer and its treatments. Of those, some were not aware of how these consequences might affect them personally. A survey of general practitioners with an interest in cancer revealed that 64% had not received any training about long-term consequences.[7]

ESSENTIALS

This book aims to improve awareness of survivorship issues among the community of acupuncturists. Acupuncturists should be aware of those in their patient list with a history of cancer and of the potential consequences.

This will help them better identify the aetiology of persistent or inexplicable symptoms that can arise, even after a period of good health, when neither the patient nor acupuncturist links them to previous cancer treatment. Furthermore, the topics and case studies throughout this book provide examples that may be used to explain the benefits of acupuncture to existing and potential patients who are cancer survivors.

This book also articulates the potential of acupuncture – and acupuncturists – to improve the wellbeing of cancer survivors. It is intended as a stimulus for developing both clinical and research approaches for this growing population with its specific, long-term healthcare needs.

By developing awareness of the needs of cancer survivors and how acupuncture can address these, I hope that acupuncturists will be empowered to build relationships with cancer care organisations. This may be through developing services, taking part in research, or simply offering ongoing clinical care to cancer survivors.

How can acupuncture support cancer survivors?

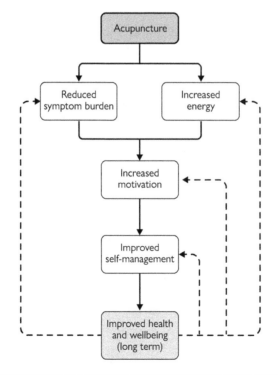

FIGURE I.4: ACUPUNCTURE AS A PROCESS FOR FACILITATING LONG-TERM HEALTHCARE

My observation of patients in research and clinical settings convinces me that acupuncture has the potential for wide-ranging and long-term benefits for cancer survivors, a view supported by feedback from patients. More than a magic bullet targeted at specific symptoms, acupuncture can be a process that leads to enduring improvements in overall wellbeing. It has the potential to empower individuals and facilitate them in managing their own health (self-management), which is essential for living with chronic conditions.

Figure 1.4 illustrates this process, showing how improvement in each of the elements can create a positive feedback loop to become a self-generating cycle of improvement. The stages are discussed below.

Reduced symptom burden
Acupuncture's key role is, obviously, to manage or eliminate symptoms. Research evidence increasingly supports acupuncture's effectiveness in managing consequences of cancer treatments, and it is recommended for symptoms which have limited biomedical solutions, such as fatigue, unresolved pain, hot flushes, xerostomia, dyspnoea (breathlessness), and anxiety.[18]

Many characteristics of acupuncture make it suitable for addressing the complex needs of cancer survivors:

- It can address multiple symptoms simultaneously. Cancer survivors often present with multiple concurrent symptoms. Biomedicine tends to address symptoms separately, leading to polypharmacy and increased risk of drug side effects and interactions.[19] The systemic nature of acupuncture (including the constitutional focus of Five Element acupuncture) facilitates treatment of multiple imbalances simultaneously. Acupuncture can be considered a form of 'one-stop shopping' to address multiple symptoms, as illustrated repeatedly in case studies throughout this book.
- Acupuncture can reduce or eliminate the need for some medications. **This applies specifically to medications that are not essential for maintaining life.** Many people wish to minimise their reliance on pharmaceutical products after cancer treatment. Acupuncture can facilitate this. For example, many survivors find acupuncture effective for managing pain, enabling them to reduce pain medications. Additional benefits of this include reduction or elimination of side effects such as dry mouth or constipation,[20] as well as having wider implications for healthcare in the face of the opioid crisis. Where pharmaceuticals are essential (e.g. adjuvant hormonal treatments to reduce risk of cancer recurrence), acupuncture can manage troublesome side effects. A study found acupuncture as effective as the antidepressant venlafaxine for managing breast cancer treatment-related hot flushes. Women in that study who had acupuncture were untroubled by the side effects of venlafaxine (nausea, dry mouth, dizziness, anxiety) and reported improvements in energy, clarity of thought, and wellbeing.[21]
- Acupuncture is generally a safe intervention. Numerous large studies demonstrate that acupuncture administered by trained acupuncturists is safe. Adverse

events, which are minimal, include transient pain, bruising or bleeding at the needle site, and tiredness after treatment.[22,23]

Increased energy

Acupuncturists are familiar with patients reporting – often with surprised delight – that their energy levels have improved, even after a few treatments. This improvement is of major importance for people recovering from cancer treatments. In my view, acupuncture's effect on vitality is a major contribution to rehabilitation for cancer survivors and I have positioned it equally with reduced symptom burden in Figure 1.4.

It's logical that energy levels improve when symptoms reduce; energy consumed by coping with those symptoms is liberated. I frequently observe that symptoms improve only after the individual's energy improves, especially when treating women with breast cancer treatment-related hot flushes. It seems the body requires its energy to be augmented before it can address troublesome symptoms. While some patients report a noticeable surge in energy following their first treatments, for others the interplay between reduced symptom burden and increased energy is a gradual, ongoing expression of the rebalancing of the body's qi. For these reasons, I have represented them as being interdependent and mutually reinforcing phases in Figure 1.4.

Increased motivation

Motivation is an important factor when living with chronic illness. A motivated patient is more likely to:

- apply a constructive approach to dealing with health problems
- seek specialist consultation
- practise preventative medicine
- adopt lifestyle practices (exercise, diet, stress management) that will enhance their sense of wellbeing.[24]

Clearly, motivation is necessary for cancer survivors to develop behaviours that enable them to live well with their chronic condition. Although complex, motivation can be described simply as the 'desire to change'.[25] Many people find they lose their motivation during cancer treatment; the process of acupuncture can act as a catalyst for change. Within the model in Figure 1.4, improved symptoms and increased energy are the foundation for improving motivation. This stands to reason: when we feel better, we are more likely to want to take actions to continue to feel better.

Improved self-management

Self-management is a key strategy in managing chronic illness and aims to empower patients to attain optimum health and wellbeing. This includes helping patients to better understand their disease and the healthcare system and support available to them, as well as developing skills in problem-solving and decision making. It encourages people living with chronic disease to engage in activities that protect and promote health, to manage the signs and symptoms of illness, and to address aspects of illness including medical and emotional management, and changes in the individual's role.[26]

Acupuncture can empower patients 'to make informed choices, adapt new perspectives and generic skills that can be applied to new problems as they arise, to practise new health behaviours, and to maintain or regain emotional stability'.[27] This is enabled partly through improving motivation, which facilitates the individual taking control of their healthcare. Lifestyle advice, an integral part of many styles of acupuncture consultation, also contributes to facilitating self-management.

Lifestyle advice is more than imparting information about healthy living to patients. It involves actively engaging the individual in making decisions about what changes to make and how to implement these in daily living to become enduring practices for good health. Changing habits can be challenging; acupuncturists can also support and encourage individuals to persevere with changes until they become habits.

Improved health and wellbeing (long term)

This model extends the discussion about the benefits of acupuncture beyond that of treating symptoms to facilitating long-term improvements in health and wellbeing. As treatment progresses and motivation increases, cancer survivors can regain confidence in their ability to take control of their health.

Feeling better is a powerful incentive to continue to feel better. This develops positive feedback mechanisms, feeding into any or all of the elements within the model (as indicated by the dotted lines in Figure 1.4) with the potential to become a self-generating process. This is a very beneficial aspect for rehabilitation of cancer survivors, and for supporting their living with cancer as a chronic condition.

What do survivors say about acupuncture?

In reviewing feedback of research participants' experiences of acupuncture treatment, it is striking how many describe this process. Repeatedly, cancer survivors report symptom reduction, often in multiple symptoms in addition to their main complaint. They delightedly note their increased 'energy', and write about being more 'motivated', giving examples of actions they have implemented to improve their self-care and long-term wellbeing. They comment on feeling able to return to work, deal with family and social commitments, and cope with cancer and the consequences of treatment.

This is demonstrated in the vignettes of Verna and Davida (below), research participants who consented to their stories being shared and whose names have been altered to protect their identity. Describing in their own words the benefits they experienced from acupuncture treatment, they illustrate a range of experiences: of the consequences of cancer and its treatments, of the possibilities that acupuncture holds for restoring health and wellbeing, and of being empowered to self-manage.

VIGNETTE: VERNA – WONDERFUL TO FEEL NORMAL AGAIN

Verna, aged 64, a breast cancer survivor with lymphoedema, wrote after 13 acupuncture treatments:

> My life has changed quite dramatically. I have very little pain from the lymphoedema and that has improved my quality of life. I am not so short tempered, I am far more tolerant with my grandchildren, and I feel much more relaxed within myself. I have taken up hobbies again that I let lapse because the lymphoedema made them difficult to do or I lacked the patience...
>
> After the first few [acupuncture] treatments I was virtually pain free. It was wonderful to feel 'normal' again and the general sense of wellbeing affected all areas of my life. I felt more energetic and able to take up the strings of my life again. I joined a swimming club and my husband and I now go out and about again...
>
> My self-confidence has never been greater. I am dealing with my weight problem in a positive manner and in 14 weeks managed to lose 30 pounds.

VIGNETTE: DAVIDA – ACUPUNCTURE GAVE ME HOPE

Davida, aged 62, a breast cancer survivor who suffered tamoxifen-related hot flushes, wrote after eight acupuncture treatments:

> [Acupuncture has] given back some 'life'. I was just existing... Constructive thinking is now possible. Fewer night sweats mean much-improved sleep. Wake with some energy. Able to relax more in evenings, couldn't do before. Pace myself better, spirits improved... even the promise of acupuncture gave me hope as I felt I was on a downward slope, sinking lower and lower.
>
> [Acupuncture] gave me fresh hope that I could slowly pick myself up...[and the] ability to start to relax and cope better with feelings of despair and panic.
>
> [Acupuncture treatment was the] first rung on ladder to dealing with problems positively. Now I attend a cancer support group to discuss experiences/fears and so on. Restarted yoga...[and] driving lessons. [Am] endeavouring not to push myself beyond my limitations; not to run myself into the ground again.

Additional benefits of acupuncture treatment

Cancer survivors appreciate features characteristic of some acupuncture frameworks, discussed in the literature as a 'complex intervention'.[28–30] These include:

- a whole-person approach to the individual
- individualisation of treatment
- creation of a safe space
- taking time out.

Whole-person healthcare

The concept of treating 'body, mind, and spirit' underpins the philosophy of many forms of acupuncture practice, and many cancer survivors appreciate this capacity to encompass more than just the physical symptoms. Maxine, a breast cancer survivor with lymphoedema, commented:

> I'd been going back and forth to the doctor and felt no one was actually listening to me, you know, how I felt. They kept saying 'go to the chemist' and I had done and nothing was improving, and I just felt that [my acupuncturist] was listening to me. And she was taking the whole, you know, looking at me as a whole, not just at the medical problems that I had.

Individualisation of treatment

It may be stating the obvious to say that tailoring treatment to the individual's changing needs is integral to practice for many acupuncturists. However, in some areas there is increasing pressure to provide standardised treatments. For example, it is common for research protocols to specify a limited selection of points, which may be relevant for answering research questions, but limits clinical practice.

Flexible, dynamic approaches are appropriate for cancer survivors, whose needs may change over time. Remaining responsive to these changes is an important aspect of treatment, appreciated by cancer survivors, as this focus group participant describes:

> [The acupuncturist] was willing to say, 'Look I think we need to move from this, what we originally said, you need to work on this emotional side as well with the acupuncture.' So she did change things as the weeks developed and then changed back when I was a bit stronger.

Creation of a safe space

For many cancer survivors, acupuncture treatment becomes a 'safe space'. This develops partly through the therapeutic relationship, as patients develop trust in their acupuncturist. Knowing they will be listened to, and their concerns acted on, is integral to this process, as is confidence in the expertise of their acupuncturist. Also important are the caring attitude and professionalism of the practitioner. In this environment, many survivors feel able to release emotions, articulate deeper concerns, and begin to make sense of their cancer experience. This safe space is described by a breast cancer participant in a focus group:

> I got to the point...of going in [to the acupuncture treatment] and I was going through a divorce at the time, and one of my close friends had just died and so forth, there were a lot of things. And I'd go in and within two minutes I'd be crying... And I just felt like I was just dumping everything, going in.

Taking time out

Making time for treatment is a commitment. For many survivors, acupuncture provides an opportunity to take time out for themselves. Work, family, and social obligations often take priority, especially for those whose energy is limited, or who may be trying to make up the time lost to cancer and its treatments. A breast cancer survivor said of having acupuncture:

> To be truthful it was really quite nice, to have an hour where I lay on the bed and didn't have to feel guilty that I wasn't doing anything else! So it was really quite nice actually, that side of it.

How can acupuncture align with the aims of survivorship programmes?
Throughout this book, I explore how acupuncture and acupuncturists can play a vital role in the multidisciplinary management of cancer as a chronic condition. I believe strongly that acupuncture can address the needs identified by the NCSI,[7] to help people treated for cancer to:

- return to as normal a life as possible, or to support changes in priorities and make a transition to a 'new normal'
- be empowered to take control of their own care
- know that the importance of consequences (e.g. hot flushes) will be recognised and help given to them
- know that their anxieties and fears will be taken seriously
- know that they will be given advice on living healthily to maximise their chance of remaining well for as long as possible.

Cancer survivors should also feel confident that their acupuncturist:

- knows what to expect and what to look out for
- is aware of the early signs of further disease or consequences of cancer
- will care for them and treat them as individuals.

How many treatments are needed?
This discussion has illustrated how acupuncture can help long-term outcomes. Many biomedical decision makers are wary of acupuncture, based on an incorrect perception that acupuncture treatment must continue long term to be effective.

Some survivors opt to continue to have long-term treatment, for example, Alauda (see Chapter 8, Cancer Treatment-Related Hot Flushes and Night Sweats) and Claire (see Chapter 11, Survivorship: Navigating the Milestones). However, as demonstrated in the preceding examples, survivors report noticeable changes after 13 treatments. Throughout this book, there are numerous examples of improvements after three, five, and eight treatments. The case study of Ann (see Chapter 14, Getting My Life Back) shows how 13 treatments gave her resources to draw on for many years after treatment ended.

Emily's story – a survivor's perspective

To exemplify the preceding discussion, it is useful to call on a survivor's story. Emily sent me this account of her experience as a spontaneous response to a question raised in a meeting. Her story is a powerful description of her experiences as a cancer survivor, and of how acupuncture helped.

Although not intended for publication, Emily agreed to its use in this book with minor edits. These comprised adding headings corresponding with the Survivorship Pathway, and some small changes to clarify meaning, indicated by square brackets.

EMILY'S STORY

Introduction

Emily, age 60, was diagnosed with breast cancer in 2005. I met her in 2009, when she received 13 acupuncture treatments as a participant in research into using acupuncture to improve wellbeing for cancer survivors with lymphoedema (see Chapter 9, Cancer Treatment-Related Lymphoedema). She had previously received eight ear acupuncture treatments for tamoxifen-related hot flushes (see Chapter 8, Cancer Treatment-Related Hot Flushes and Night Sweats). After the lymphoedema study, Emily participated in developing funding proposals to continue research into using acupuncture for cancer survivors with lymphoedema. The following text is Emily's own words.

Background

The background is necessary to put the improvement into perspective. This is my experience and that of others may be completely different. This…is not intended to be a 'moan' about the way I was treated [in the medical system]. Everyone is treated the same and there are a lot of people to treat. They do their best in the time available but they do keep you waiting for an inordinate length of time when you go to the hospital appointments, when you are already in an anxious state.

Diagnosis

I found a lump and was seen the same day by the GP. They arranged an appointment with the consultant the following week. The appointment involved a number of tests; biopsy, ultrasound, mammogram, and so on. It was fairly obvious to me then that there was something wrong. A further appointment was made to give the biopsy results. I had to have more tests during the following week; ECG, whole body scan, CAT scan, and so on.

By this stage, you are reduced to a sleepless, quivering jelly. The operation was scheduled for the next week. The whole thing took less than four weeks and you are just taken along with the flow and don't really think straight at all, so it is difficult to ask the right questions. Your feet never touch the ground. I was fortunate to have the support of my husband.

Primary treatment

The operation was on Monday and I was sent home on Thursday morning – this was the day before the Easter holiday weekend. I was not given any medical support (except for a long bandage to replace the one in place. I could not possibly put it on as I was immo-bilised on one side) but I was told that I could go back to the hospital in an emergency.

I had to return in ten days to have the stitches removed. I had been seen [by] the physiotherapist, for about five minutes, two days after the operation but, as I had tubes protruding from several orifices, she couldn't do much. I did not see her again. The sister on the ward gave me a sheet with exercises on it but no one went through it with me. I was issued with a 'pad' to replace the missing breast. It was about half the size of the remaining breast. What a morale booster. Everyone would know! (I did not get a prosthesis properly fitted until the first silicon one ruptured and I *finally* saw the person who knew how to fit them.)

By this stage, you feel mutilated, uninformed, terrified, and isolated. Nothing has really been explained. I found that it was like walking around with a book under my arm. You could feel both sides but not where the arm touched the ribs. No one mentioned that might/would happen. There was, and is, lack of sensation in large areas. They give out a book but I suppose they have [to] address the lowest common denominator and I found it of little use. I took to the internet and quickly found that there was conflicting information. Trust Mayo Clinic, reject Wikipedia.

Just as you are starting to pull yourself together, an appointment is arranged with the consultant oncologist. I was spared the chemotherapy and radiotherapy – that is kept in reserve for a possible future event, somewhat like a sword of Damocles.

Remission

I was set on a course of tamoxifen. This caused tremendously bad hot flushes. They are far, far worse than menopausal flushes. They happened in the day as well as at night. It seemed as though the body thermostat had stopped working. It also causes the skin to become so dry that it starts to resemble reptilian scales. Sleep is also adversely affected. Great for the self-esteem and energy levels!

No one tells you of the side effects so you think it is only you and you should be grateful for being saved and not moan. After a year of this I saw the consultant and begged for something else. Arimidex® was prescribed. This has much the same effect but was less severe.

Every time you mention a side effect they look at you quizzically and treat you as though this is the first they have heard of it. The dry skin causes severe itching – all over. The medication makes you feel tired and by 7.30 in the evening you really cannot hold up any longer. You try, but by 8.30 you are off to bed. Sleep for a few hours and wake up with hot flushes, profuse sweating and itching. Wakeful for some hours and, with luck but not always, drop off for another hour or so. Go to the GP and ask for something to help you sleep and get a lecture about addiction to sleeping tablets and nothing to help. Comments about going to bed too early are thrown in for good measure. So, with self-confidence at rock bottom, you face life.

Faced with the situation there are basically two choices: give in and submerge in the misery or fight your way out. I chose the latter. I went back to teaching, albeit on a part-time basis, and went to several groups in the U3A [University of the Third Age].

Long-term effects

So, there you are, body image at an all-time low, isolated, demoralised and feeling generally very tired and low, when your arm suddenly swells up. Short of getting a metastasis, this is the worst. Eventually I found [the lymphoedema nurse] who makes you an active participant in the treatment, and explains things. There is, however, the sleeve. Old people wear elastic bandages. I am not old. I have an elastic bandage and, ergo, must be old. … There are other bad problems but the sleeve is…a horror for me.

Fight back again, but it is wearying. Further demoralised, I realised that I had not been out in the evening for five years. My poor husband had been left sitting alone every evening during the majority of that time.

How acupuncture helped

Someone asks if I would like to participate in a research project to remove hot flushes – anything to make *some* symptoms disappear: why not try?

You go along to the [ear acupuncture treatments]… Go along to the fifth [treatment] with no hope, as no improvement has been felt. I suppose they must have some people for whom it does not work. Fifth treatment and unbelievably, symptoms start to subside. Will it continue? Only one more visit to go. Well, yes it did and has continued and what a blessed relief it was and is. It was a truly amazing improvement.

The next research project was very specifically not to reduce the lymphoedema but to promote wellbeing. Well, the ear one worked well so maybe this would too.

This was a totally different approach, being completely tailored to the individual. The specific things that bothered each person were addressed and heeded. That in itself was an enormous help. The acupuncture was aimed at specific problems. As a slow responder the last time, I did not hope for a swift change but gradually found that the sleep was improving. The sleep pattern was, after four years, established and, even now (after 2010), after cessation of the medication, is difficult to change effectively but the acupuncture helped a lot. Acupuncture effectively stopped the itching which, in turn, helped with the sleep. What a blessed relief.

The other main effect of the acupuncture was to help emotionally. The whole view of life improved: the body image, self-confidence, which, in turn, helped with social intercourse. The feeling of isolation vanished. It was unfortunate that while the treatment progressed I had a few problems. My mother became ill, my husband was fighting his employers for unjust dismissal due to age, and a few other things. These could have skewed the results and could have caused regression but I was able to cope with the difficulties much more effectively than I would have anticipated just a few months earlier.

I also started to take an interest in the décor at home. I had, I realised, just got on with the cleaning and ignored everything else but now I was more interested.

Emily's summary of her biomedical treatment

Insufficient attention is paid to the side effects which are dismissed so readily by some health professionals. If a person feels isolated, self-conscious, too tired to be bothered and, maybe due to these effects and lymphoedema, unable to go out or mingle with other people, their mental state will deteriorate, they will become introverted and maybe head for dementia when it is not necessary. The NHS [National Health Service] would effectively save money by investing in helping people to cope with these debilitating side effects instead of ignoring them or, worse still, pretending that they are of no consequence or do not exist.

CHAPTER SUMMARY

To conclude, I will let Emily speak. In reviewing this chapter, she wrote:

> This…represents both the problems faced by cancer survivors and the beneficial effect which can be obtained, by the use of acupuncture, in the relief of the many side effects associated with the various treatments. The view needs to be seen as twofold: the removal of the immediate threat of cancer, and the following treatments. The patient is very grateful for the first but would like more support and information about the second, which can be very debilitating. This chapter shows clearly the two sides of the coin.

References

1. Bell K, Ristovski-Slijepcevic S Cancer survivorship: why labels matter. J. Clin. Oncol. 2013;31(4):409–411.
2. Macmillan Cancer Support Throwing light on the consequences of cancer and its treatment. Macmillan Cancer Support; 2013. Available from: www.macmillan.org.uk/Documents/AboutUs/Research/Researchandevaluationreports/Throwinglightontheconsequencesofcanceranditstreatment.pdf
3. American Cancer Society The cancer atlas. Atlanta, GA: American Cancer Society; 2019.
4. Macmillan Cancer Support Statistics fact sheet. London: Macmillan Cancer Support; 2021. Available from: www.macmillan.org.uk/_images/cancer-statistics-factsheet_tcm9-260514.pdf
5. Cancer Research UK Cancer statistics report: cancer survival in the UK up to 2011. London; 2014. Available from: www.cancerresearchuk.org/health-professional/cancer-statistics/survival#heading-Zero
6. Macmillan Cancer Support Living after diagnosis: median cancer survival times. London: Macmillan Cancer Support; 2012.
7. Department of Health, Macmillan Cancer Support, NHS Improvement The National Cancer Survivorship Initiative Vision. London: Department of Health; 2010.
8. Mullan R Seasons of survival: reflections of a physician with cancer. N. Engl. J. Med. 1985;313:270–273.
9. Ahmed RL, Prizment A, Lazovich D, et al. Lymphedema and quality of life in breast cancer survivors: the Iowa women's health study. J. Clin. Oncol. 2008;26(35):5689–5696.
10. Office of Cancer Survivorship Definitions. 2014. Available from: http://cancercontrol.cancer.gov/ocs/statistics/definitions.html
11. Glare P, Aubrey K, Gulati A, et al. Pharmacologic management of persistent pain in cancer survivors. Drugs 2022;82(3):275–291.
12. Macmillan Cancer Support The burden of cancer and other long-term health conditions. Macmillan Cancer Support; 2015. Available from: www.macmillan.org.uk/documents/press/cancerandother-long-termconditions.pdf
13. National Cancer Institute Facing forward: life after cancer treatment. National Institute of Health; 2018. Available from: www.cancer.gov/publications/patient-education/life-after-treatment.pdf
14. Jefford M, Rowland J, Grunfeld E, et al. Implementing improved post-treatment care for cancer survivors in England, with reflections from Australia, Canada and the USA. Br. J. Cancer 2013;108:14–20.
15. Jacobsen PB, Mollica MA Understanding and addressing global inequities in cancer survivorship care. Journal of Psychosocial Oncology Research and Practice 2019;1(1):e5. DOI:10.1097/OR9.0000000000000005.
16. National Cancer Survivorship Initiative The Recovery Package. 2014. Available from: www.macmillan.org.uk/documents/aboutus/health_professionals/macvoice/sharinggoodpractice_therecoverypackage.pdf

17. Konno R, Gyi AA Use of acupuncture and moxibustion in the control of anticancer therapy-induced nausea and vomiting. In: Cho WCS, editor. Acupuncture and moxibustion as an evidence-based therapy for cancer. Dordrecht: Springer; 2012. pp. 121–152.

18. Towler P, Molassiotis A, Brearley SG What is the evidence for the use of acupuncture as an intervention for symptom management in cancer supportive and palliative care: an integrative overview of reviews. Support. Care Cancer 2013;21:2913–2923.

19. Stone J, Greene S, Johnstone P Acupuncture for the treament of symptoms associated with radiation therapy. In: Cho WCS, editor. Acupuncture and moxibustion as an evidence-based therapy for cancer. Dordrecht: Springer; 2012. pp. 183–198.

20. de Valois B, Peckham R Treating the person and not the disease: acupuncture in the management of cancer treatment-related lymphoedema. Eur. J. Orient. Med. 2011;6(6):37–49.

21. Walker EM, Rodriguez AI, Kohn B, et al. Acupuncture versus venlafaxine for the management of vaso-motor symptoms in patients with hormone receptor-positive breast cancer: a randomized controlled trial. J. Clin. Oncol. 2010;28(4):634–640.

22. MacPherson H, Thomas KJ, Walters S, et al. The York acupuncture safety study: prospective survey of 34 000 treatments by traditional acupuncturists. BMJ 2001;323:4876–4877.

23. Witt CM, Pach D, Brinkhaus B, et al. Safety of acupuncture: results of a prospective observational study with 229,230 patients and introduction of a medical information and consent form. Forsch. Komplementarmed. 2009;16:91–97.

24. Shulman LM The effect of motivation on living with chronic illness. In: Factor SA, Weiner WJ, editors. Parkinson's disease: diagnosis and clinical management. New York: Demos; 2002.

25. Golay A, Lagger G, Giordan A Motivating patients with chronic disease. J. Med. Person 2007;5(2):57–61.

26. McCorkle R, Ercolano E, Lazenby M, et al. Self-management: enabling and empowering patients living with cancer as a chronic illness. CA. Cancer J. Clin. 2011;61(1):50–62. Available from: https://doi.org/10.3322/caac.20093

27. Lorig K Self-management of chronic illness: a model for the future. Generations 1993;Fall:11–14.

28. Paterson C, Britten N Acupuncture as a complex intervention: a holistic model. J. Altern. Complement. Med. 2004;10(5):791–801.

29. Paterson C, Dieppe P Characteristic and incidental (placebo) effects in complex interventions such as acupuncture. BMJ 2005;330(21 May 2005):1202–1205.

30. Rugg S, Paterson C, Britten N, et al. Traditional acupuncture for people with medically unexplained symptoms: a longitudinal qualitative study of patients' experiences. Br. J. Gen. Pract. 2011;June:306–315.

Chapter 2

The Consequences of Cancer Treatments

Introduction

That surviving cancer can have both favourable and unfavourable outcomes, and that acupuncture can support people living with the long-term effects of cancer treatment is encapsulated in these quotations:

> Put simply, the better we get at treating and curing cancer patients, the more people we will have living with the long-term effects of cancer and its treatment. In other words, progress is a double-edged sword. (Professor Jane Maher, Chief Medical Officer, Macmillan Cancer Support)[1]

> You've got to learn to live with it, and…[acupuncture] helps you to get on with life really, accepting it as what you've got. (Head and neck cancer survivor)

We might assume that the end of cancer treatment is a time for celebration for an individual diagnosed with cancer. However, this is often a time of stress and disappointment. Many people feel 'abandoned' when treatment ends, lost in the transition from patient to survivor.[2] Expectations that health and life will return to what they were before the cancer diagnosis are disappointed. Many continue to feel unwell; fear of cancer recurrence is common.

Cancer survivors report poorer health and wellbeing than the rest of the population, comparable with that of people with chronic conditions such as diabetes or arthritis.[3] Survivorship has been described as being 'disease-free, but not free of your disease'.[4]

Consequences of cancer treatment may continue after treatment ends, and new cancer treatment-related symptoms may emerge soon after or many years later. This chapter examines some of those consequences and their potential impact on the lives of cancer survivors, arranged according to these anti-cancer treatment modalities:

- surgery
- radiotherapy
- systemic anti-cancer treatments, including chemotherapy, hormonal therapies, targeted therapies, and immunotherapies.

ESSENTIALS

Acupuncturists should be aware of:

- who in their patient list has been diagnosed with cancer
- what cancer treatments they had or continue to have
- what drugs they had or continue to have.

They should be aware of the long-term and late effects of cancer treatments, to identify aetiologies of symptoms that may present – sometimes long after a patient has put their cancer experience behind them.

They should also be aware that acupuncture often is more effective at treating some late effects than biomedicine, as will be explored later in this book.

Consequences of cancer and its treatments

As introduced in Chapter 1, 'consequences' is a term that encompasses 'the wide range of long-term physical and psychosocial changes that seem to be associated with cancer and its treatment, however long ago the diagnosis and treatment might have been given'.[5] Many other terms are used in relation to these changes.

TERMINOLOGY

'Consequences' also refers to:

- adverse effects
- chronic effects
- consequences of treatment
- late effects
- long-term effects
- side effects
- toxicity, toxicities.

'Long-term' and 'late effects' are terms used to denote chronic problems that may arise during, soon, or a long time after treatment ends ('late onset'). For most patients, consequences that develop during treatment resolve. For others, those consequences may worsen and become chronic (such as lymphoedema affecting head and neck cancer survivors). The possible consequences are many and varied; all have the potential to affect quality of life.

Consequences are associated with any of the modalities used in cancer treatment, such as surgery, radiotherapy, and systemic anti-cancer therapies (SACTs), and other treatments (such as bisphosphonates to manage bone-related conditions).

Most people with a cancer diagnosis undergo one or more of these treatment modalities. The treatments administered to any individual depend on the type of cancer, its stage, and other factors. Each of these therapies has the potential for multiple physical and psychosocial consequences for a patient, affecting individuals differently.

A common configuration is a trio of surgery, radiotherapy, and SACTs, increasing the potential opportunities for consequences to develop. Survivors may also experience several types of SACTs; for example, a pre-menopausal woman with breast cancer might be treated with chemotherapy, endocrine therapy (e.g. tamoxifen), and targeted therapy (Herceptin®), in addition to surgery and radiotherapy.

Physical and psychosocial consequences

TERMINOLOGY

Psychosocial refers to factors that influence an individual psychologically and/or socially. Such factors can describe individuals in relation to their social environment and how these affect physical and mental health.[6]

Physical and/or psychosocial consequences may be triggered by the treatments, as well as the significant changes and challenges associated with a cancer diagnosis, and these may be intertwined. For example, consequences may physically affect how the body looks or functions, leading to possible embarrassment, loss of confidence, and changes in sexuality and relationships. Fear, anger, shock, and grief are common emotional reactions to the unwanted changes that cancer brings (see Chapter 3, Cancer Survivorship and the Emotions). People with a cancer diagnosis face the possibility of dying. Anxiety, fear of recurrence, and uncertainty about the future are common issues for survivors, as well as for those around them.[5,7]

The 'new normal'

Cancer and the consequences of its treatments may impact the way survivors live their lives. Relationships with partners, family, and friends may change. The ability to work may suffer, leading to financial concerns. Survivors' ability to self-manage may diminish, leading to greater reliance on other people, or on health or social services. Life after cancer treatment may never be the same as life before. Many survivors face the challenges of establishing this new and different life, often called the 'new normal'.

Possible permutations of consequences

Just as there are many possible routes through the Survivorship Pathway, there are many possible permutations of the consequences of cancer treatments. Some cancer survivors do not experience long-term consequences. Others describe a process of personal growth triggered by diagnosis, reporting positive effects such as improved relationships, greater appreciation of life, and increased resilience.[8] An American study reported that breast cancer survivors experienced significant improvements in outlook on life, love for their partner, religious satisfaction, and spirituality, compared with women with benign breast problems, in spite of having poorer health and physical functioning.[9]

Box 2.1: Examples of consequences of cancer and its treatments

Of 1152 people with breast, colorectal, haematological, and gynaecological cancers:

- 30% reported more than five moderate to severe unmet needs at the end of treatment
- 60% of these individuals reported no improvement in the six months after the end of primary treatment
- the most common unmet needs were psychological needs and fear of recurrence.[11]

Of 332 men undergoing hormone therapy for prostate cancer:

- 70% reported fatigue that impacted their ability to work, conduct household chores, and pursue hobbies
- 80% reported erectile dysfunction, of whom 25% reported that they found this difficult to cope with
- 50% reported issues related to mental wellbeing (depression, loss of confidence, cognitive problems).[12]

Of breast cancer survivors surveyed:

- 84% reported experiencing at least one physical health problem within the previous 12 months. The main physical consequences experienced were fatigue, nerve damage, hot flushes, early menopause, lymphoedema, pain, and cognitive and sexual problems.[13]

Of cancer survivors who had undergone pelvic radiotherapy:

- 50% experienced bowel problems that impacted quality of life
- 30% of these reported that these bowel problems had a moderate or severe impact.[14]

Cancer survivors, in the 12 months prior to being surveyed:

- required greater access to healthcare services than the wider population, with 90% visiting their general practitioner and 45% visiting a specialist doctor, compared with 68% and 15% of the wider population
- 78% had experienced physical health problems
- 71% of those who finished treatment ten years previously had experienced physical health problems.[13]

All statistics cited in *The National Cancer Survivorship Initiative Vision* (2010), pages 12–15.[14]

Significant numbers of survivors do experience consequences that impact quality of life, which also have potential to become permanent. Furthermore, survivors may experience multiple consequences simultaneously, or over time. These may be relatively minor problems that collectively become debilitating over time.[10] Some consequences may not arise until many years after the end of treatment. Box 2.1 illustrates how wide-ranging and long-term consequences can be for many cancer types.

Some common consequences associated with specific cancers

Moving from the general to the specific, Table 2.1 and Table 2.2 present common consequences of cancer treatments, linking them to specific cancers and treatments.

In contrast to the physical consequences, psychosocial long-term and late effects (Table 2.2) are not the consequences of any specific cancer or treatment modality. Rather they are a response to the experience of having cancer and its treatments. They may manifest during active treatment and may persist, or they may arise after treatment ends.

Increasing the complexity – symptom clusters

Table 2.1 presents consequences as they relate to specific treatments for specific cancers, perhaps giving the impression that these are single, stand-alone effects. However, a consequence can be related to, or give rise to other consequences. For example, a breast cancer survivor may experience hot flushes, which lead to fatigue, poor sleep, and depressed mood. That survivor might also have lymphoedema, bringing with it pain, anxiety, and body image issues.

Presentations of multiple, concurrent symptoms experienced by many cancer survivors are beginning to be explored in research identifying 'symptom clusters', defined as: 'a stable group of two or more concurrent symptoms that are related to one another, but independent of other symptoms or symptom clusters'.[15]

Some examples of cancer treatment-related symptoms that occur together and are regarded as symptom clusters include:

- pain/fatigue/sleep
- nausea/vomiting
- dyspnoea/cough.

Table 2.1: Physical long-term and late effects related to cancers and treatments[16]

Consequence	Cancers commonly associated with	Resulting from treatment with	When arises
Bone health	Breast Haematological Prostate	• Bone marrow transplantation • Chemotherapies that cause premature ovarian failure • Hormonal treatments including aromatase inhibitors, androgen deprivation therapy, gonadotrophin-releasing hormone • Radiotherapy	Can arise during cancer treatment and persist long term, or develop years after treatment completion.
Cancer (subsequent primary cancers)	Many cancers	• Radiotherapy • Chemotherapy agents including alkylating agents, topoisomerase II inhibitors and anthracyclines are all associated with acute myeloid leukaemia	Risk of developing subsequent primary cancers related to treatments can last years after completion of a first primary cancer (see Chapter 13, Reducing Risk of Recurrence and Subsequent Primary Cancers).
Cancer treatment-induced metabolic syndrome: Central obesity Dyslipidaemia (high cholesterol) Hypertension Insulin resistance	Breast Childhood malignancies Colorectal Gynaecological Haematological Neurological Prostate Testicular Thyroid	• Anti-oestrogen and androgen deprivation therapies • Chemotherapies such as platinums or anthracyclines • Radiotherapy including cranial, thyroid or total body • Surgery including pituitary or hypothalamic, orchidectomy, or salpingo-oophorectomy	Can arise during cancer treatment and persist long term, or develop years after treatment completion.
Cancer-related fatigue	49% in all cancers; 25–33% experience fatigue for up to ten years after cancer diagnosis	'A distressing, persistent subjective sense of physical, emotional and/or cognitive tiredness or exhaustion related to cancer and/or cancer treatment that is not proportional to recent activity and significantly interferes with usual functioning'.[17] Can extend months to years after treatment, and can negatively affect mood, relationships, ability to work, activities of daily living, quality of life.	
Cardiac dysfunction: • Arrythmias • Cardiomyopathy • Coronary artery disease • Valvular disorders	Breast Haematological Sarcoma	• Chemotherapy – anthracyclines • Immunotherapy – trastuzumab (Herceptin®) • Radiotherapy – high dose, ≥ 30Gy when heart is in the treatment field	Can arise during cancer treatment and persist long term or develop years after treatment completion.

Chemotherapy-induced peripheral neuropathy (CIPN)	Breast Colorectal Gynaecological Head and neck Prostate	• Chemotherapies including taxanes (e.g. paclitaxel and docetaxel), platinums (e.g. cisplatin and oxaliplatin), vinca alkaloids, eribulin, and proteasome inhibitors	Arises during cancer treatment and may persist long term.
Cognitive impairment	All cancers	• Chemotherapy • Radiotherapy	Arises during cancer treatment and may persist months to years after treatment completion.
Infertility[18]	Bladder Breast Gynaecological Prostate Testicular	• Chemotherapy agents that may impact fertility include the alkylating agents (e.g. cyclophosphamide, ifosfamide, procarbazine, and busulfan) and platinums • Radiotherapy taking in the pelvic area, or cranial irradiation which can damage the hypothalmus, pituitary and associated vasculature, with consequent impact on sexual development and fertility • Pelvic surgery may directly impair or remove reproductive structures or may affect sexual performance	
Lymphoedema	Bladder Breast Gynaecological Head and neck Melanoma Prostate	• Surgery, especially lymph node dissection • Radiotherapy when lymph nodes are within the field of radiation • Some chemotherapies, e.g. taxanes	Can arise during cancer treatment (e.g. after surgery or radiotherapy) or arise months or years after treatment completion.
Menopausal symptoms: • Hot flushes and night sweats (HFNS) • Vaginal dryness	Breast Gynaecological Prostate	• Chemotherapies that cause premature ovarian failure • Hormonal treatments including aromatase inhibitors, androgen deprivation therapy, gonadotrophin-releasing hormone • Surgery, e.g. oophorectomy	Arises during cancer treatment and may persist months to years after treatment completion.
Pain (chronic)	All cancers	Multiple types and causes, including: • Osteoporotic fractures in people on long-term steroids, anti-androgens, aromatase inhibitors, radiotherapy to area of pain • Arthralgia and myalgia due to selective oestrogen receptor modulators or aromatase inhibitors for breast cancer • Post-surgical pain syndrome, including post-mastectomy pain and post-amputation phantom pain	Pain can arise during cancer treatment, become chronic and persist long term or develop some time after treatment completion. **NOTE: New or acute pain should be assessed for cancer recurrence or disease progression.**
Sleep problems	All cancers, 25–60%; common up to five years after diagnosis		Includes insomnia, excessive sleepiness, and sleep-related breathing difficulties.

Table 2.2: Psychosocial long-term and late effects[16]

Consequence	Estimated prevalence	Notes
Anxiety and depression	Anxiety reported to affect up to 18% of survivors; depression affects 13%	Highest occurrence is during and immediately after treatment but may persist for many years.
Fear of cancer recurrence	Mild to moderate in 49% of survivors, severe in 7%	Manifests as constant, intrusive thoughts about cancer; conviction that cancer will recur regardless of prognosis; inability to plan for the future. Can adversely affect quality of life, especially when severe. Also affects health service usage and adherence to follow-up.
Sex and intimacy	Estimated 40–100%, depending on population, treatment, aetiology, and manifestation	Can occur after surgery, chemotherapy, radiotherapy, or hormonal therapy. A common yet overlooked concern, which may manifest as: • Physical: erectile dysfunction, painful intercourse (dyspareunia) • Psychological: body image • Interpersonal: change in relationships. Consequences of hormonal therapies may include: • Men: gynaecomastia (breast enlargement) and reduced body hair because of androgen deprivation • Women: vaginal dryness associated with oestrogen deprivation • Women and men: hot flushes and night sweats, arthralgia and myalgia.
Financial hardship	28%	Cancer survivors experience greater financial hardship than people without a cancer diagnosis. In some countries, insurance may not cover all aspects of cancer-related healthcare; in countries with universal care there may still be treatment-associated expenses to be met. Treatments and their consequences may affect a survivor's ability to work in the short and long term.
Returning to work	37% relative risk of not returning to work compared with population without a cancer diagnosis	Approximately 35% of survivors are aged 40–64, and potentially interested in returning to work. Return to work may be hampered by physical limitations, or workplace issues such as stigma or inflexibility in assigning new roles that accommodate a survivor's changed functional capacity. Cancer may trigger a change in an employee's priorities, including bringing forward retirement.

A brief guide to cancer treatments
A note about treatments
Availability of treatments and how they are administered are related to national health guidelines and licensing determined by governmental and other health agencies, plus factors such as health economics. Specific details of treatments for different types of

cancers, or the availability of treatments in different countries or regions are available on the websites of national cancer information providers and cancer charity websites.

Some essential terminology

Terms used in oncology may be used differently in different contexts (e.g. from country to country), they may be used interchangeably, or have nuanced meanings. Table 2.3 lists some frequently used terms and defines how they are used in this book.

Table 2.3: Definitions of some cancer-related terms

Term	Definition
Active treatment	Treatment with curative intent or to manage the disease.[19]
Adjuvant	Additional cancer treatment given after the primary treatment to lower the risk that the cancer will come back. Adjuvant therapy may include chemotherapy, radiation therapy, hormone therapy, targeted therapy, or biological therapy.
Local	The site of the tumour and sometimes the cells immediately surrounding it. A local treatment may involve excision of the tumour, removal of the entire organ, or removal of the of the regional tissues at risk of tumour involvement.[19]
Loco-regional or regional	The area of the body surrounding the tumour. May also include the local lymph nodes.
Metastatic	Metastatic cancer, also called metastatic disease, secondary cancer, or distant recurrence, is cancer that has spread from the primary site to another part of the body.
Neoadjuvant	Radiotherapy, chemotherapy, or hormonal therapy administered prior to active treatment (usually surgery). The aim is to reduce the size of a tumour or extent of local spread prior to radical treatment, to make surgery less invasive.
Palliative	Treatment to improve quality of life and has no implied impact on the patient's survival.[19] Palliative care, sometimes called 'supportive care' can happen any time of the cancer trajectory, from diagnosis onward, and aims to keep the patient comfortable. The term encompasses 'end-of-life care', which is specifically for people thought to be in the last year of their life.[20] May or may not involve anti-cancer therapies.
Primary	Has two meanings in cancer: 1) originating site of the tumour, 2) initial curative intent treatment, in which case it may also be called first-line therapy, induction therapy, and primary therapy.
Radical treatment	Treatment that is given with long-term control or curative intent. May also be referred to as active, primary, or first-line treatment.[19]
Recurrence or relapse	Cancer that returns after it has been in remission is defined as a recurrence or relapse of that cancer.
Remission	Decrease in or disappearance of cancer signs and symptoms. Partial remission means some, but not all, signs and symptoms of cancer have disappeared. Complete remission means all signs and symptoms of cancer have disappeared, although cancer still may be in the body.
Systemic	Treatment that circulates throughout the body via the blood and lymphatic systems.

TERMINOLOGY

Curative intent

The hope for all cancer treatment is that it will 'cure' the condition, meaning the cancer disappears and does not return. Medically, the term 'cure' is not used except to describe a possibility or intent and is applied to treatment as being 'curative', or with 'curative intent' or 'intent to cure'.

It may be impossible to know if a cancer is 'cured', and cancer may return months or many years after treatment.

Surgery

About 45–60% of people diagnosed with cancer will undergo surgery,[21,22] which has several applications in cancer management including diagnosis, treatment, repair and restoration of function, and palliative care. A local treatment, it is often the primary treatment for cancer. While it may be used as the sole treatment, it is often combined with other therapies, most frequently radiotherapy.

Types of surgery[21]

The type and extent of surgery is determined by the tumour type, its anatomical location, and the degree of spread of cancer outside the tumour. Patient-related factors include age, performance status (ability to perform certain activities of daily living), and comorbidities. Three main types of surgery include:

- Surgery of the primary tumour: this aims to remove the tumour and a clear margin of normal tissue. Prognosis is good if the cancer has not already spread and can be completely removed along with a border of healthy tissue. Where complete removal of a tumour is not possible, a partial removal may be undertaken to alleviate symptoms and delay further spread.
- Surgery of regional lymph nodes: some tumours spread to the regional lymph nodes in a predictable fashion. In these cases, the regional lymph nodes and lymphatics may be removed with the tumour. Screening is often carried out to assess whether there is already pathological involvement of the lymph nodes. For example, sentinel lymph node biopsy (SLNB) is used to assess whether cancer has spread from the tumour. Dyes or radioisotopes identify the first single (sentinel) node, to which the cancer would spread before spreading onwards to other lymph nodes. If no cancerous cells are found in the sentinel node, cancer is unlikely to have spread; if cancer cells are found, additional lymph nodes may be removed.
- Reconstructive (oncoplastic) surgery: extensive surgery may affect normal anatomy, with consequent cosmetic and/or functional damage. Plastic surgery may be used to correct anatomical defects, for example breast reconstruction, and restore function (e.g. restoring bone structures or the tongue in head and neck cancers).

Some consequences of surgery

The consequences of surgery depend on the location and extent of the intervention; some potential consequences are presented in Table 2.4.

Table 2.4: Potential consequences of surgery

Physical consequences may include	Psychosocial consequences may include
• Changes in or loss of function resulting from tissue damage to or loss of an organ or part of the body, e.g. removal of tongue • Cosmetic effects including visible scarring, change in body shape • Incisional hernia • Infertility • Lymphoedema (chronic swelling) • Pain, including phantom limb pain and scar pain • Scarring/adhesions • Sensory changes, such as loss of smell or taste • Sleep disturbance • Tiredness	• Adjustment to change and loss • Adjustment to change in body image • Aversion to ostomy (the incision made in the body to allow for passage of wastes) • Effects on libido, sexuality, fertility • Embarrassment, guilt, inhibition • (Hyper-)awareness of (perceived) attitudes of others • Impact on ability to work • Lack of desire or ability to continue with usual role • Relationship issues • Scar may be a reminder of cancer

Radiotherapy

Radiotherapy is the use of high energy electromagnetic radiation (X-rays, gamma rays, electrons, or protons) to destroy cancer cells. It is a local treatment, where the beam of radiation is focused on the tumour and surrounding tissue and may be a regional treatment when aimed at surrounding lymph nodes as well. It is often combined with surgery (used pre- or post-operatively), as well as with chemotherapy (called chemoradiation or chemoradiotherapy). Approximately 50% of people with cancer undergo radiotherapy as part of their treatment.[20]

Dose and radiosensitivity[20]

Radiotherapy also affects normal cells, especially rapidly dividing cells such as skin and stem cells. The balance between causing serious damage to normal tissue and curing a tumour (the 'therapeutic ratio') is an important consideration in determining dose. New radiotherapy techniques such as intensity modulated radiotherapy (IMRT) aim to increase the dose delivered to the tumour while reducing that to nearby healthy tissue.

Dose is measured in a unit called a Gray (Gy), which is a measure of absorbed energy (1Gy = 1J/kg). The total dose, which is planned by specialists, is subdivided into smaller units, called fractions, and this determines the number of treatments required to deliver the total dose. 'Fractionation' is calculated to allow normal cells to recover between treatments to minimise adverse effects. The area of the body the radiation is directed at is called the 'field'.

A dose given in a shorter time (that is, fewer fractions) has a greater effect than the same dose given over a longer time in many fractions. Small fractions require a longer course of treatment with a higher total dose to have the same effect. To ensure cancer cells do not recover, delays and interruptions in treatment should be avoided, and overall treatment time should not exceed six to seven weeks.

The response of a cancer to radiotherapy is described as its radiosensitivity. In highly radiosensitive cancers (such as leukaemias) cancer cells are destroyed rapidly with low doses of radiation. Radioresistant cancers (such as renal cell cancer and melanoma) require higher doses of radiotherapy to effect cell death, and these higher doses cause more damage to normal tissues.

Some consequences of radiotherapy
Consequences of radiotherapy are classified as:

- early (or acute) effects that occur during treatment: they may resolve when radiotherapy is completed, or they may become chronic
- late effects, which do not occur until months or years after treatment.

Early effects
Fatigue and skin irritation are the most common side effects:

- Fatigue usually sets in midway through a course of radical radiotherapy (during the second and third weeks of a five- to six-week course) and may last for several weeks after treatment ends. Many factors contribute to fatigue, including radiation exposure, travelling to treatment every day, other treatments such as surgery or chemotherapy, and emotional reactions, including anxiety and depression.
- Skin sensitivity, like mild to moderate sunburn, may develop at the treatment site. It often resolves once radiotherapy is complete and epithelial cells have recovered their normal capacity for cell division, although the skin may discolour or lose its elasticity. Medical teams advise patients on skin care. This includes avoiding perfumed products that may exacerbate sensitivity, and using specific emollients to moisturise the area. It is important not to use products apart from those recommended.

Nausea and vomiting are not generally a side effect of radiotherapy, although they may be associated with radiotherapy to the stomach, abdomen, or the nausea-producing structures in the head (such as the vestibules of the inner ears during treatment for some head and neck cancers). Some patients may experience anticipatory nausea and vomiting as a psychological response. Other early effects are specific to the site of treatment and are presented in Table 2.5.

Table 2.5: Early effects of radiotherapy treatment

Consequences	Notes
Bladder problems	Urination flow problems, painful urination, infections in the treatment of bladder cancer or other pelvic cancers.
Bowel discomfort	Includes soreness and/or diarrhoea because of direct radiation to the colon, rectum, or anus, or exposure to other pelvic structures that fall within the field of radiation, including the prostate, bladder, and female genital tract.
Fertility	Radiotherapy fields encompassing the ovaries, and high-dose radiotherapy affecting the uterus, may impact fertility.

Lowered sperm counts, retrograde ejaculation, and limited quality and quantity of seminal fluid may be the consequences of radiotherapy for prostate and bladder cancers and affect fertility. |
| Mouth and pharynx sores | Soreness and ulceration, which if severe can affect swallowing, in the treatment of head and neck cancers.

Soreness of the oesophagus can result from direct treatment of oesophageal cancers, or as collateral damage in the treatment of lung cancer. |
| Oedema | General inflammation may cause swelling of soft tissues, which is of concern in the treatment of brain tumours and metastases. |
| Sexual effects | Libido may be affected temporarily or permanently.

Narrowing of the vagina may result from radiotherapy to the vaginal area.

Impotence may be temporary or permanent because of treatment for male bladder, rectal, or prostate cancer. |

Late effects

Late effects rarely emerge before six months after treatment, and typically start to appear two to three years after radiotherapy. They are more serious than early effects, as they tend to be progressive and irreversible. They are the result of damage to the blood vessels, and from stem cells losing their potential to recover.

Radiation is a potential cause of cancer, so with radiation therapy, there is a risk of inducing a second cancer at a new distant site. This risk is low, usually less than 1/1000, and is outweighed by risk from the established malignancy for which treatment is administered. For most solid tumour cancers, second malignancies rarely occur before ten years and may develop 30 or more years after exposure. Other late effects are usually local to the area treated, and are listed in Table 2.6.

Table 2.6: Late effects of radiotherapy treatment

Consequences	Notes
Cognitive decline	Associated with radiation to the head and may especially affect young children.
Dryness	Dry mouth (xerostomia) and dry eyes (xerophthalmia) are associated with radiation for head and neck cancers and can severely affect quality of life.

Sweat glands in treated areas may cease functioning.

Vaginal mucosa may become dry following radiation to the pelvis. |
| Fibrosis | Irradiation may cause hardening and thickening of tissues, and can affect the skin, lungs, ureters, bladder, and urethra. |

cont.

Consequences	Notes
Hair loss	Epilation may occur on hair-bearing skin in the radiation field, and may be permanent depending on radiation dose.
Heart disease	A radiation field encompassing the heart confers risk for damage to the heart (cardiotoxicity) and can manifest as pericardial, valvular, myocardial, or coronary heart disease many years after treatment. This is worsened in breast cancer if treatment includes anthracyclines and Herceptin®.
Lymphoedema	Chronic swelling can result from radiation damage to the lymphatic system and is a frequent complication of radiation to the axillary lymph nodes in treatment for breast cancer.
Menopause and infertility	Radiotherapy to the pelvis usually affects the ovaries, bringing on the menopause and affecting fertility.
Osteoradionecrosis	A complication of radiotherapy occurring most commonly in the mouth during treatment of head and neck cancer and may arise over five years after treatment. Associated with pain, difficulty chewing, restricted mouth opening (trismus), and non-healing ulcers.
Radiation proctitis	Inflammation and damage to lower parts of the colon may manifest as rectal bleeding, diarrhoea, and urgency.
Urinary tract damage	Includes conditions such as cystitis, bleeding, urinary frequency, urgency, stress and other incontinence.

Psychological effects

These may include anxiety, depression, shock, fear, and body image problems. Many cancer patients find the hardest time to cope is after radiotherapy finishes. Expectations of the patient, their family, and friends are that life can return to normal now treatment is over. However, this is a time when many survivors feel very low. The end of daily visits to the treatment centre can leave patients feeling abandoned and isolated.

Systemic anti-cancer therapies (SACTs)

SACTs encompass a wide range of therapies, including cytotoxic chemotherapy and hormonal therapies, as well as new and emerging therapies such as molecular therapies and immunotherapies. The aims of SACTs can be curative, palliative, adjuvant, and neoadjuvant.

Chemotherapy

Chemotherapy refers to drug therapies for cancer which are cytotoxic (toxic to cells). Chemotherapy drugs travel via the bloodstream to destroy cancer cells throughout the body and are therefore a systemic treatment as they reach all systems within the body. Cancer chemotherapy may be used as:

- neoadjuvant treatment, to shrink a tumour prior to local treatment
- radical treatment with curative intent
- adjuvant treatment after surgery or radiotherapy to reduce the risk of recurrence

- palliative care in late-stage or advanced cancer, when shrinking a tumour might palliate a symptom in the short term, leading to improved quality of life.

About 28% of people with cancer have chemotherapy,[22] which usually is used in conjunction with surgery and/or radiotherapy to enhance local and regional treatment, to target sites of metastases, and to attack micrometastases.

Chemotherapy agents kill cells that divide rapidly, a characteristic of cancer cells and of many normal cells such as those in the bone marrow, digestive tract, and hair follicles. Cytotoxic drugs cannot differentiate between cancer and normal cells, and damage to the normal cells means the treatment is highly toxic with the potential for unpleasant side effects (toxicities).

Treatment requires finding the balance between destroying the cancer cells to control the disease, and minimising destruction of normal cells to limit side effects. New developments focus on anti-cancer drugs called 'targeted therapies', designed to attack cancer cells more specifically with fewer toxic side effects.

Some consequences of chemotherapy

The consequences of chemotherapy depend on the type of agent(s) used in treatment (there are nearly 100 chemotherapy agents in use), as well as the patient's age, underlying health, and other factors. Many toxicities are managed during treatment or resolve when treatment ends or shortly thereafter, for example chemotherapy-induced nausea and vomiting, and hair loss associated with breast cancer treatment.

Long-term and late effects

Some early effects of chemotherapy may not be fully reversible and persist well beyond the end of treatment. Fatigue, a common symptom of cancer and its treatments, is a widely experienced side effect of chemotherapy and may be severe and persistent. It may be cumulative, peaking towards the end of treatment, and can be disabling and frustrating. It may ease after treatment ends or may continue for months or in some cases for years following the end of treatment.

Risks for long-term and late effects are affected by multiple factors, including age, gender, pre-existing or hereditary disease, combination therapy, and cumulative effects of other cancer treatments, including surgery, radiotherapy, and hormone therapies. Long-term and late effects of chemotherapy depend on the chemotherapy agents used (Table 2.7). Second primary cancers may develop as a consequence of some chemotherapy agents; for example, leukaemia is a late consequence of alkylating agents used to treat childhood cancers.

Psychological effects

These may include anxiety, depression, shock, fear, body image problems. Antidepressants or cognitive behavioural therapy (CBT) may be prescribed to manage the psychological effects.

Table 2.7: Some potential late effects of chemotherapy by body system[23]

Body system	Toxicity	Chemotherapy agent/notes
Cardiovascular	Cardiotoxicity	Anthracycline, cisplatin
	Hypertension, increased weight, elevated lipid profile	Cisplatin and bleomycin in treatment of testicular germ cell tumours
Pulmonary	Pulmonary fibrosis	Alkylating agents (primarily busulfan), nitrosoureas (e.g. lomustine, carmustine), bleomycin
Endocrine	Gonadal toxicity	Alkylating agents such as cyclophosphamide
	Testicular damage with azoospermia	Mechlorethamine, cyclophosphamide, cytosine arabinoside, and high-dose cisplatin and etoposide
	Chemotherapy-related amenorrhea, premature menopause	Alkylating agents
Neuromuscular	Sensory neuropathy, including pins and needles or sensory loss, loss of balance; hand-foot syndrome (palmar-plantar erythrodysesthesia)	Platinum compounds (cisplatin, carboplatine), vinca alkaloids (vincristine, vinblastine), antimitotics (taxanes, ixabepilone)
	Motor neuropathy, including weakness, foot drop, gait disturbance	Capecitabine
	Tinnitus, hearing loss	
Cognitive function	Deficits in executive function, verbal memory, information processing speed, attention, learning	Cognitive dysfunction is greater in cancer patients who receive chemotherapy compared with both those who do not and healthy controls. Higher chemotherapy dose is a risk factor.
Genitourinary	Cystitis; reduced bladder capacity and contractility; fibrosis of the ureters, bladder, urethra; nephritis	Cyclophosphamide, ifosfamide, cisplatin
Head and neck	Hearing loss, especially in the high tone range	Cisplatin
	Conjunctivitis, keratitis, retinopathy, retinal haemorrhage, optic neuritis, blurred vision. May or may not be reversible.	

New developments in chemotherapy treatment

Given the toxicity of these drugs, there is a continual search to find methods of destroying cancerous cells or suppressing their growth more effectively while minimising damage to normal cells and improving tolerance to treatment. Research into chemotherapy agents continues to modify existing drugs and find new combinations of drugs and new delivery techniques. Targeted therapies are directed to a specific target on cancer cells and may have fewer side effects associated with them.

Hormone therapies

Growth of some tumours is stimulated by sex hormones produced naturally in the body. Oestrogen and progesterone can promote the growth of some breast and endometrial cancers, while testosterone stimulates prostate cancer. Growth of these hormone-dependent cancers can be slowed or halted by inhibiting the supply of the hormones to the tumour. Surgical removal of the ovaries (oophorectomy or ovariectomy) or testes (orchidectomy or orchiectomy) is a permanent way of achieving this. Drug therapies allow for temporary suppression of hormone production, and this form of treatment is called hormone therapy, hormonal therapy, hormone treatment, or endocrine therapy.

Hormone therapy may be used in a neoadjuvant setting with curative intent, as an adjuvant therapy, in palliative care, and more recently as a prophylactic treatment for women at high risk of developing breast cancer. A systemic treatment, hormone therapy may be used on its own or in combination with other hormone therapies, as well as with surgery, radiotherapy, chemotherapy, and or/other treatments.

Hormone therapies for breast cancer

TERMINOLOGY

'Hormone therapy' for breast cancer should not be confused with menopausal hormone therapy (MHT) or female hormone replacement therapy (HRT), where medicines are administered to *increase* levels of female sex hormones to reduce the symptoms associated with the menopause.

Consequences of hormone therapies for breast cancer

The most common of the wide range of potential side effects are displayed in Table 2.8. Individuals will be affected differently. The most frequently occurring symptoms are:

- hot flushes associated with tamoxifen
- muscle and joint pains (arthralgia) associated with aromatase inhibitors (AIs).

For many survivors, these consequences subside after a few months of taking the drugs; for others, side effects may continue for as long as treatment lasts, and even longer. This can be up to and beyond ten years for some cancer survivors. The continuous troublesome consequences often motivate patients to take 'holidays' from their hormone therapy or stop taking the therapy altogether. This has potential negative impact on survival rates, as these therapies are usually used to reduce risk of cancer recurrence.

Hormone therapies for womb cancer (endometrial cancer)

Hormonal therapies are most usually prescribed to manage recurrent or metastatic endometrial cancers, with consequences as listed in Table 2.8.

Table 2.8: Hormone therapies for breast and endometrial cancers[24]

Hormone therapy	Cancers used to treat	Some common consequences
Aromatase inhibitors (AIs) • Anastrozole • Exemestane • Letrozole	Breast Endometrial	• Bone loss and a higher risk for fractures (osteoporosis) • Decreased sexual desire • Fatigue
Oestrogen receptor antagonists • Fulvestrant • Toremifene	Breast	• Higher risk of other types of cancer, stroke, blood clots, cataracts, and heart disease • Hot flushes, night sweats
Luteinising hormone-releasing hormone (LHRH) agonists • Goserelin • Leuprolide • Triptorelin	Breast Endometrial	• Nausea • Pain in muscles and joints (arthralgia) • Vaginal discharge, dryness, or irritation
Progestins: • Medroxyprogesterone acetate (Provera®) • Megestrol acetate (Megace®)	Endometrial	• Weight gain Note: Men with breast cancer who undergo hormone therapy may also experience many of these same side effects, as well as erectile dysfunction.
Selective oestrogen receptor modulators (SERMs) • Tamoxifen • Raloxifene	Breast Endometrial	

Hormone therapies for prostate cancer

Hormone therapy is used to control levels of the male hormone testosterone, which is made in the testes, and which stimulates growth of prostate cancer. While surgery (orchidectomy) can reduce testosterone levels, it is more common to manage testosterone levels with drug therapies. Use of hormone therapies for prostate cancer is determined by stage and grade of cancer. Treatment may be short term (for as little as three months) or may last many years.

Consequences of hormone therapy for prostate cancer

Potential side effects of hormone therapies for prostate cancer (Table 2.9) affect individuals differently. The most common side effects are erectile dysfunction, hot flushes, reduced libido; others include breast growth (gynaecomastia) and tenderness, increase in body fat around the waist, and increased blood sugar levels. These symptoms are likely to be long term, and cause physical and emotional distress.

Table 2.9: Hormone therapies for prostate cancer[24]

Hormone therapy	Some common consequences
Anti-androgens (also called androgen deprivation therapy or ADT): • Apalutamide • Enzalutamide • Darolutamide • Bicalutamide • Flutamide • Nilutamide	• Bone loss and a higher risk for fractures (osteoporosis) • Decreased sexual desire • Erectile dysfunction • Fatigue • Gynaecomastia (growth of breast tissue) • Hot flushes, night sweats • Increased risk of other health problems • Memory problems • Weight gain (especially around the belly), with decreased muscle mass • Muscular weakness
CYP17 inhibitors: • Abiraterone • Ketoconazole	
Luteinising hormone-releasing hormone (LHRH) agonists • Goserelin • Leuprolide • Triptorelin • Degarelix	

Hormone therapies for adrenal cancer

Hormonal therapies used to treat adrenal cancer, with consequences as listed in Table 2.8, include:

- adrenolytics, such as mitotane
- oestrogen receptor antagonists, such as fulvestrant and toremifene
- selective oestrogen receptor modulators (SERMs), such as tamoxifen and raloxifene.

New therapies

Priorities for cancer research include developing treatments that maximise damage to the tumour while limiting damage to normal tissues. This has led to investigating the use of the body's immune system to fight cancer, a category of treatment that encompasses new technologies, including:

- biological therapy
- immunotherapy
- biological response modifier therapy
- biotherapy
- targeted therapies.

This relatively new group of cancer treatments is designed to repair, stimulate, or enhance the immune system's responses. The therapies work in a variety of ways, including:

- making cancer cells more recognisable, and therefore more readily eliminated by the immune system (e.g. cytokine therapy, gene therapy)
- boosting the destructive powers of immune system cells (e.g. interferons, interleukins, monoclonal antibodies, cytokine therapy, gene therapy)
- altering the way cancer cells grow, so that they behave more like normal cells (e.g. interferons, monoclonal antibodies)
- interfering with the processes that convert a normal cell to a cancerous cell
- improving the body's ability to repair and replace normal cells damaged by other cancer treatments (e.g. colony stimulating factors (CSFs), also known as hematopoietic growth factors)
- preventing cancer cells spreading to other parts of the body (cancer vaccines).

These therapies may be used on their own, in combinations with each other, and with other treatments including surgery, radiotherapy, and chemotherapy. Many of these therapies are still in the experimental stages. In some cases, they may be only available as part of a clinical trial; others may be recently licensed and await approval by national agencies. For details about these therapies, refer to national sources for cancer information.

The long-term consequences of these new therapies are not yet known. Two therapies discussed below are:

- Herceptin®, a monoclonal antibody used widely in the treatment of breast cancer
- immune checkpoint inhibitors.

Trastuzumab (Herceptin®)

Trastuzumab is a monoclonal antibody used in the management of HER2 positive cancers, most commonly of the breast, but also some gastrointestinal cancers. About 20% of women with breast cancer are prescribed Herceptin®.[25]

Trastuzumab is administered by intravenous infusion at frequencies of once a week or once every three weeks for early breast cancer, and once every three weeks for stomach cancer. Treatment duration for early breast cancer is one year; for other cancers treatment continues for as long as it effectively controls the cancer.

Flu-like symptoms are experienced by many patients immediately following administration of the drug, especially on initial treatment. Potential later side effects include diarrhoea, headaches, nausea, fatigue, weakness, hot flushes, skin rashes, pain, and changes in blood pressure.

Cardiovascular problems may be experienced and may be minor and reversible (palpitations, irregular heartbeat), or may include long-term weakening of the heart muscle leading to chest pain, breathlessness, cough, heart fluttering, and swelling of the arms or legs. These consequences are likely to be more severe if cancer treatment includes anthracycline chemotherapy. Other occasional side effects occurring in 1–10% of patients include infections (which may be life threatening), anaemia, and bruising and bleeding. One per cent of patients may have long-term lung changes (difficulty breathing, cough), liver problems, amenorrhoea, and loss of fertility.

Immunotherapy and immune-related adverse events[16,26]

Immune checkpoint inhibitors, a form of immunotherapy which stimulates the immune system to fight disease, are beneficial for treating a range of cancers (Table 2.10).

Table 2.10: Some immune checkpoint-blocking antibodies and the cancers they are used to treat[26]

Drug	Cancers used to treat
Atezolizumab	Non-small-cell lung cancer, urothelial carcinoma
Avelumab	Merkel-cell carcinoma, urothelial carcinoma
Dostarlimab	Endometrial cancer, rectal cancer, other solid tumours
Durvalumab	Urothelial carcinoma
Ipilimumab	Melanoma
Nivolumab	Melanoma, non-small-cell lung cancer, classic Hodgkin lymphoma, squamous-cell carcinoma of the head and neck, urothelial carcinoma, gastric cancer, some solid tumours
Pembrolizumab	Melanoma, non-small-cell lung cancer, renal-cell carcinoma, hepatocellular carcinoma, classic Hodgkin lymphoma, squamous-cell carcinoma of the head and neck, urothelial carcinoma, some colorectal cancers

Acute and long-term consequences

These drugs have potential inflammatory side effects, called 'immune-related adverse events' (Table 2.11).[26] Acute events associated with active treatment, their occurrence can be severe enough to warrant discontinuation of treatment in 13% of patients.[16] It is not known why they affect some patients and not others. Some of these adverse events constitute a medical emergency; patients are informed of the symptoms to look out for and the requirement for urgent treatment from the oncology team if they arise.

> ### RED FLAG
>
> It is not currently known how long after completion of immunotherapy the associated adverse events may occur; however, they may surface during the year after treatment ends.[16] For this reason, acupuncturists should:
>
> * be aware of who in their patient list is having or has received these treatments
> * know that the appearance of adverse events should be referred immediately to the oncology team, even if the patient has completed treatment some time previously.

Table 2.11: Immune-related adverse events from immune checkpoint inhibitors[16,26]

Cancers commonly associated with	Important symptoms that should prompt consideration of an immune-related adverse effect	When arises
Bladder Lung Melanoma Renal	• Watery diarrhoea with blood or mucous and severe abdominal pain (suggests colitis) • Headaches with nausea or visual symptoms (hypophysitis (inflammation of the pituitary gland)) • Photophobia and neck stiffness (meningitis) • Confusion (encephalitis) • Fatigue with weight change (thyroid disorder, hypophysitis, or adrenal insufficiency) • Cough and shortness of breath (pneumonitis) • Joint aches, muscle aches and pains (arthritis or myositis) • Skin rashes with itching	Usually occurs within weeks to months of treatment commencement. However, they can be delayed and may occur after discontinuation of treatment.[26]

The complexity of consequences and comorbidities

Cancer is a condition associated with ageing, with over half of all diagnoses occurring in people 65 years and over.[27] This means cancer survivors will simultaneously experience the conditions of ageing, thus increasing the complexity of the symptom burden.

Cancer survivors are also more likely to experience additional chronic conditions. They are 31% more likely to be living with one or more other long-term conditions than the population of people who have never had a cancer diagnosis.[28] An estimated 29% of people with cancer in the UK have three or more potentially serious chronic health conditions as well as cancer (Table 2.12). The impact of these comorbidities may be more damaging to quality of life than the cancer itself, and lead to increased needs.[29,30]

Table 2.12: Five most common comorbidities experienced by cancer survivors in the UK[28]

Note:
The top four conditions are also the most common chronic conditions affecting people without cancer.

Comorbidity	% cancer survivors reporting
Hypertension (high blood pressure)	42
Obesity	31
Mental health problems	21
Chronic heart disease	19
Chronic kidney disease	17

CHAPTER SUMMARY

This chapter focused on the potential consequences of many of the modalities used in cancer treatment. It does not aim to be an exhaustive list of all treatments, nor of all possible consequences.

Acupuncturists should be aware of the complexities of the symptom burden that cancer survivors may present, including physical and psychosocial consequences that may arise many years after cancer treatment has ended. They should also be aware of the increased possibility of non-cancer comorbidities in this patient group, including conditions associated with ageing.

References

1. British Journal of Family Medicine Half a million UK cancer survivors faced with disability and poor health; 2013. Available from: www.bjfm.co.uk/half-a-million-uk-cancer-survivors-faced-with-disability-and-poor-health
2. Hewitt M, Greenfield S, Stovall E From cancer patient to cancer survivor: lost in transition. Washington DC: National Academies Press; 2005.
3. Elliott J, Fallows A, Staetsky L, et al. The health and well-being of cancer survivors in the UK: findings from a population-based study. Br. J. Cancer 2011;105:S11–S20.
4. National Cancer Institute Facing forward: life after cancer treatment. National Institute of Health; 2018. Available from: www.cancer.gov/publications/patient-education/life-after-treatment.pdf
5. Macmillan Cancer Support Throwing light on the consequences of cancer and its treatment. Macmillan Cancer Support; 2013. Available from: www.macmillan.org.uk/Documents/AboutUs/Research/Researchandevaluationreports/Throwinglightontheconsequencesofcanceranditstreatment.pdf
6. Thomas K, Nilsson E, Festin K, et al. Associations of psychosocial factors with multiple health behaviors: A population-based study of middle-aged men and women. Int. J. Environ. Res. Public Health 2020;17(4).
7. Jefford M, Rowland J, Grunfeld E, et al. Implementing improved post-treatment care for cancer survivors in England, with reflections from Australia, Canada and the USA. Br. J. Cancer 2013;108:14–20.
8. Carlson LE, Speca M Managing daily and long-term stress. In: Feuerstein M, editor. Handbook of cancer survivorship. New York: Springer; 2007. pp. 339–360.
9. Ganz PA, Desmond K, Leedham B, et al. Quality of life in long-term, disease-free survivors of breast cancer: a follow-up study. J. Natl. Cancer Inst. 2002;94(1):39–49.
10. Maher E, Makin W Life after cancer treatment – a spectrum of chronic survivorship conditions. Clin. Oncol. 2007;19:743–745.
11. Armes PJ, Richardson A, Crowe M, et al. Patients' supportive care needs beyond the end of treatment: a prospective and longitudinal survey. J. Clin. Oncol. 2009;27:6172–6179.
12. The Prostate Cancer Charity Hampered by hormones? Addressing the needs of men with prostate cancer Campaign Report: The Prostate Cancer Charity; 2009.
13. Macmillan Cancer Support Health and wellbeing survey: Macmillan Cancer Support; 2008.
14. Department of Health, Macmillan Cancer Support, NHS Improvement The National Cancer Survivorship Initiative Vision. London: Department of Health; 2010.
15. Miaskowski C, Barsevick A, Berger A, et al. Advancing symptom science through symptom cluster research: expert panel proceedings and recommendations. J. Natl. Cancer Inst. 2017;109(4).
16. Emery J, Butow P, Lai-Kwon J, et al. Management of common clinical problems experienced by survivors of cancer. Lancet 2022;399(10334):1537–1550.
17. Berger AM, Mooney K, Alvarez-Perez A, et al. Cancer-related fatigue, Version 2.2015. J. Natl. Compr. Canc. Netw. 2015;13(8):1012–1039.
18. Kort JD, Eisenberg ML, Millheiser LS, et al. Fertility issues in cancer survivorship. CA. Cancer J. Clin. 2014;64(2):118–134.
19. Neal AJ, Hoskin PJ Clinical oncology: basic principles and practice. 3rd ed. London: Arnold; 2003.
20. Marie Curie What is palliative care? London: Marie Curie; 2022. Available from: www.mariecurie.org.uk/help/support/diagnosed/recent-diagnosis/palliative-care-end-of-life-care
21. Ajithkumar T, Barrett A, Hatcher H, et al. Oxford desk reference: oncology. Oxford: Oxford University Press; 2021.

22. Cancer Research UK Cancer treatment statistics. London: Cancer Research UK; 2017. Available from: www.cancerresearchuk.org/health-professional/cancer-statistics/treatment#heading-Two

23. Stricker CT, Jacobs LA Physical late effects in adult cancer survivors. Oncology (Williston Park) 2008;22(8 Suppl. Nurse Ed.):33–41.

24. American Cancer Society Hormone therapy. 2020. Available from: www.cancer.org/treatment/treatments-and-side-effects/treatment-types/hormone-therapy.html

25. UT Southwestern Medical Centre What new research on Herceptin® could mean for breast cancer patients. Dallas; 2018. Available from: https://utswmed.org/medblog/herceptin-treatment-update/#:~:text=Approximately%20237%2C000%20cases%20of%20breast,%2Dpositive%20 (HER2%2Dpositive

26. Postow MA, Sidlow R, Hellmann MD Immune-related adverse events associated with immune checkpoint blockade. N. Engl. J. Med. 2018;378(2):158–168.

27. National Cancer Institute Age and cancer risk. National Cancer Institute; 2021. Available from: www.cancer.gov/about-cancer/causes-prevention/risk/age

28. Macmillan Cancer Support The burden of cancer and other long-term health conditions. 2015. Available from: www.macmillan.org.uk/documents/press/cancerandotherlong-termconditions.pdf

29. Denlinger C, Barsevick A The challenges of colorectal cancer survivorship. J. Natl. Compr. Canc. Netw. 2009;7(8):883–894.

30. Rohan E, Townsend J, Fairley T, *et al.* Health behaviours and quality of life among colorectal cancer survivors. J. Natl. Compr. Canc. Netw. 2015;13(3):297–302.

Chapter 3

Cancer Survivorship
and the Emotions

Introduction

The emotional burden of a cancer diagnosis and the support that acupuncture can provide are expressed in these quotations:

> Newly diagnosed patients embark on a journey with an uncertain destination, laden with stress and anxiety, and desperate for hope and support. (Drew & Fawcett)[1]

> You have given me hope! (Colorectal cancer survivor's comments about acupuncture treatment)

Cancer can generate strong emotions. From the initial shock and fear of diagnosis, to worry and anxiety about treatment success and possible recurrence, survivors may also experience anger, grief, and sadness. Emotional distress may continue after treatment ends. Drew and Fawcett's description applies equally to both newly diagnosed patients and to long-term survivors.

This chapter discusses the emotional challenges that may arise in the aftermath of cancer treatment. This is a time when many survivors feel their cancer experience is 'over' and they should be able to deal with their emotions.[2] They may be perplexed to find that emotions remain strong and complex.

An important role for acupuncturists working with cancer survivors is to develop awareness of the possible emotional challenges facing their patients. These may be concurrent and intertwined with physical symptoms. The case study of Fleur at the end of this chapter illustrates the powerful interrelationship of emotional states and physical symptoms.

This chapter focuses on:

- the emotions as viewed in Chinese medicine and their relationship to cancer survivorship
- some societal attitudes to cancer and the pressures they exert on survivors
- how acupuncture practitioners can support cancer survivors in the acknowledgement and appropriate expression of emotions.

This chapter does not imply any relationship between emotions and causes of cancer.

Emotional challenges of survivorship

When active treatment ends, survivors may feel uncertain, isolated, and vulnerable, especially as their long contact with medical staff comes to an end. Emotional challenges may also continue into the long term. For some, these can be powerful and long-lasting; they may ebb and flow, changing according to an individual's emotional landscape. Such feelings may take the survivor by surprise. 'I thought I had got over that' or 'It's time that I got over that' are comments I often hear from survivors when strong feelings relating to their cancer surge, sometimes months or even years after diagnosis and treatment.

In addition to the physical and physiological consequences of treatment, cancer survivorship involves coping with 'extra-physical' issues. These are defined as emotional, social, occupational, and financial concerns that accompany and extend beyond acute treatment.[3] These may have long-lasting effects on an individual's emotional health, with consequent impacts on resilience and quality of life.

An American study surveyed 1024 respondents, 73% of whom were two or more years from diagnosis.[4] Over half found dealing with 'emotional needs harder than physical needs', and one third felt resources for dealing with emotional needs were inadequate. Depression and relationship problems were also reported (by 72% and 60% respectively).

Surprisingly, respondents were also upbeat about having cancer:

- 62% were currently experiencing 'good' health
- 59% were optimistic they would die from something 'besides cancer'
- 47% said dealing with cancer made 'life better'.

Levels of psychological health were found to be similar in the majority (80%) of cancer survivors studied compared with healthy population-based studies in the UK.[5] However, a subset of survivors showed poor adjustment severe enough to require psychiatric treatment. The study identified factors associated with successful adaptation to illness, including perceived social support from spouse/partner and a positive active coping style. Other factors contributing to resilience include optimism, finding a positive meaning from the cancer experience, maintaining self-esteem and 'normal' life roles, and expression of emotions.

This last factor, expression of emotions, is the focus of this chapter.

Cancer survivorship and the emotions in Chinese medicine

Emotions are an essential aspect of human life. Feeling joy, worry, sadness, fear, and anger is part of the experience of living. Life events may provoke strong emotional responses that are entirely appropriate to the circumstances; for example, it is natural to feel grief on losing a loved one. When experiencing cancer and its treatments, it is also appropriate for a survivor to feel strong emotions.

The emotions as internal causes of disease

In Chinese medicine theory, emotions are categorised as 'internal' causes of disease. Emotions can become pathological when they are very intense or very long lasting. This can impact circulation of qi and disturb the mind (*shen*), ethereal soul (*hun*) and corporeal soul (*po*), and through these alter the balance of the internal organs and the harmony of Blood and qi. The interaction between the emotions, internal organs, and unity of body and mind is 'one of the most important and distinctive aspects of Chinese medicine'.[6]

Historical Chinese medical texts discuss this, providing lists of emotions that have evolved to comprise seven emotions commonly cited in modern texts: shock, fear, anger, worry, sadness, pensiveness, and joy (Table 3.1).[6] Contemporary commentators extend this list to encompass emotions common to modern Western culture, such as guilt and shame.[6,7] Exploring these in relation to cancer survivorship provides insights into the emotions survivors may experience.

Table 3.1: Emotions in Chinese medicine and descriptions

Emotion	Description
Shock	Sometimes translated as 'fright', can result from physical or emotional trauma. Can cause disorientation, emotional volatility, agitation, fatigue, and unpleasant heart sensations.[8]
Fear	Chronic state of fear, anxiety, or a sudden fright.
Anger	May include resentment, repressed shame, feeling aggrieved, frustration, irritation, rage, indignation, animosity, bitterness.
Worry	Preoccupation, or in its extreme form, obsession; can become a major part of a person's stream of consciousness.[8]
Sadness and grief	Common and important causes of disease in modern Western society; encompass loss and regret.
Pensiveness	Brooding, constantly thinking about certain events or people, nostalgic hankering after the past, generally thinking intensely about life rather than living it.
Joy	Excessive excitement and craving; also, reaction akin to shock to sudden unexpected good news.
Modern additions relevant to cancer survivorship	
Guilt	Self-reproach for actual misdeeds or an inborn feeling of guilt totally disconnected from any misdeeds.
Shame	The feeling that one must hide because one has done something wrong, something that society frowns on, something 'dirty'.

Adapted from The Psyche in Chinese Medicine, pages 116–159,[6] except descriptions of shock and worry.

Ground rules pertaining to emotions as internal causes of disease

Emotions are healthy and appropriate responses to life; the emotions described in the Chinese medical literature are natural reactions to external and internal stimuli. Mostly, they become pathological when they are excessive or prolonged.[9]

To curb the impression that experiencing emotions inevitably leads to developing disease, it is important to establish some 'ground rules' about the emotions as internal causes of disease.

Duration and intensity

An emotional state risks becoming a cause of disease when it is experienced for a long time (months or years). However, extremely intense emotions (such as extreme shock) may become a cause of disease in a short time.

Maciocia posits that emotions become causes of disease when 'they take over our mind, when we no longer possess them but they possess us', a state he describes as 'mental suffering'.[6]

Free expression

Suppressed or blocked emotions may become pathological; thus, the free expression of appropriate emotions should be encouraged.[10] This contradicts belief systems that promote the practice of detachment from feeling or expressing emotion.

Emotional health means resilience. This involves avoiding the extreme positions of falling prey to emotions or striving for lack of emotion. In the words of Larre and de la Vallee:

> In treating people, we are not asking them to be emotionless, or not be taken over by emotions, but just as far as possible to be able to come back to a state where the emotion will be felt inside their quietness.[11]

Exploring the emotions of survivorship through Chinese medicine

The emotions in Chinese medicine provide a useful filter to explore the emotional states of people living with and beyond cancer.

Shock

Shock in Chinese medicine

Discussions of shock are often derived from the classical texts on fright (*jing*):[8]

> When there is starting with fright the qi is in disorder...the heart no longer has a place to rely on, the spirits no longer have a place to refer to..., planned thought...no longer has a place to settle. This is how the qi is in disorder.[11]

Shock scatters the qi, affecting the Heart and Kidney. Sudden depletion of Heart qi affects the Kidney, as the body draws on Kidney-essence to supplement this depletion.[6] While the 'heart is the first victim of *jing*', the Liver, Spleen, and Stomach are also implicated, and occasionally the Gall Bladder and Lung.[11]

Symptoms arising from shock include extreme fearfulness, anxiety, nightmares, insomnia, depression, and fear of leaving the house,[7] as well as night-sweating, dry mouth, dizziness, and tinnitus.[6] Disordered qi causes anarchy:

> ...no one knows how to cope with the situation or how to make connections...there is no basis from which to express yourself or make thinking work.[11]

Shock in cancer survivorship

A cancer diagnosis invariably engenders a profound sense of shock, even when an individual 'knows' that something is physically amiss. Newly diagnosed patients may be unable to take in information. Some may cope by avoiding thinking about cancer; others by constantly thinking or talking about it.

In recounting her reaction to the shock of diagnosis, Emily (see Chapter 1, Cancer Survivorship and the Role of Acupuncture) describes a state of disordered qi. She was 'reduced to a sleepless, quivering jelly' unable to 'really think straight at all'. With treatment rapidly following diagnosis, there is little time to assimilate shock. As she says, once this process starts 'your feet never touch the ground'.

My sense is that this shock, often unprocessed and unresolved, may contribute to the severity of symptoms arising during and after cancer treatment.

Fear

Fear in Chinese medicine

Fright (see Shock above) is a sudden and acute response to a threat. In contrast, fear (*kong*) is a prolonged, continuous response to a real or perceived stimulus. This chronic nature gives fear its pathologic status in Chinese medicine; the fear response itself is a necessary survival mechanism to generate appropriate behavioural responses to threats, namely the 'fight or flight' response to danger.

While fright causes qi to become chaotic, fear causes qi to sink. However, a more complex action is described in *Su Wen*, Chapter 39:

> When there is fear, kong, the qi descends... When there is fear, the essences withdraw; withdrawing, the upper heater closes; closing, the qi leaves; leaving, the lower heater is swollen. This is how the qi does not circulate.[11]

This impaired circulation disrupts communication between the upper and lower burners, severing the Kidney–Heart axis. Blocking of the upper burner causes the qi of the lower burner to descend; it also causes qi stagnation in the upper burner. Maciocia observes that when the Heart is strong, fear causes qi to descend; when the Heart is weak, qi rises.[6] Thus, fear can give rise to symptoms associated with:

- sinking Kidney qi, such as nocturnal enuresis in children, urinary incontinence in adults, diarrhoea, and malar flush
- imbalance in the Heart qi, such as palpitations, insomnia, dry mouth, and dizziness.

Fear can also affect the Stomach, Spleen, Lung, and Liver.[11]

Fear in cancer survivorship

Fear understandably accompanies a cancer diagnosis. Cancer is potentially life threatening, raising fears about suffering and mortality. During active treatment, cancer survivors may experience fear about cancer treatment and its impacts on their body, independence, role, quality of life, and their very survival.

Fear of recurrence is a major concern for many people when active treatment ends. For Dee, a colorectal cancer survivor, fear and anxiety set in after her treatment was pronounced successful. During active treatment, her attitude was 'what will be, will be'. On receiving the 'all clear' from her consultant, Dee 'didn't believe it' and subsequently lived in fear of cancer recurrence.[12]

As discussed in Chapter 11, Survivorship: Navigating the Milestones, fear of recurrence is common and can occur at any time. For Rose, its constant presence seriously impacted her quality of life. For Claire, it arose suddenly and unexpectedly eight years after active cancer treatment ended. For Alauda, fear of recurrence emerges at anniversaries of diagnosis, significant treatment dates, and routine follow-ups. Throughout this book, case studies illustrate how fear of recurrence affects individuals.

Anger
Anger in Chinese medicine
Anger (nu) in its healthy state is an impetuous violent force, a creative energy that has the 'kind of violence proper to all beginnings'.[11] This is movement that engenders change. In its pathological state, it encompasses resentment, repressed anger, frustration, irritation, rage, animosity, bitterness, and indignation.[6]

Anger is associated with the Liver and its movement is to make qi rise. In its pathological state, this manifests in headaches, tinnitus, dizziness, red face, red eyes, thirst, bitter taste, and a red tongue with red sides. The behaviour is violent, shouting, and aggressive.

However, there are two sides to anger.[11] Contrasting with this bursting, violent movement of anger is a more subdued form wherein the energy is blocked, suppressed, and bottled up. In this state, the person presents as subdued, pale, and quiet, with slow movements. While this suggests depletion of qi and Blood deriving from sadness or grief, it may be depression due to suppressed anger.[6]

While anger is commonly associated with its violent manifestation, suppression of anger has 'enormous and unhappy effects on the psychological balance'.[13] It is the basis of numerous conditions including depression, insomnia, psychiatric disorders, headaches, and disorders of the chest, stomach, bowels, and reproductive organs.[7]

Anger in cancer survivorship
Anger is commonly experienced by cancer survivors; one study reported that 14% of breast cancer patients experienced feelings of anger following surgery.[14] It is quite normal for cancer survivors to feel angry about their condition. This anger may be directed at people close to them, their medical team, God or fate, or healthy people: 'Why has this happened to me?'

Anger is generally perceived as negative by society, researchers,[15] and other cancer survivors, and may be one of the most challenging emotions to deal with. Author Barbara Ehrenreich recounts how she was rebuked by other cancer survivors for her 'bad attitude' and 'anger and bitterness' when she posted comments about her cancer experience on a message board under the subject line 'Angry'.[16] Cultural and societal attitudes contrive to inhibit the expression of anger; repression may result in turning the emotion inward, or in anger bursting out inappropriately or directed at an inappropriate target.

For Miriam, diagnosis and treatment of a gynaecological cancer triggered powerful feelings of anger – towards fate, her medical team, and the medical system. Her feelings were so strong that she chose to stop cancer treatment (as a senior oncology health professional she was aware of the risks associated with her decision). She told me how this anger was rekindled, years later, on receiving a letter inviting her participation in cancer research. (Fortunately, many years on, Miriam remains well.)

In my experience, such overt expressions of anger are rare. It is more common for cancer survivors to suppress feelings of anger, making recognition of this emotion clinically challenging.

Worry
Worry in Chinese medicine
Worry is the pathological counterpart of the Spleen's capacity for thought (*si*). There are many interpretations of worry in contemporary discussions of Chinese medicine:

- Macicocia views it as one of the most common causes of disease in modern Western society, brought about by rapid and radical changes that have created a climate of insecurity in all aspects of life.[6]
- Rossi equates *si* with obsessive rumination, whereby thought circles endlessly, failing to transform or result in action. She notes that patients may describe this as being anxious.[13]
- Deadman equates worry with anxiety, positing that worry is a necessary skill evolved by humans to deal with the world, to anticipate difficulties and plan strategies to deal with them. In their pathological state, worry and anxiety fixate on what might happen in the future, consuming energy and impairing clear judgement and action.[17]

These commentators agree that worry knots the qi, stopping circulation and causing stagnation, and prevents people from transforming thought into effective action.

Worry commonly manifests in Spleen symptoms including poor appetite, epigastric discomfort, abdominal pain and distension, tiredness, and pale complexion. It may affect other organs including the:

- **Lung** – manifesting as shallow breathing, discomfort in the chest, slight breathlessness, tensing of the shoulders, dry cough, and pale complexion
- **Liver** – causing Liver qi stagnation or Liver yang rising; may cause stiffness and aching in the shoulders and trapezius muscles
- **Heart** – manifesting in palpitations, chest tightness, and insomnia.

Clear judgement is impaired, and other symptoms include headaches, chronic muscle tension, dizziness, shortness of breath, fatigue, palpitations, and hyperventilation.[17]

Worry in cancer survivorship

In the cancer literature, worry is frequently discussed in terms of worries about cancer coming back; in this sense, 'worry' is another expression for fear of recurrence.

My view is that it may be difficult to differentiate between fear, worry, and anxiety, which may all be intertwined for some individuals. I situate worry in the practical issues that cancer survivors may face. These include the extra-physical concerns, such as social, occupational, and financial issues – the very real, practical problems for which solutions may be difficult or non-existent.

Samson is a colorectal cancer survivor whose treatment left him unable to work. As well as experiencing chronic fear of recurrence, Samson is extremely concerned about his financial state. Inability to work has also affected his self-regard, as he has lost his role as provider for his family. His concerns are well founded and insoluble, and manifest as insomnia, chronic muscle pain, fatigue, and digestive issues.

Sadness and grief

Sadness and grief in Chinese medicine

Sadness and grief derive from loss. Loss may be experienced as the break-up of a relationship, a death, or when life does not match up to a person's expectations.[8] Experiencing sadness or grief in such circumstances is not harmful; rather it is a part of the cycle of life. The potential to become pathological happens when these emotions are suppressed or prolonged, or when the emotional trauma caused by loss is so great that it can scarcely be borne.

Sadness and grief affect the Lung and the Heart. Citing *Simple Questions*, Chapter 39, Maciocia observes that sadness primarily affects the Heart; the Lungs suffer as a consequence of their proximity to the Heart in the upper burner.[6]

Sadness depletes qi, particularly Lung qi, manifesting in a weak voice, pale complexion, breathlessness, weeping, and oppression in the chest.[6] Tiredness may be extreme – the qi is exhausted and the person may feel they have nothing left.[13]

In grief, the qi sinks and drains away, causing postural changes such as drooping shoulders and collapsing chest, which injures the Lungs, respiratory system and qi.[7] Prolonged sadness and grief can also lead to stagnation of qi. In addition, these emotions may affect the Liver, causing mental confusion, forgetfulness, and reduced vitality.[6,11]

Sadness and grief in cancer survivorship

It is appropriate for cancer survivors to experience sadness and grief. There may be sadness about the loss of good health, about being unable to do things as before, or that the future may not be as planned. Survivors may need to grieve these losses.

Sadness is a natural part of loss, grief, change, or disappointment, and the feeling may be constant or may come and go. It is important to distinguish the normal feelings of sadness from depression. Medical advice is that if a patient feels sad for more than two weeks and finds it hard to feel good about anything, they may be depressed rather than sad.[18]

In my clinical experience, cancer survivors often cope with multiple concurrent losses. Frequently, death of a loved one complicates the emotional picture, particularly if it coincides with the survivor's cancer diagnosis and treatment. For Ann (see Chapter 14), a significant bereavement at the time of her diagnosis prevented her coming to terms with her cancer. Simultaneously, coping with her cancer treatment prevented her grieving that loss. In Ann's case, an unusual pattern of deaths occurring at Christmas over many years further added to her burden of grief. The accumulation of this suppressed emotion developed into patterns of fear and anxiety.

Similarly, Franceszka was a breast cancer survivor whose diagnosis and treatment coincided with her mother's death and impeded her grieving process. At the anniversary one year later, Franceszka experienced a relapse of symptoms – worsening hot flushes and muscle pains were accompanied by breathlessness and chest pains, typical manifestations of sadness and grief in Chinese medicine.

Guilt and shame

Pensiveness and joy may be less applicable to cancer survivorship than shock, fear, anger, worry, sadness, and grief. Maciocia notes that guilt and shame are two emotions commonly experienced by Western patients that are absent from Chinese medicine texts.[6] I have included them as they are experienced by cancer survivors.

Guilt and shame in Chinese medicine

A fundamental difference between these two emotions is that:

- feelings of guilt are the result of a negative judgement of one's own behaviour
- feelings of shame are the result of fear of being negatively judged by others.[19]

Guilt is a subjective feeling and is independent of any status of actual guilt (e.g. breaking the law). It is directed inwardly at the self, and Maciocia calls it the opposite of anger, which is usually directed outward. Guilt affects people differently and can lead to:

- **qi stagnation:** affecting any organ, especially the Lung, Heart, Liver, and Kidney
- **Blood stasis:** resulting from qi stagnation; can occur anywhere in the body but particularly in the Lung, Heart, Spleen, and Liver
- **Kidney qi sinking:** leading to urinary or menstrual problems.[6]

Shame may be a feeling about our own behaviour; more commonly it is a feeling of worthlessness or an absence of feelings of self-worth. It is related to our place in society and what people think of us. There is a feeling of needing to hide something that we have done 'wrong', something 'dirty' that society disapproves of.

Like guilt, shame is inwardly directed, and contrasts with the rising movement of anger. It can lead to qi sinking and damp, manifesting in prolapse of the organs and a range of chronic persistent conditions, including persistent vaginal discharge, slight urinary incontinence, and excessive menstrual bleeding resulting from sinking of Spleen and Kidney qi. Shame is often expressed as feeling 'dirty', and 'dirtiness' is a characteristic of damp.[6]

Guilt and shame in cancer survivorship

Guilt and shame are commonly experienced in cancer survivorship. Survivors may feel guilty that they are alive when others have died of their disease. Ann (see Chapter 14) experienced survivor guilt on the death of her young neighbour. Guilt may also manifest as:

- a need for survivors to justify their existence – 'to give something back'
- inability to enjoy life
- comparisons with someone they know who has died or had a more difficult experience of cancer.

Guilt may trigger symptoms such as anxiety, poor sleep, hypervigilance, or feelings of depression, worthlessness, hopelessness, and self-blame.[20]

Shame may be felt by survivors who feel their behaviour caused their cancer, for example through smoking or poor diet. It has been suggested that such feelings of shame make it more difficult for cancer survivors to adhere to good lifestyle practices. Shame is also associated with psychological conditions such as low self-esteem, anxiety and depression, eating disorders, post-traumatic stress disorder, and suicidal thoughts.[19]

Societal pressures on cancer survivors

We have seen that cancer survivors may experience profound, complex emotions from the time of diagnosis to long after treatment ends. As acupuncturists, we can support patients to acknowledge, express, and process these emotions.

There are also powerful inhibitors to having, acknowledging, or discussing strong emotions related to cancer. Embedded into societal attitudes to cancer, practitioners and patients may be unaware of the influence these exert over us all.

Language of struggle

The language of struggle and 'battle mentality' underpin the way cancer is discussed in Western societies, affecting attitudes to cancer and its treatments: an aggressive disease requires aggressive treatment.[21] Military and sporting expressions are frequently employed, such as:

- war against cancer
- crusade
- fight or battle cancer
- win (or lose) the battle against cancer
- destroy the cells
- fighting spirit, bravery.[22]

This may cause distress and be detrimental for people with cancer, making them feel they must battle on against all odds. One young mother with gynaecological cancer, who opted for aggressive treatments despite their discomfort and poor prognosis, told me she was doing this to show her children she had done everything possible to defeat the disease.

Tyranny of positive thinking

Attitudes to cancer have changed drastically since the mid-20th century when it was referred to in hushed tones as the 'Big C'. Today, there is much more openness about cancer. Information is freely available, with daily coverage in the media. So much attention is focused on cancer, it is difficult to remember that heart disease is the major cause of mortality globally.

Concurrent with these changes was the development of ideas about the power of positive thinking, which became interwoven into attitudes to cancer. Over recent decades, much has been written about the importance of positive thinking when faced with cancer and its treatments. While many people with cancer have found this to be beneficial and life affirming, the need to 'be positive' may be burdensome for others.

The pressure to always have a 'good attitude' can come from within the individual, from other people, or both. Some people feel guilty or blame themselves when they can't 'stay positive', adding to their emotional burden. There is also a problem when positive thinking 'fails' and the cancer spreads or eludes treatment. Then the patient bears the blame – the perception is that by failing to be sufficiently positive, their negative attitude caused their disease.[23] A colleague told me of a woman who, in spite of doing 'all the right things' suffered a breast cancer recurrence. In despair, she committed suicide.

So far, research has not found convincing links between personality type and likelihood of cancer[24] or impact of optimism on cancer survival.[25,26] Encouraging a positive outlook may even have detrimental effects, as cautioned by the lead author of a study investigating optimism in lung cancer survival:

> We should question whether it is valuable to encourage optimism if it results in the patient concealing his or her distress in the misguided belief that this will afford survival benefits ... If a patient feels generally pessimistic ... it is important to acknowledge these feelings as valid and acceptable.[25]

Expectations about the end of treatment

Cancer treatment has finished. Life can now get back to normal. This is the expectation and hope of cancer patients at the end of primary treatment. It is an unexpected and often cruel blow when life does not return to what it was before the intrusion of the cancer diagnosis and treatment.

What surprises and disappoints many people is that they now face physical and emotional changes that are the consequences of the life-saving treatment. Furthermore, unintended pressure may be exerted by family and friends, who are relieved to see the end of treatment, and who also share expectations that life can now return to normal. These expectations can cause distress. A breast cancer survivor, two years post treatment, told me that she was still having trouble coming to terms with having cancer, yet her family felt she should 'move on'.

The pressure to return to normal may come from the survivor's own expectations or may be generated by family, friends, or workplace expectations. In my experience, there is a tendency for many cancer survivors to 'overdo' things at this stage – to return to work too soon, to take on rigorous exercise regimes, to make up for time lost to cancer and its treatments. This can lead to frustration and feelings of inadequacy, especially if home or work life is threatened.

Summary of societal pressures

These are three underlying pressures that may affect individuals' attitudes and ability to cope with survivorship. They are often unconscious, engrained in the fabric of societal expectations. Contributing to unrealistic expectations, they may increase the emotional burden of individuals as they navigate life after cancer treatment. It is useful for us, as acupuncturists, to be aware of these influences and their potential impact.

The importance of acupuncture

In 1997, eminent UK cancer researcher Dame Jessica Corner proposed a model for a 'counter-culture' against the then (and still) current biomedical construction of cancer treatment.[21] Intended for the nursing profession, her four keystones for this alternative model of care (Box 3.1) strike me as being fundamental to what acupuncture can, and often does, offer to cancer survivors. Embedded into many of the theoretical frameworks of acupuncture is the view of the whole person: body, mind, and emotions, as expressed in this chapter.

Box 3.1: An alternative model of care

- Offers an environment which is participative, collaborative, and empowering of people with cancer, their families, and carers.
- Adopts an integrated view of the person (that is an understanding of the inseparable nature of mind and body in the experience of cancer-related problems and needs).
- Shifts the dominant construct in cancer management from 'survival' to the here and now, and to the problems and needs individuals are facing. This need not be played out as a heroic struggle that all parties are engaged in but is rather an experience which needs to be shared and understood, where mutual decisions are made to determine the future, which may involve containing, or for some, curing the disease.
- Seeks to move individuals towards healing and health in the broadest sense.[21]

Cancer survivors who opt to have acupuncture value this capacity to encompass the emotional aspect of their experience, as evidenced by these quotations from participants in a research study of acupuncture to improve wellbeing for people with cancer treat-ment-related lymphoedema (see Chapter 9, Cancer Treatment-Related Lymphoedema):

> She was just easy to talk to and easy to offload and easy to cry in front of. And it just happened for that one hour in there each time and it was lovely. (011 BC)

> When we have sickness like this, talking at home doesn't generally help. Because it's a depressing thing to talk. But when you're talking with somebody like [name of acupunc-turist]...it's more professional and at the same time you are able to tell them what you would otherwise not want to unnecessarily depress the rest of the family. So you are very open, and she is receptive, and she is also counselling, because that part is very important, besides the needles, the counselling part, and then supported by the acupuncture and everything else. (007 HNT)

> I don't know...whether it's the acupuncture or not, but...whatever happened to me during that period of time, I'm in a much better emotional place than before. And physical as well, because of the hot flushes and so forth. (018 BC)

CASE STUDY: FLEUR AND THE POWER OF EMOTIONAL RELEASE

This case study is an in-depth examination of the interrelationship of emotional states and physical symptoms in cancer survivorship, and demonstrates the power of releasing pent-up emotions.

Introduction

Fleur's oncologist referred her for acupuncture in November 2011 to manage breast cancer treatment-related hot flushes and night sweats (HFNS).

Background

Fleur, aged 51, was diagnosed with a tumour in the left breast in 2011. A lumpectomy in March 2011 showed no spread of cancer to the lymph nodes. Radiotherapy was completed at the end of May 2011.

Main complaints

In April 2011, adjuvant hormonal treatment with tamoxifen commenced and was accompanied by the immediate onset of 'horrendous' HFNS. Fleur had experienced night sweats during natural menopause; however, the tamoxifen-related incidents were 'vicious', occurring four to five times per night and leaving her 'dripping wet'. She also got very hot during the day. 'Morning is a struggle': profuse sweating triggered by blow-drying her hair hampered her attempts to prepare for the day.

Palpitations and chest pain began during cancer treatment. These were thought to be anxiety-related, and Fleur was prescribed beta blockers while undergoing further investigations with a cardiac specialist.

Questioning the systems

Sleep: Prior to cancer diagnosis, Fleur had been a good sleeper. Now sleep was 'awful'. Although she had no problem getting to sleep, night sweats woke her as often as five times a night. She was 'drenched and hot', needed to change sheets often, and protected the mattress with a liner. Experiencing frequent dreams that were 'vivid and exciting', Fleur also talked and walked in her sleep. However, she did not have nightmares.

Appetite: This was 'fine'. Fleur ate well but skipped breakfast on weekdays. Lunch could be sushi or pasta salad, and her home-cooked evening meal relied on a variety of fresh vegetables, fish, and lean meat. At weekends, she ate more 'unhealthy' foods, such as a bacon sandwich for breakfast or a scone with afternoon tea. Because of her work, Fleur ate out often. Although she had a sweet tooth and enjoyed desserts, she did not snack between meals. She did not experience any digestive discomfort and maintained an appropriate weight.

Drink: Fleur drank six to eight cups of fluid daily, consisting of hot water on rising, followed by herbal teas throughout the day. Although she drank socially, alcohol triggered HFNS.

Bowels: Fleur had a bowel movement most days; 'a bit more effort' was needed for these since her diagnosis.

Urine: Flow had become less forceful since a recent gynaecological investigation; she woke twice nightly to empty her bladder.

Temperature: Fleur described herself as a 'chilly person', with hands, feet, and back especially cold. She had a 'tendency to Reynauds'.

Gynaecological: She had used oral contraceptives for most of her adult life and stopped because of migraines, which subsequently subsided. Periods had ceased on diagnosis of cancer. Prior to this, they occurred every two to three weeks, and while accompanied by a 'dragging' pain, they were light and lasted two to three days. Fleur had never been pregnant.

Head, body, ears, eyes: Although Fleur had a history of migraines, she had only experienced one since her cancer diagnosis nearly six months previously. Dizziness experienced after surgery due to low blood pressure corrected itself and was no longer a problem.

Numbness and pain: Fleur sometimes experienced numbness in her fingers and tingling in her arms and legs. Joint pain 'comes and goes'; this had started in her twenties.

Health history: Laser treatment to the cervix for precancerous cells (age 25), laparoscopy for endometriosis (no date), and varicose vein surgery (age 35).

Additional information: Fleur lived with her husband in the country at weekends; during the week they lived near her work in the city. Fleur was a director of a successful company she had established and developed over the years. Following her diagnosis, she had 'done all the right things', taking six months off work to recuperate. Now she was back at work and not coping.

Physical examination: Tongue: Pale overall; pale and wet at sides; no coating, no cracks. **Pulses:** Deep and weak on the first and third positions on the right side, and especially so on the third position on the left side. The middle positions on both sides were the dominant pulses. Rhythm and rate were regular.

Diagnoses
CM diagnosis: A history of Spleen qi not holding the Blood compounded by shen disturbance and Heart qi deficiency.

CF diagnosis: Fire, probably on the Pericardium side.

Treatment approach
Fleur's treatment priority was to relieve the HFNS. Given her cardiac symptoms and my diagnosis of her CF as fire, the treatment plan that evolved focused on:

- regulating Heart qi
- calming the shen
- treating the CF.

She attended for five treatments, outlined in Table 3.2. However, the significant feature of this case – the impact emotional release had on Fleur's symptoms – is recounted below.

The power of emotional release on HFNS
During her second treatment, Fleur told me about her career, describing her transition from secretary to manager of her own public relations company. Entertaining clients was a major activity, which Fleur said she enjoyed greatly. I was struck by the disparity between the woman she described performing this role and the woman I saw before me: outgoing, vivacious, lively, enthusiastic, motivated, and energetic compared with the pale, vulnerable, listless, and dispirited woman in my clinic.

At her third treatment, we discussed Fleur's emotional life. During this discussion, I reassured her that it was okay to cry and important to express emotions, saying 'emotions are like wind, better out than in'. Fleur gave me such a strange look that I resolved to rethink my comparison of emotional release with flatulence!

The following week, I greeted a transformed woman! Fleur related how my comparison had captured her attention. On returning to work and home, she warned her secretary and her husband she was likely to disappear at times during the week; if they found her in tears, it was alright and to let her get on with it. She reported that she had locked herself in the toilet several times that week and cried her eyes out. And she felt better.

Transformation was apparent. Fleur's colour was good, her eyes clear and sparkling; now I could see the lively and vivacious entrepreneur she had described previously. Furthermore, she reported improvements in her symptoms. Night sweats reduced to two per night, her sleep improved, she could blow-dry her hair in the morning, and the chest pain was less intense. She felt 'like a different person'.

At her fifth treatment the following week, she confirmed she had 'turned a corner'. With fewer disturbances at night, Fleur was more cheerful. She had experienced three flush-free days; at night she was 'a bit sweaty'. Chest pain was intermittent and so I changed treatment priorities to regulating Heart qi.

This was prior to the Christmas break. Fleur travelled a considerable distance through trying traffic conditions to have treatment. In the New Year, she opted to stop seeing me; her symptoms were sufficiently reduced for her to discontinue treatment.

Table 3.2: Fleur's five acupuncture treatments

Notes:

Details of how to administer these treatments are in Chapter 5, Toolkit.

Fleur, as a breast cancer survivor, was at risk of lymphoedema and consequently needling was avoided in the limb on the at-risk side, in her case the left side. For details see Chapter 9, Cancer Treatment-Related Lymphoedema.

Abbreviations: Tx treatment; **RS** right side; **LS** left side; **bi** bilateral; **(n)** shows number of direct moxa cones applied

2011	Treatment principles	Points	Notes
Tx 1	**16 Nov:** Give acupuncture-naive patient experience of needling; monitor reactions.		
	Harmonise qi	Three Gates: LI-4 *Hegu* (RS) LIV-3 *Taichong* (bi)	
Tx 2	**23 Nov:** Fleur said she was comfortable with acupuncture needling. Reported having fewer severe flushes during the previous week, no night sweats on night of treatment. Chest pain became intermittent rather than constant.		
	Treat HFNS	Open *Ren Mai*: LU-7 *Lieque* (RS) KID- 6 *Zhaohai* (LS) HE-6 *Yinxi* (RS) KID-7 *Fuliu* (LS)	
	Regulate Heart qi	BL-14 *Jueyinshu* (7) (RS)	
	Calm shen	M-HN-3 *Yintang*	
	Support spirit	KID-24 *Lingxu* (5) (RS) REN-17 *Shanzhong* (5)	Direct moxa only.

Tx 3

7 Dec: Two weeks since previous treatment. Fleur felt calmer after last treatment, found it restful. However, was experiencing four to six sweats per night and feeling 'grotty' with tiredness. Had two nights' good sleep prior to today's treatment, with no flushes today. Last week saw cardiac consultant, 24-hour monitor fitted; rhythm irregular and palpitations; beta blocker dosage increased. Experienced pain in stomach and left arm. (*Discussed emotional release at this treatment.*)

	'Toasted Pericardium Sandwich' to nourish organs and calm shen	BL-43 *Gaohuangshu* (15) (RS) REN-17 *Shanzhong* (5)	Direct moxa only.
	Regulate Heart qi Calm shen Support the spirit Treat CF (Pericardium)	BL-14 *Jueyinshu* (RS) P-3 *Quze* (RS) P-6 *Neiguan* (RS) P-7 *Daling* (RS) REN-15 *Jiuwei*	
Tx 4	**14 Dec:** Feeling much better! Sweats down to two per night, can blow-dry hair in the morning. Chest pain and palpitations less intense. Slept very well after last treatment. Experiencing tingling up and down legs.		
	As per Tx 3	With additionally: KID-24 *Lingxu* (5) (RS)	Direct moxa only.
Tx 5	**20 Dec:** Felt as if she had turned a corner. Three hot-flush-free days; slightly sweaty at night. More cheerful as less disturbed during night. Sleeping better. Chest pain intermittent although overall improved. Experiencing pain in left arm.		
	Regulate Heart qi Calm shen Support the spirit Treat arm pain	P-2 *Tianquan* (RS) P-3 *Quze* (RS) TB-11 *Qinglengyuan* (RS) TB-12 *Xiaoluo* (RS)	Needled right arm to treat pain in left arm.
	Treat CF (Luo-connecting points of Pericardium)	P-6 *Neiguan* (RS) TB-5 *Waiguan* (RS)	

Long term follow-up and summary

I followed Fleur's progress over the next year courtesy of her oncologist's review letters. During the summer of 2012, Fleur had a recurrence scare; investigations confirmed all was normal. HFNS were bothersome again (perhaps in response to this scare?) and she was prescribed venlafaxine. Fleur disliked the side effects, which made her feel sick and 'hungover'. The oncologist noted that she had found acupuncture helpful and would seek a practitioner locally. At her December follow-up, the oncologist made no mention of HFNS. Fleur was cancer free.

CHAPTER SUMMARY

As acupuncturists working with cancer survivors, we can:

- be aware of the of the potential emotional burden, and of the inhibitors to allowing those emotions (e.g. positive attitude)
- create a safe space for patients to express or discuss these emotions
- help patients to recognise emotional patterns and their impact on physical symptoms.

References

1. Drew A, Fawcett TN Responding to the information needs of patients with cancer. Prof. Nurse 2002;17(7):443–446.
2. Macmillan Cancer Support. After cancer treatment: a guide for professionals. London: Macmillan Cancer Support; no date.
3. Lent RW Restoring emotional well-being: a theoretical model. In: Feuerstein M, editor. Handbook of cancer survivorship. New York: Springer; 2007. pp. 231–247.
4. Wolff S The burden of cancer survivorship: a pandemic of treatment success. In: Feuerstein M, editor. Handbook of cancer survivorship. New York: Springer; 2007. pp. 7–18.
5. Alfano C, Rowland J Recovery issues in cancer survivorship: a new challenge for supportive care. Cancer J. 2009;12(5):432–443.
6. Maciocia G The psyche in Chinese medicine. London: Churchill Livingstone; 2009.
7. Deadman P Live well live long: teachings from the Chinese nourishment of life tradition. Hove: The Journal of Chinese Medicine; 2016.
8. Hicks A, Hicks J, Mole P Five element constitutional acupuncture. Edinburgh: Churchill Livingstone; 2004.
9. Mast ME Survivors of breast cancer: illness uncertainty, positive reappraisal, and emotional distress. Oncol. Nurs. Forum 1998;25(3):555–562.
10. Flaws B, Lake J Chinese medical psychiatry: a textbook and clinical manual. Boulder, CO: Blue Poppy Press; 2001.
11. Larre C, Rochat de la Vallee E The seven emotions. Cambridge: Monkey Press; 1996.
12. de Valois B, Glynne-Jones R Acupuncture in the supportive care of colorectal cancer survivors: Four case studies, Part 1. Eur. J. Orient. Med. 2017;8(6):34–43.
13. Rossi E Shen: psycho-emotional aspects of Chinese medicine. Edinburgh: Churchill Livingstone; 2002.
14. Schubart JR, Emerich M, Farnan M, et al. Screening for psychological distress in surgical breast cancer patients. Ann. Surg. Oncol. 2014;21(10):3348–3353
15. Carreira H, Williams R, Müller M, et al. Adverse mental health outcomes in breast cancer survivors compared to women who did not have cancer: systematic review protocol. BioMed Central 2017;6(162).
16. Ehrenreich B Smile! You've got cancer. London; 2010. Available from: www.theguardian.com/lifeandstyle/2010/jan/02/cancer-positive-thinking-barbara-ehrenreich
17. Deadman P, Al-Khafaji M, Baker K A manual of acupuncture. Hove: The Journal of Chinese Medicine; 2007.
18. Cancer Research UK Coping with sadness. London: Cancer Research UK; 2019. Available from: www.cancerresearchuk.org/about-cancer/coping/emotionally/cancer-and-your-emotions/coping-with-sadness
19. Arian M, Masoumi R, Shojaei SFR Feelings of shame and guilt in patients with cancer and their family caregivers. Int. J. Cancer Manag. 2021;14(8):e117159.
20. Glaser S, Knowles K, Damaskos P Survivor guilt in cancer survivorship. Soc. Work Health Care 2019;58(8):764–775.
21. Corner J Inaugural lecture. Nursing and the counter culture for cancer. Eur. J. Cancer Care 1997;6(3):174–181.
22. Seale C Sporting cancer: struggle language in news reports of people with cancer. Sociol. Health Illn. 2001;23(3):308–329.
23. Ehrenreich B Smile or die: How positive thinking fooled America and the world. London: Granta; 2009.
24. Nakaya N, Bidstrup PE, Saito-Nakaya K, et al. Personality traits and cancer risk and survival based on Finnish and Swedish registry data. Am. J. Epidemiol. 2010;172(4):377–385.
25. Schofield P, Ball D, Smith JG, et al. Optimism and survival in lung carcinoma patients. Cancer 2004;100(6):1276–1282.
26. Whitfield JB, Zhu G, Landers JG, et al. Pessimism is associated with greater all-cause and cardiovascular mortality, but optimism is not protective. Sci. Rep. 2020;10(1):12609.

Part II

USING ACUPUNCTURE TO SUPPORT CANCER SURVIVORS

Chapter 4

Offering Complex Patients a Simple Piece of Heaven

Introduction

The scope for managing complicated conditions using uncomplicated approaches, and the empowerment acupuncture can bring to cancer survivors is expressed in the following quotes:

> Keep it simple so complicated things can happen. (Dr Michael Smith)[1]

> I think the underlying feeling is that you are actually able…you're doing something to help yourself, where prior to [having acupuncture], you felt quite useless. There was nothing you could do to aid your recovery, really. (Breast cancer survivor with lymphoedema)[2]

Supporting people who have been treated for cancer lies within the scope of qualified acupuncturists. The remaining chapters of this book describe some of the issues cancer survivors bring to clinic and illustrate how acupuncture can help them. As well as exploring approaches to these issues, we hear the voices of patients who share their experiences of acupuncture treatment in the quotations and case studies presented throughout.

Acupuncture is a diverse and flexible discipline, within which each practitioner brings their own approach to provide the best patient care. Apart from the section on safety, the guidance in this chapter is intended to be illustrative rather than prescriptive, to help and not hinder. It stems from my style, which evolved from my training, experience, continuing professional development, and the different contexts I have worked in. It illuminates how I have applied the techniques described throughout this book and informs the treatment approaches detailed in the case studies.

Guidelines for treating cancer survivors following active treatment

ESSENTIALS

I have three basic guidelines to approaching treatment:

1. Keep it simple.

2. Treat what you see.
3. Understand cancer and cancer treatments and their consequences.

1. Keep it simple

In 2008, I discovered a paper bearing the title of this chapter.[3] The title was immediately appealing. So was Daniel Schulman's discussion of the challenges of treating patients whose complex presentations frustrated his attempts at pattern differentiation.

These were patients whose presentations he described as 'daunting, overwhelming and intimidating all at once'. Diagnosis was complicated by the patients' inability, due to their 'multi-symptomatic and medication-induced confusion' to provide 'consistent and informative answers to the finer questions' Daniel liked to ask.

His eventual solution was to devise a simple, adaptable treatment strategy for complex patients based on the 'Early Heaven – Later Heaven' framework. This simultaneously engages the patient's pre-heavenly or constitutional essence (*xian tian zhi jing*, or congenital, prenatal, or inherited jing) by addressing the Kidney while generating the post-heavenly or acquired constitutional essence (*hou tian zhi jing*) by addressing the Stomach, to offer the patient a connection between their past and their present. This informed his approach and his compelling title.

This paper spoke to me. I had completed two research studies investigating using acupuncture to manage breast cancer treatment-related hot flushes and night sweats.[4] In the first of these, using a semi-individualised protocol, I felt I stretched acupuncture to the limit to address the complex presentations of the study participants. In the second, I witnessed how an apparently simple standardised ear acupuncture protocol could achieve remarkable results. I was poised to start my third research study, investigating acupuncture in the management of lymphoedema, a condition resistant to treatment and presenting alongside complex comorbidities.

Although I did not adopt Schulman's protocol, his ethos of keeping treatment simple for complex patients wove itself into my approach to treatment. It was a timely reminder of what I had been taught at the College of Integrated Chinese Medicine – minimal interventions give the best feedback to the practitioner while giving the patient the opportunity to thrive.[5] In my early years of practice, it was all too easy to forget this! I was fortunate to also work with the National Acupuncture Detoxification Association (NADA). I benefitted from Dr Michael Smith's admonition to 'keep things simple so complicated things can happen'.

It takes courage to keep things simple, especially when faced with a patient who is desperate for relief from troubling symptoms. I am grateful to the many teachers over the years who encouraged me to administer a simple treatment, observe and reflect, and then adapt as required. Most importantly, they encouraged me to have patience.

Cancer survivors are likely to have experienced trauma on many levels – physical, emotional, and spiritual as well as financial and social. Respecting this, I treat gently, starting with a simple treatment to assess the individual's response.

This 'simple' approach has enabled me to learn; to see more clearly what I have done and why. This in turn makes it easier to assess what may or may not have worked and informs how to move forward. As I learn about the person, what they need, and how they respond to treatment, I adjust the treatment accordingly.

This also gives the patient time to process treatment. Cancer survivors often need stability and time to process the changes they have experienced before they can move on. Adopting a simple treatment approach minimises the risk of overwhelming or overstimulating the patient.

Simplicity has become a mainstay of my style. When I stray from this principle, I notice the results are less good and I must simplify again.

2. Treat what you see
Qualified acupuncturists can observe, diagnose, and develop a treatment plan within the theoretical framework(s) for which they are trained.

There are patterns, syndromes, and generalisations that are understood to be associated with cancer treatments. Experience has taught me that these can be incorrect.

Questioning the received wisdom
When I designed the protocol for my first hot flush study, I consulted the textbooks, journals, and leading practitioners at the time. (There is far more information available about hot flushes and acupuncture than there was in 1999–2000.) The consensus was that Kidney yin deficiency was the key syndrome underlying hot flushes. Consequently, I designed my protocol around this. When my research clinic started, I expected to see patients with the tongue presentation associated with Kidney yin deficiency – red, dry, and peeled in patches. Yes, there were some of those, but there was a range of other presentations, causing me to question the received wisdom (see Chapter 8, Cancer Treatment-Related Hot Flushes and Night Sweats).

This taught me to treat what was presenting, regardless of the theory. While theory can *inform*, patients rarely *conform*. Understanding this liberated my practice. Eventually, it helped me understand that moxa can be an appropriate modality for treating hot flushes, a symptom for which moxa is generally contraindicated.

The diversity of cancer survivors as a patient group
Cancer survivors are a hugely diverse patient group. They have different tumour types, have undergone different treatment regimens, are of differing ages, come from a range of ethnicities and socioeconomic groups, and have widely varying comorbidities for which they may be taking any number of medications. Cancer survivorship as a study is also a relatively new phenomenon and will constantly change as medical treatments for cancer evolve and survivors live longer. These are all cogent reasons for treating what you see, within the context of your theoretical framework(s).

3. Understand cancer and cancer treatments and their consequences
To work with cancer survivors, it is essential to understand cancer and its treatments. It is vital to recognise signs and symptoms of cancer, understand the course of the disease, be realistic about prognoses, and be able to refer.

It is also important to understand the rationale for the biomedical advice given to patients and be conversant with specialist terms used in oncology. This facilitates better understanding and communication with both cancer survivors and their healthcare professionals.

At a minimum, find an introductory course about cancer and its treatments; it does not need to be acupuncture related. Many cancer centres provide introductory training to their new employees or volunteers, which may be open to others to attend. This book provides background and insight into the challenges facing cancer survivors who are shaping their lives to accommodate the 'new normal' of life after cancer treatment. For specific and more detailed information, there are also many good sources of information about cancer and its treatments. See the Further Information and Resources section in the Appendices online for examples.

How acupuncture can help cancer survivors

Chapter 1 introduced some of the benefits of acupuncture for cancer survivors. This chapter continues the discussion.

Something can be done!

Many patients say their health professionals tell them 'Nothing can be done' about some of the uncomfortable consequences of cancer treatments. Survivors may be told that symptoms will disappear over time (which they often do). Sometimes they are advised to accept the consequences and be satisfied their life has been saved.

This is disheartening for the individual, as Emily's story in Chapter 1 testifies. While acupuncture is not a 'cure all', it can improve quality of life for cancer survivors. Something can be done! As these breast cancer survivors reported:

> They [hot flushes] were intense and they had been for months. And I kept going... I'd been to my doctor saying, 'There must be something that you can do!' I couldn't believe that this was a condition that couldn't be treated. And when [name of lymphoedema nurse]...said, 'Oh you should go and see [name of acupuncturist]'...I just jumped at the chance to do anything to get rid of that. (018 BC)

> I also have this ongoing thrush which was driving me bonkers, because I went to the doctor and I had medication and I had the pessaries and I said, 'What's causing this?' and she [acupuncturist] treated that and that went! Which was really good... I just mentioned it on the off-chance and she said, ' I have a remedy for that' and I said, 'Well you could try it' and it worked. I was so pleased. (005 BC)[2]

Understanding acupuncture's potential can give hope and help to cancer survivors. It can also help oncology health professionals, many of whom are actively searching for more effective means to manage the challenging consequences their patients experience.

Single symptom vs multiple effect

Cancer survivors and their healthcare professionals may be unaware of the multiple effects that acupuncture can have – a usual expectation is that treatment targets a single symptom. Acupuncturists trained in styles of East Asian medicine (EAM) expect treatment to have multiple, wide-ranging effects, made possible through rich and diverse means:

- Chinese medicine (CM) acupuncture achieves this through pattern differentiation, choosing effective treatment principles, and judicious point selection (one point has many functions).
- Five Element Constitutional Acupuncture aims to strengthen a person's underlying constitution, which leads to symptom relief, rather than targeting the symptoms themselves. Addressing the patient at the levels of body, mind, and spirit is a fundamental principle of this approach.[5]
- The NADA ear acupuncture protocol also has wide-ranging effects. These are attributed to its action of promoting homeostasis to improve an individual's endocrine and autonomic function, leading to improvements in overall wellbeing.[6]

These are just a few examples of the many styles of acupuncture available around the world.

Symptom clusters

Acupuncture works well to address the multiple, concurrent symptoms presented by many cancer survivors. Biomedical research is beginning to explore 'symptom clusters', defined as: 'a stable group of two or more concurrent symptoms that are related to one another, but independent of other symptoms or symptom clusters'.[7]

Examples of cancer treatment-related symptom clusters include pain/fatigue/sleep, nausea/vomiting, and dyspnoea/cough/fatigue.[8]

EAM practitioners are already trained to think in terms of clusters of symptoms, especially those practising Eight Principles or TCM styles, wherein the practitioner identifies group of signs and symptoms that together form patterns of disharmony. While these may differ from cancer-related symptom clusters, the concepts are similar. For example, in CM pattern identification, insomnia, anxiety, poor memory, and dizziness 'cluster' together as signs of Heart Blood deficiency.[9] These symptoms are also often presented by breast cancer patients experiencing hot flushes.

Getting my life back!

Cancer survivors appreciate the restorative nature of acupuncture. They frequently remark how it has 'given my life back' and they feel 'normal' again. This is expressed by two research participants treated for different cancers, using different acupuncture approaches, who reported far-reaching benefits:

> ...was feeling very 'down' and tired before the treatment... As I have said my quality of life has improved dramatically and I am back to feeling my 'old' self. (Alfred, prostate cancer survivor, after eight NADA treatments)[10]

It gave me so much confidence, I even changed my job! Which was incredible under the circumstances, you know, and I've done so well with my job... I just started feeling so much better after the acupuncture. And I've gone back full-time, I was only doing part-time at the time, so all-in-all I've really got my life back. (017 BC, breast cancer survivor with lymphoedema, after 13 acupuncture treatments)[2]

These reports bear witness to acupuncture's supportive role in helping cancer survivors navigate the transition to life after cancer treatment. Ann's case study in Chapter 14 is a detailed example of how one woman with very complex consequences of cancer and its treatments 'got her life back' through having acupuncture.

Enabled coping and acceptance

My research into cancer treatment-related lymphoedema crystallised my understanding of acupuncture as a catalyst to facilitate change that can lead to improved long-term healthcare for people with chronic, often comorbid, conditions. The research participants described symptom reduction and improved energy levels as perceived benefits of acupuncture and moxibustion treatment.[2]

In research exploring acupuncture for early breast cancer patients undergoing chemotherapy, Dr Sarah Price discusses 'enabled coping'. For the acupuncturists in her study, enabling coping was a long-term outcome that they intended. It was achieved through the combined actions of relieving symptoms and increasing the patient's strength through 'fortifying', 'increasing the vitality', and 'tonifying the Qi' of the person. As Dr Price concluded, this strengthening enables the person to both withstand emotional distress and manage physical discomfort.[11,12]

Figure 4.1 illustrates the cycle of enabled coping inserted into the model for acupuncture facilitating long-term health improvement, introduced in Chapter 1. While Price's research focused on women undergoing primary treatment, cancer survivors post active treatment also require 'enabled coping' to deal with the aftermath of treatment. That acupuncture can facilitate this is expressed by this breast cancer survivor, who participated in the hot flush study:

I felt more able, I think, to cope with things. (Participant 16)[13]

For others, acupuncture enables a state of acceptance, as reported by this woman with breast cancer treatment-related lymphoedema (BCRL):

But actually now it [lymphoedema] doesn't bother me quite so much. I just think 'do you know what, this is what I've got' and it might be as a result from the [acupuncture] treatment now, I think it is in a way, but I think I've tried whatever I can try and I'll carry on trying other things to reduce it. But I think it did make me more positive to it. (023 BC)[2]

There are instances where a condition might not be resolved. Nevertheless, acupuncture can help the survivors reach a stage of acceptance that enables them to live more comfortably with their condition. This is expressed by this woman with BCRL:

And I mean really and truly, it's just maybe being able to cope with it better because it definitely doesn't rule me as it did. (004 BC)[2]

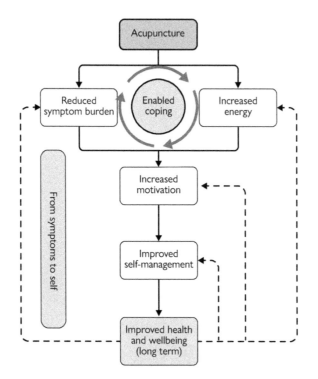

FIGURE 4.1: ACUPUNCTURE AS A CATALYST FOR LONG-TERM HEALTH IMPROVEMENT
SHOWING ENABLED COPING AND MOVING FROM SYMPTOM TO SELF

Facilitating wellbeing – moving from symptom to self

Moving from symptom to self is an important stage of acupuncture treatment. It marks a milestone in a person's relationship to their condition, where they experience a shift from:

- symptoms, where the focus is on aspects of discomfort to
- self, where the focus is on overall wellbeing.

This is a concept taught by Angela and John Hicks at the College of Integrated Chinese Medicine, but it has not been published and I thank the Hicks for their kind permission for me to discuss it here.

Patients generally come for acupuncture focused on a particular symptom (often physical). As discussed above, they are unlikely to be aware of acupuncture's capacity to improve multiple symptoms and overall wellbeing. This applies not only to patients, but to their healthcare professionals and some acupuncturists. Understanding this fuller potential enables a broader view of what acupuncture can achieve.

Acupuncturists aware of this process can help a person make the transition from symptom to self, a process called 'moving the orientation'.

ESSENTIALS

Moving the orientation involves educating the patient, and can be achieved by following these guidelines:

- Introduce the concept of wellbeing, ideally at the first acupuncture treatment, as this quotation illustrates:

  I thought it was to treat the lymphoedema, but when I went in there [name of first acupuncturist] explained and she said, 'It isn't to treat the lymphoedema, it might affect the lymphoedema, it might make it better, but it's really just to give you just a sense of wellbeing.' This was when we were having the initial discussion. (005 BC)

- Encourage the patient to think beyond their presenting symptom: ask, 'How will you know when you are really well?'
- Check at the next visit if they have noticed a change in how they feel about themselves. Some patients will report this spontaneously, for example, 'I can't explain it, I just feel better in myself.'
- Give examples of other patients feeling better.

Often a patient's orientation will move naturally as their symptoms improve. It is important not to attempt to move orientation if:

- a patient resists
- their symptom is acute.

It is common for people to experience changes in wellbeing and not realise this is the result of acupuncture treatment. Thus, it is important to draw their attention to this. Once patients are aware of this connection, they may be more committed to their acupuncture treatment as well as to taking action to maintain their wellbeing.

The importance of wellbeing

What is wellbeing? Women with BCRL provided these views:[2]

Wellbeing is just waking up in the morning feeling that I can carry on with my everyday life and not feeling debilitated in any sense. (016 BC)

It's feeling joyful about the world, I think, you want to go out and do things. (019 BC)

That you're more in control of what's happening to you. (018 BC)

Improved wellbeing has the potential to facilitate long-term health benefits. For some patients it improves self-care, enabling the patient to take the initiative in self-managing their health. These are important benefits for people living with chronic conditions and especially for those experiencing multiple comorbidities.

VIGNETTE: FROM 'SYMPTOM TO SELF' TO IMPROVED SELF-MANAGEMENT

These quotations illustrate one woman's movement from symptom to self, from her despair at receiving a BCRL diagnosis, through her acupuncture treatment, to being able to self-manage her condition:[2]

> When I was diagnosed with breast cancer, it was like the worst thing ever, and I had, obviously, the radiotherapy and the chemotherapy and then I developed lymphoedema, and it was as if I'd hit rock bottom, it was horrible. (004 BC)

> And as somebody else said, you've tried everything and when [the lymphoedema nurse] suggested acupuncture, I mean I would have jumped at anything, I really would have done, because I was just so low, so depressed. (004 BC)

> When I came back in January, this was for the second [course of treatments], I said to her [the acupuncturist] 'I've joined Weight Watchers, I'm really being positive about this and I'm really working on my exercises for the lymphoedema, I'm really working hard... and I can honestly say this is the acupuncture and the moxibustion.' ...it changed the way I thought about myself. (004 BC)

> I just feel so much more in control of myself. I feel a happier person and I've got far more time, far more patience with the grandchildren, you know. We go out and we do things far more now than what we used to do, even this time last year I didn't have the energy that I have now, it's marvellous. (004 BC)

The importance of enabled coping and moving from symptom to self

Figure 4.1 illustrates how acupuncture facilitates enabled coping and moving from symptom to self, with the potential to improve motivation and self-care.

These processes, valuable for any person, are particularly so for cancer survivors who have one or more chronic conditions. They are especially helpful for people with lymphoedema, for whom successful management of their chronic condition is crucially dependent on the quality of their daily self-care (as discussed in Chapter 9, Cancer Treatment-Related Lymphoedema).

Important features of acupuncture care
The 'whole-person' approach
In extensive research into using acupuncture to manage a range of chronic conditions, Dr Charlotte Paterson highlights the importance to patients of the 'whole-person' approach to healthcare.[14,15] People with medically unexplained symptoms valued 'talking to a friendly/empathic practitioner who listened, understood, provided explanations, and sometimes gave advice and "treated me as a whole"'.[15]

Cancer survivors also appreciate these features of acupuncture, especially after having cancer treatment:[2]

> When you go to the hospital and you go to anybody, they're only looking at the bit they're looking at, and nobody actually asks how you're feeling generally. I thought that was really helpful. (001 BC)

> Coming and associating with somebody who is caring about you, gave a tremendous positive vibe; that there are people who want to really try and help you, so that itself was a positive thing. (007 HNT)

While not the exclusive preserve of acupuncture, this 'whole-person' approach to patient care is taught and prized by many acupuncture schools and appreciated by many acupuncture patients. (It is also important to recognise that dry needling may be administered within a context of whole-person care that informs other therapeutic approaches.)

The importance of time and attention
Regularly, when I discuss acupuncture with oncologists, even those who practise acupuncture remark that its effects are simply due to time and attention. While this is dismissive of the specific effects of acupuncture, it does acknowledge that time and attention are valuable components of treatment, appreciated by patients:

> She was always very unhurried, she always seemed as if she had all the time in the world to speak to you. (023 BC)

> They were both very sympathetic and listened to what you had to say and acted upon it in what was appropriate today. (019 BC)[2]

This is an important aspect of supporting cancer survivors to process their experience and enable them to move on. I acknowledge that I have worked with oncologists who truly envy the time I can spend with patients as well as the in-depth knowledge that it has been my privilege to gain in those encounters.

Empowering the patient
Cancer survivors have undergone unpleasant interventions, where the choices given may have felt like having no choice at all:

> What I felt, when I was diagnosed with the cancer and everything, was that everything happens so fast and you're on this conveyor belt, which I was very grateful for, thank you, you know, didn't have to make decisions, they were all made for me, and that was it. (015 BC)[2]

Because of this, I deliberately seek to create opportunities for them to make choices about their acupuncture treatment. In clinic, I attempt to give patients a sense of control by involving them in decision making about their treatment and giving them choice. This includes discussing my treatment plan with them, talking through the treatment, and encouraging their participation:

> She was really very helpful and if there was anywhere that I was not going to be comfortable having the needle, she would never say, 'We need to put it in here', we always discussed it at length but she always managed to put them a bit further away... And then, as I got more used to them, she'd say, 'Would you mind if I put one in here because I think it would help?' (001 BC)[2]

Often, I am guided by their feedback and preferences and through this I learn. For example, listening to patient feedback is how I learned that an Aggressive Energy Drain (see Chapter 5, Toolkit) can be effective for managing hot flushes.

Lifestyle advice

For many acupuncturists, lifestyle advice is an integral part of treatment, and the means by which they encourage patients to engage in self-care.[16] In research into communications in acupuncture consultations, Paterson found 'self-care talk' interwoven through the consultation, highlighting that it is essential to some styles of acupuncture.[17]

Lifestyle advice is an extensive topic and I recommend Peter Deadman's *Live Well, Live Long* for a full discussion of the subject.[18] In this book, I discuss aspects of lifestyle advice appropriate for cancer survivors.

Practical considerations for working with cancer survivors

I have discussed ways that acupuncture can help cancer survivors. In the remainder of this chapter, I discuss practical aspects to consider when working with this patient group.

Practicalities: Working as part of a multidisciplinary team

Acupuncture is an intervention that can be used alongside other interventions in the multidisciplinary care of cancer survivors. It is desirable for acupuncturists to work as part of the multidisciplinary oncology healthcare team to enable the best possible care for the cancer survivor.

ESSENTIALS

In this sphere, it is important to acknowledge responsibilities. While acupuncturists have a vital role to play in the supportive care of cancer survivors, the responsibility for the treatment of cancer itself falls to the oncology team. It is therefore prudent for acupuncturists to:

- avoid making any claims about acupuncture as an intervention to treat cancer, with any implication of cure
- be aware of the key signs and symptoms of cancer and refer patients presenting with these to the appropriate medical practitioner
- be aware of the consequences of cancer and its treatments and refer patients to the relevant healthcare professionals when appropriate.

Reinforcing messages

Acupuncturists can also reinforce messages. The case study of Linda in Chapter 9 shows that people with cancer may be too preoccupied with the demands of active cancer treatment to take in information offered by their medical team. Again, as illustrated by Linda, when treatment finishes, they may just wish to put the experience behind them. For Linda, this meant losing valuable time in understanding that lymphoedema was a potential consequence of her breast cancer treatment.

Acupuncturists can play a vital role in reinforcing healthcare messages and practices. When all members of the healthcare team reinforce the same messages, patients are more likely to adopt recommended practices. This includes such things as reinforcing the importance of wearing compression garments for lymphoedema, encouraging routine carrying out of prescribed exercises, taking required medications, moisturising scars, maintaining a healthy weight, and being physically active.

Supporting biomedicine

As an acupuncturist working in a cancer centre, my role is to support cancer survivors treated within the biomedical system, and I am supportive of biomedical treatments for cancer.

Most cancer survivors I meet are extremely grateful for their cancer treatment and enjoy good relationships with their oncology healthcare team. They may be overwhelmed and surprised by the late and long-term consequences of their life-conserving treatment. I endeavour to avoid giving mixed messages to cancer survivors, or undermining their relationship with their oncology team.

Occasionally, I may experience a conflict with my own beliefs or the theories of EAM. In such situations, my priority is to ensure I do not cause a patient conflict over what their medical team have advised, nor engender lack of confidence in their oncology team.

Practicalities: Tips on interacting with other members of the oncology team

I am often asked for advice on how to interact with the members of the oncology team. I find this almost impossible to answer. With patients who have completed anti-cancer treatment, I may never have contact with their oncology healthcare professionals.

In working with many oncologists, I have encountered attitudes to acupuncture that span a spectrum from utter disdain to actively seeking and promoting acupuncture for their patients. Organisations and the individuals working within them have different approaches to practice and communications, making it difficult to generalise. Fundamentally, it is about cultivating professional relationships with individuals from other professions.

ESSENTIALS

Some tips for interacting with oncology health professionals:

- Act in a professional manner and to encourage mutual respect; treat others as you wish to be treated by them.
- In general, biomedical healthcare professionals are rarely interested in the 'qi paradigm' or EAM theories. I find it best to talk to them in their language, using the terms they use.
- Citing the evidence base is often the most effective means of communication.
- 'How does acupuncture work?' or 'What is the mechanism for acupuncture?' are questions invariably asked by biomedical healthcare professionals. It is wise to be conversant with at least one of the latest evidence-based theories to answer such questions.
- It may depend on who you are dealing with and where they are in the medical hierarchy. I find it easier to talk about using acupuncture to improve wellbeing with specialist nurses, speech therapists, and other allied health professionals, who seem to understand this approach and who want help with their patients' insoluble problems. This also applies to some oncologists.

Practicalities: Needling techniques
Each style of acupuncture has its own guidelines for needling and every practitioner will have their own techniques. Here are the methods and preferences I have evolved over my years of practice and research.

ESSENTIALS

As with many aspects of this book, the discussion below is intended for guidance rather than prescription. It is to illustrate the approach used in the case studies throughout this book. These techniques are based on my experience and may differ greatly from what is taught or published.

Adopting a gentle approach
My clinical experience is that cancer survivors respond well to gentle, light needling techniques. This accords with their potential vulnerability resulting from trauma they have experienced as well as any damage to their qi, Blood, body fluids, essence, and shen due to cancer and its treatments. As discussed previously, many will also have complex

presentations with multiple comorbidities. In addition, I adopt aspects of Five Element acupuncture, especially the use of fine and gentle techniques, which are appropriate to treating at the level of the spirit.[5]

I also employ gentle needling techniques using a minimum number of needles. Many survivors have an aversion to needles, especially after having chemotherapy, as expressed by these breast cancer survivors:

> Well I was nervous, because I'm not good with needles, and although I'd seen the acupuncture needles at the meeting, you still think 'well a needle's a needle and it's going to hurt!' (003 BC)

> My first reaction was, I don't think I can cope with the needles, because after chemotherapy I now have this awful time giving blood, it's dreadful, my veins. (Participant 10)[13]

Clean technique

I assume all practitioners will use clean techniques and work according to the guidelines for safety and clinical practice as specified by their local professional and legal guidelines.

Number of needles

I aim to limit the number of needle insertions in a single treatment to about six to ten.

Exceptions are treatments such as an Aggressive Energy Drain (using up to 15 insertions) or Seven Dragons followed by the source points (11 insertions) (see Chapter 5, Toolkit).

Needles, gauge, and length

Practitioners have their preferred needle types, gauge, and length. Hicks *et al.* recommend very fine needles for Five Element acupuncture, usually #36-gauge (0.20mm).[5]

For years, I used Acuglide #34-gauge (0.22mm diameter) needles. When Acuglide became unavailable in the UK, I changed needle size to the much finer #40-gauge (0.16mm diameter). I now prefer the finer needle, which seems more sensitive.

This fine gauge does not support long needle lengths; 40mm is the maximum and at this length I find the #40-gauge difficult to use. However, the use of relatively short needles accords with my needling style, which is quite superficial insertion. Thus, my preferred needle lengths are:

- 25–30mm (1–1.2 inch) for the majority of points
- 13–14mm (0.5–0.6 inch) for points such as nail points, or where the flesh covering is thin (e.g. extra point *yintang*, and some head and face points, fingers, and toes).

I mostly use these sizes for the cancer survivors I treat. I also keep a supply of #36-gauge needles in these lengths for patients who seem more robust. And of course, a good long strong needle – either #28–#30-gauge (0.30–0.35mm) 50–75mm (2–3-inch needle) is essential for needling GB-30 *Huantiao* when sciatica presents.

Needle technique

I find cancer survivors respond well to even technique. To needle using even technique:

- Insert the needle perpendicular to the skin surface at the location of the point.
- Obtain deqi.
- Leave the needle in place for about 20 minutes, without further manipulation.

I also use tonification technique, particularly when working in a Five Element style. To needle using this technique:

- Insert the needle 10° off the perpendicular in the direction of the flow of qi.
- Obtain deqi.
- Turn the needle clockwise 180°.
- The needle may be removed or left in situ for the remainder of the treatment.

Breathing

With all needle insertions, I ask the patient to:

- inhale while I position the needle
- exhale as I insert the needle.

Needle sensation (deqi)

I aim for needle sensation, or deqi, the feeling that the patient has when the needle contacts the qi as well as the sensation the acupuncturist may feel.

Needle sensation is often described as a dull ache, soreness, heaviness, a pulling sensation, heat, or other sensations around the needle. Patients new to acupuncture may find these descriptions confusing or off-putting. I describe needle sensation as a 'feeling of contact' that they will experience in their own unique way. I reassure them that this will be an instantaneous, fleeting sensation – here and then gone.

I encourage each person to:

- experience needle sensation in their own way
- develop their own way of describing this sensation.

This avoids some of the potentially negative connotations of the usual descriptions of deqi (e.g. ache, soreness). It also alleviates patients' anxieties about whether they are experiencing the 'right' sensation. Removing the pressure some patients feel to have a 'typical' or 'normal' experience of needle sensation validates the individuality of their response. This is another way of supporting the cancer survivor to regain control, and often contributes to establishing greater rapport with the patient.

As the acupuncturist, I may simultaneously experience the arrival of the qi, recognisable through a distinct sensation on the needle. While this doesn't always happen for me, I find it beneficial to discuss with the patient when it does.

My needle technique is delicate, and my intention is to obtain a gentle sensation, rather than elicit strong sensation. This again respects the possible fragility of the cancer survivor.

Pain, bleeding, and bruising

I find patients who experience chronic pain or anxiety or were extremely traumatised by their cancer experience may be very sensitive to needle insertion and sensation. With some patients in my clinics, each needle becomes a negotiation. In extreme cases, I find it necessary to abandon needles for an alternative intervention, such as moxa, tuning forks, or even referral to another form of treatment. Usually, I plan treatments using as few needles as possible and seek to avoid areas the patient finds sensitive.

Cancer survivors may be more prone to bruising and bleeding at the needle site than non-cancer patients. I find this is especially common during the first year after active treatment ends. Some patients do not appreciate being bruised, especially when the bruise persists, as it sometimes does for these individuals. If a patient is prone to bruising, I explain that this can be a usual consequence of cancer treatment, and acupuncture helps address this.

Practicalities: Positioning, comfort, and privacy

As for all patients, cancer survivors should feel comfortable during treatment. Care should be taken with positioning and support, with attention paid to scars, lymphoedema swelling, mobility restrictions, or medical devices such as stomas for breathing, bowel, or bladder.

Some patients may say they are so accustomed to stripping off for their medical interventions and examinations that they are not bothered removing clothing for acupuncture. Others may be sensitive about exposing scars or disfigurements to the acupuncturist. Offering gowns, careful covering, and privacy for disrobing are helpful for these individuals. It may be useful, prior to the first treatment, to discuss any potential requirements for undressing and how this will be handled in clinic.

This can prevent rude surprises, such as those expressed in this exchange between breast cancer survivors in a focus group. These research participants were asked to disrobe (apart from underpants) for their first treatment, an Aggressive Energy Drain (using points on the back) and for their second treatment, Internal Dragons, using points on the front of the torso and legs (see Chapter 5, Toolkit). They were offered gowns to wear, and during the second treatment towels were carefully draped to protect modesty and warmth. They expressed their shock at being asked to disrobe for these acupuncture treatments:

- 005 (BC): 'That came as a bit of a shock because I expected to be only taking off a part of my clothes and when she said to strip down, "oh I don't know if I want to strip right down". Because as I said, when my husband went for his treatment all he took off was his shirt... It came as a bit of a surprise because I wasn't prepared for it...'
- 006 (BC): 'Actually, were you given warning about that? Because I wasn't.'
- 005 (BC): 'I wasn't, that's why.'
- 006 (BC): 'I didn't realise we'd have to take all our clothes off.'

My learning from this was two fold:

- Patient information leaflets need to be explicit about disrobing.
- My practice changed; it contributed to me changing from an Aggressive Energy Drain to using Four Gates as a first treatment (see Chapter 5, Toolkit). This eliminated any need for disrobing at the first treatment, a time when developing trust and rapport is in its initial, vulnerable stage.

Practicalities: Safety of acupuncture treatment

Many cancer survivors have acupuncture during primary treatment, as it is an intervention offered increasingly in oncology settings. The use of acupuncture in integrative oncology is growing in Europe, North America, and Australasia, where it is recommended by official oncology organisations for a growing number of cancer treatment-related symptoms.[19]

Some practitioners may be nervous about treating people who are living with and beyond cancer. Patients, and some oncology health professionals, may also have concerns about the safety of acupuncture, at whatever stage of the survivorship continuum.

Thanks to large-scale studies in many countries including the UK, Japan, Sweden, and Germany, a large body of evidence supports the safety of acupuncture for the general population. Serious adverse events are rare. A German study, in the largest acupuncture research series to date, reported only six potentially serious adverse events in 760,000 treatments given to 97,733 patients. These included one case each of asthma attack, exacerbated depression, hypertensive crisis (severe increase in blood pressure), and vasovagal reaction (fainting) and two incidents of pneumothorax. These were rated according to the likeliness of being caused by acupuncture:

- Pneumothorax was *directly* due to acupuncture needling.
- Vasovagal reaction was *likely* to be caused by acupuncture.
- The remainder were *possible* reactions to acupuncture.[20]

The most commonly reported minor adverse events of acupuncture treatment are bleeding and transient pain at the needling site, occurring in fewer than two in 1000 treatments.[21] Mild bruising, drowsiness, headache, local skin irritation may also occur, as well as dizziness and fainting in about 1% of treatments.[22]

There is growing consensus among cancer information websites and clinical practice guidelines that acupuncture performed by experienced, well-trained practitioners is safe for people with cancer.[22-25] One leading integrative oncology team in the USA recommends that clinicians cultivate relationships with local qualified acupuncturists to make acupuncture accessible to their patients.[26]

Clinical practice guidelines for using acupuncture

At the time of writing, no published guidelines specifically address safety issues for cancer survivors who have completed active cancer treatment (surgery, radiotherapy, chemotherapy).

The Society for Integrative Oncology (SIO) publishes evidence-based guidelines for integrative oncology on its website[*] and on that of the National Center for Complementary and Integrative Health.[**]

These clear guidelines for acupuncture are intended for cancer patients undergoing active treatment. Nevertheless, they provide a good starting point for discussing guidelines for safe practice for treating people living beyond active treatment.

ESSENTIALS

Evidence-based clinical practice guidelines for integrative oncology: acupuncture[21]

Recommendations:

Acupuncture should be performed only by qualified practitioners and used cautiously in patients with bleeding tendencies.

It is prudent to avoid acupuncture:

- at the site of the tumour or metastasis
- in limbs with lymphoedema
- in areas with considerable anatomic distortion from surgery
- in patients with severe thrombocytopenia, coagulopathy, or neutropenia.

Cancer patients require certified practitioners who are experienced in treating patients with malignant diseases.

Using these guidelines as a starting point, I would recommend the following guidelines for treating cancer survivors post active treatment (my adaptations are presented in *italics*):

ESSENTIALS

Modified acupuncture guidelines for cancer survivors post active treatment

Recommendations:

- Acupuncture should be performed only by qualified practitioners and used cautiously in patients with bleeding tendencies.
- *Acupuncturists cannot advertise or claim that they can 'treat' cancer (in the UK, this is law under the Cancer Act 1939).*
- Sterile single-use needles should be used, and clean needle technique should be always observed.
- *Acupuncturists should follow their local guidelines and laws for practice as well as the clinical practice guidelines of their professional organisation.*

---

[*]   https://integrativeonc.org/practice-guidelines/guidelines
[**]   www.nccih.nih.gov/health/providers/clinicalpractice

- *Practitioners should have training to understand cancer and its treatments to understand the disease, its processes, and treatment.*
- *Practitioners should be able to interact with a multidisciplinary oncology team, knowing how to work as part of that team and when to refer a patient to other services.*[21,24,27]
- For cancer survivors post active cancer treatment, it is prudent to avoid acupuncture:
    - at the site of the tumour or metastasis
    - in *areas* with or *at risk of* lymphoedema *(this may include limbs, lymph nodes that have been exposed to radiotherapy, or areas on the torso, head, or neck)*
    - in areas with considerable anatomic distortion from surgery, *for example* breast reconstructions* or extensive surgeries for head and neck cancers.
- *Be aware of patients who have undergone immunotherapy; side effects of treatment can occur up to one year after the end of treatment and patients should be referred to their oncology team for treatment if these occur.*

* Some acupuncture schools contraindicate needling in breast tissue. Others, for example Western medical acupuncturists, actively promote needling around breast scars. I find this quite confusing, as the general advice for needling cancer patients is to avoid needling over a tumour site.

Practicalities: Moxibustion

Where clinics allow, I use moxa (copiously), especially for patients who enjoy its aroma and the warmth, as discussed in Chapter 5, Toolkit. Patients vary in their views of moxa, as these comments from research participants with cancer treatment-related lymphoedema illustrate:

> I really liked that, especially the smell and the warmth, it's incredible... But I thought the effect was brilliant ... I loved having that treatment. (001 BC)

One participant asked for a moxa stick to take home, she loved the smell so much! Others were less enthusiastic:

> I don't know whether that [moxibustion] helped me or not. (009 HNT)

> I felt myself being a bit cynical. It struck me as a bit sort of...gosh what do you call those... witchdoctor-ish...they put it on and set it alight and whip it off. ...I would have preferred pure acupuncture. (014 BC)

I accept that patients may not like it, so I do not press it on them. For those who like moxa, I use it liberally if it appears beneficial.

When working in clinics that do not allow moxibustion, I may explore other options such as:

- heat lamps or electric moxa devices

- teaching people to self-administer moxa in their own homes
- seeing patients in an alternative clinic that allows moxa.

When these are not possible, I accept that in the circumstances, moxa is not a treatment option.

Safety of moxibustion

There has been less research into the safety of moxibustion for people living with and beyond cancer.

A 2010 systematic review of the effectiveness and safety of using moxibustion in cancer care noted that none of the five included randomised controlled trials reported adverse events. The authors did identify three papers in the literature that reported adverse events; these were mild or non-existent, although one study discussed possible health hazards of moxa smoke. Summarising, the authors said adverse events were mild, infrequent, and perhaps negligible, especially when compared with the adverse events associated with biomedical treatments, and concluded further research is needed.[28]

By contrast, Xu *et al.* conducted a systematic review examining case reports of moxa-related adverse events.[29] Twenty-four papers from six countries (China, USA, South Korea, Spain, Japan, and Israel) reported 64 adverse events. Burns were the most common adverse event, caused either by direct contact with moxa or from the radiant heat of indirect moxa.

These authors discuss whether a moxa burn is an adverse event: in 'scarring' or 'suppurative' moxibustion, local burns are the norm among doctors who maintain that 'where there is a moxibustion scar, there is a cure'.[29] In some cultures, patients accept the resulting skin lesions and the authors suggest that whether a burn or scar is an adverse event depends on the expectations and acceptance of both the doctor and patient.

Other adverse events reported in the review include allergies and infections in patients receiving moxibustion treatment, as well as chronic laryngitis reported in both patients and practitioners caused by moxibustion smoke in five hospitals in Guandong province.

Moxibustion is not entirely risk free; it is, after all, working with fire and there is potential for injury to patients and damage to property. The acceptability of burning and scarring is related to cultural expectations; while they may be a mainstay of treatment in some countries and cultures, they are unacceptable in others. Some UK insurers of acupuncturists do not provide cover for direct moxibustion because of the risk of burns.

Risks may be negligible and avoidable. In our study that taught chemotherapy patients to self-moxa ST-36 *Zusanli* daily for the duration of their chemotherapy treatment,[30] there were no reports of burns in 1975 self-administered treatments carried out by 25 participants. Three participants reported mild skin sensitivity on occasion (unpublished data). We found that patients need to be well trained and need clear instructions not to self-moxa when in a hospital or near medical gases. A potential nuisance factor to consider is that smoking moxa will set off smoke alarms.

Clinical practice guidelines for using moxibustion

Sagar and Wong have published guidelines for using moxibustion for cancer patients undergoing active treatment.[31] The following guidelines are an abridged version.

ESSENTIALS

Guidelines for using moxibustion with cancer patients

- Explain the slight risk of burns and obtain informed consent.
- Do not leave a patient alone with burning moxa.
- Contraindications include sensitive areas of the body, including the face, nipples, and genitals.
- The smoke of regular moxa can be avoided by using smokeless moxa or other methods of heating (e.g. infra-red heat lamp).
- When using moxa on herb-slice or cake, punch holes in the material to allow heat to penetrate. The thickness of the slice should be 0.2–0.3 centimetres. For practical purposes, ginger slices may be the most convenient.
- *Effective moxibustion should cause significant local heating and an inflammatory response, and should be done for a prolonged period, such as 10–20 minutes. Chinese medicine practitioners typically administer moxa daily for several treatments or more.
- Warming a broader region is an acceptable treatment for relaxing tension and moderating pain at the site.
- **Risks of exposure to smoke are probably like those for any other smoke, and total exposure time, especially if prolonged, is the key concern. Adequate ventilation is important, especially when moxa is done regularly. There is no evidence that moxa smoke contains any unusually harmful substances, but long-term data is incomplete.
- Female patients are unlikely to be pregnant during anti-cancer treatment; however, they may become pregnant during follow-up. In these cases, observe the usual contraindications for acupuncture and moxibustion during pregnancy.

*This is an approach very specific to modern TCM practice. Methodologies observed by other types of East Asian medicine may be different and also be very effective.

**Sagar and Wong[31] caution that although rare, arsenic may be present in some preparations from China, and should be avoided.

CASE STUDY: OFFERING A COMPLEX PATIENT A SIMPLE PIECE OF HEAVEN

Rosa's case study illustrates the approach of treating a complex presentation using a simple approach.

Rosa was actively involved in writing the original version of this case study published in the *European Journal of Oriental Medicine*, of which this is an abridged version.[32] She gave written consent for publication of her anonymised data, chose her pseudonym, and contributed her written perceptions of acupuncture treatment.

Background

Rosa's oncologist referred her to the hospital outpatient acupuncture clinic for colorectal cancer survivors in September 2016. Bowel 'problems' and anxiety were troublesome consequences of a colorectal anastomosis for Stage II (low risk) sigmoid colorectal cancer two years previously.

Rosa, aged 63, attended for 72 acupuncture treatments over two and a half years, during which she presented with increasingly complex health problems. These included a diagnosis of (possible) thyroid cancer, an aortic valve replacement, onset of Type 2 diabetes, and recurrence and metastatic spread of the primary cancer, for which she had further surgery and chemotherapy.

An estimated 29% of people with cancer have three or more chronic conditions in addition to cancer.[33] Rosa had hypertension, obesity (a body mass index (BMI) greater than 30), and chronic heart disease, three of the five most common long-term comorbidities for people with cancer (the others are mental health problems and chronic kidney disease). Her pre-existing conditions included asthma and hiatus hernia. Overlying this was her fear of cancer recurrence.

We will meet Rosa again in Chapter 5 to discuss the treatment of the constipation and anxiety for which she was originally referred for acupuncture, and which were well managed to this point.

This case focuses on the nine months following an aortic valve replacement, a very difficult time for Rosa. This was partly due to the after-effects of the surgery, including pain, insomnia, constipation, mood swings, anxiety, and depression.[34] Major life events at this time included early retirement and concerns about her aged mother who lived abroad. Throughout this eventful time, Rosa found acupuncture beneficial and supportive.

Managing post-surgery recovery and chronic anxiety

Resuming acupuncture treatment five weeks after aortic surgery, Rosa reported high levels of anxiety, fear of going to sleep (she needed to keep a light on during the night), and dream-disturbed sleep. Physical symptoms included scar pain and numbness and tingling in her left arm and fingers.

Rosa's psychological symptoms equate with shen disturbance, characterised by insomnia, agitation, mental restlessness, and anxiety.[35] Shen is related to the Heart energy in CM theory, affecting mental activity (including emotions), consciousness, memory, thinking, and sleep.[9]

My treatment plan was to calm the shen and regulate the Heart. Points on the Heart and Pericardium channels perform these functions, and also address pain and discomfort in the chest, arm, and hand.[36] The following points formed the mainstay of Rosa's treatment, chosen for their dual function of addressing emotional and physical symptoms: HE-3 *Shaohai*, HE-7 *Shenmen*, HE-8 *Shaofu* and P-3 *Quze*, P-7 *Daling*, P-8 *Laogong*.

As treatment progressed, I gradually added other points such as the back shu points of the Heart and Pericardium channels: BL-14 *Jueyinshu*, BL-15 *Xinshu*, and BL-44 *Shentang*. Extra point M-HN-3 *Yintang* was used in most treatments for its calming effect.

I used this approach in 13 of the 20 treatments during this period, examples of which are shown in Table 4.1. Variations included:

- Treatment 1, where I used External Dragons post-operatively to restore the shen after the physical shock of surgery (see Chapter 5, Toolkit).
- Other treatments (not shown), to address acute problems, including hip pain, a cold, and breathing difficulties.
- Treatments 19 and 20, to address Rosa's hernias, using points indicated for prolapse. This decreased discomfort and enabled Rosa to be more physically active.

Table 4.1: Examples of Rosa's treatments

Calm shen, regulate the Heart, relieve pain in the chest and left arm and hand

Tx	Treatment principles	Points*
1	External Dragons	DU-20 *Baihui* BL-11 *Dazhu* BL-23 *Shenshu* BL-61 *Pucan*
2, 3, 7	Calm shen and clear channels (Pericardium, Heart) to relieve arm pain	Extra point M-HN-3 *Yintang* HE-3 *Shaohai* (LS) HE-8 *Shaofu* (LS) P-3 *Quze* (LS) P-7 *Daling* (LS)
9, 13, 14, 15, 16	Calm shen**	Extra point M-HN-3 *Yintang* HE-8 *Shaofu* (LS) P-3 *Quze* (LS) BL-14 *Jueyinshu* BL-15 *Xinshu* BL-44 *Shentang*
11	Calm shen as per Tx 15 and 16 Strengthen the spirit	KID-24 *Lingxu****
19, 20	Calm shen Treat hernias: raise qi Treat prolapse	Extra point M-HN-3 *Yintang* HE-7 *Shenmen* (LS) HE-8 *Shaofu* (RS) or P-3 *Quze* (RS) DU-20 *Baihui* REN-6 *Qihai* and SP-6 *Sanyinjiao*

*Points needled unilaterally are indicated **LS** for left side and **RS** for right side. Needle technique is even, with needles retained for 20 minutes.

**This treatment was repeated with variations, choosing from HE-3 *Shaohai*, HE-7 *Shenmen*, HE-8 *Shaofu* and P-3 *Quze*, P-7 *Daling*, P-8 *Laogong*. Usually, I select four of these points, which are needled unilaterally.

***Rosa had received news of possible thyroid cancer; this point is indicated when 'a person is resigned and depleted by the vicissitudes of life.'[5]

Progress through treatment

Tx 1: Rosa reported feeling much better after the External Dragons administered at Treatment 1 and was cheerful and positive.

Tx 2, 3, 7: Pain in the scar and chest were bothersome, as were sensations of numbness along the Pericardium channel and tingling in her wrist and fingers. Constipation returned when she stopped taking the laxatives prescribed post-operatively. Disturbed sleep and anxiety continued, but she managed to sleep without a light on for one night.

To alleviate the pain, I used wrist and elbow points on the Pericardium and Heart channels to clear the channels. These points were also used to address the insomnia and anxiety. By the fifth treatment, Rosa reported she had 'turned a corner'. Arm sensations were less bothersome, bowel performance had improved, and she reduced her painkillers. The anxiety was diminishing, and she no longer slept with the light on, although she expressed anxieties about having a car accident on her next trip abroad.

Tx 9: Rosa continued to improve gradually, with minor setbacks. By treatment 9, she was sleeping well with no lights on, and feeling more uplifted. She was physically active, walking daily and doing a cardiac rehabilitation programme of aerobic exercise. She also attended weekly yoga and tai chi classes.

Tx 11: Three weeks later, she was distressed by a diagnosis of possible thyroid cancer. This triggered a significant setback, manifesting in breathlessness and evening palpitations. She returned to sleeping with the light on, and her imagination was pervaded with fears about traffic accidents and other misfortunes. This distress was worsened by a diagnosis of borderline diabetes.

Tx 13–16 and beyond: This period was filled with medical investigations. Rosa felt 'engulfed by hospitals', 'overwhelmed' by the frequency of appointments, and described her table at home covered with letters from numerous hospital departments. At treatment 14, she said:

> Three years ago I considered myself a healthy woman, very active...now I feel like I am grabbing the side of a hole to get myself up, and things push me down all the time.

Rosa felt desperate and I requested a referral from her medical team for counselling. She found acupuncture supportive during this turbulent period, writing:

> When I was first introduced to acupuncture I did not know what to expect but I was only too happy to try it out as I wanted to achieve some improvement in my bowel movements and stop using laxatives ... I am now fully supportive of acupuncture and would strongly recommend it to anyone ... The benefits of this treatment are endless. My bowel movements have improved beyond recognition and without the aid of any laxatives. Breathing has also improved and I have also gained a general feeling of calmness.

Her oncologist also noted the difference, writing:

> She has found the acupuncture extremely helpful and it seems to have regularised her bowels quite effectively, so she is coping much better with that aspect of things and it also seems to keep her rather calmer.

Longer-term follow-up

Rosa, a vibrant, determined woman, was diligent in observing good health practices. Her struggle with the consequences of cancer and its treatments, the increasing burden of other health conditions, and cancer recurrence with metastases continued. Acupuncture was clearly supportive in helping her cope with increasingly complex health issues.

Sadly, this acupuncture clinic ended. In our final appointment, she said that acupuncture had helped in great moments of stress – the heart surgery and the cancer recurrence. That it had normalised her bowel functions was 'a gift from heaven'. She knew she would always sleep well on the night of treatment, and her breathing would improve.

Conclusion

Rosa's journey following initial cancer diagnosis and treatment was not towards better health and is traced by the shaded boxes in Figure 4.2. She experienced metastatic spread, had surgery and chemotherapy, and died recently. She once remarked that 'cancer loves me more than I love it'. In the face of these challenges, a simple approach to acupuncture treatment helped her on many levels. I was privileged to be able to support her.

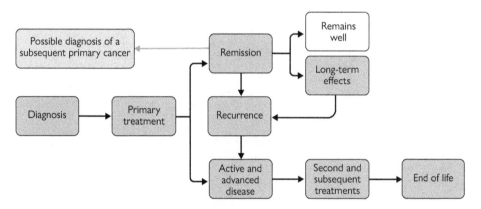

FIGURE 4.2: ROSA'S PROGRESS THROUGH THE SURVIVORSHIP PATHWAY

CHAPTER SUMMARY

- Have the courage to keep treatment simple and the patience to allow time for complicated things to happen.
- Remain mindful that acupuncture has the potential to enable coping and move the patient's orientation from symptom to self.
- Acupuncture and moxibustion are safe interventions for cancer survivors when administered by trained and qualified acupuncturists.

References

1. National Acupuncture Detoxification Association Compilation of Michael Smith's writing. Laramie, WY: National Acupuncture Detoxification Association; 2021. Available from: https://acudetox.com/compilation-of-michael-smiths-writing
2. de Valois B, Asprey A, Young T 'The monkey on your shoulder': a qualitative study of lymphoedema patients' attitudes to and experiences of acupuncture and moxibustion. Evid. Based Complement. Alternat. Med. 2016;Article ID 4298420.
3. Schulman D Offering complex patients a simple piece of heaven. J. Chinese Med. 2007;85:36–37.
4. de Valois B Using acupuncture to manage hot flushes & night sweats in women taking tamoxifen for early breast cancer: two observational studies: Thames Valley University; 2006.
5. Hicks A, Hicks J, Mole P Five element constitutional acupuncture. Edinburgh: Churchill Livingstone; 2004.
6. Smith MO Acupuncture for the treatment of cocaine addiction. Vancouver, WA: J & M Reports LLC; 2001.
7. Miaskowski C, Barsevick A, Berger A, et al. Advancing symptom science through symptom cluster research: expert panel proceedings and recommendations. J. Natl. Cancer Inst. 2017;109(4).
8. Thompson L, Johnstone PA Acupuncture for cancer symptom clusters. Alexandria, VA: American Society of Clinical Oncology; 2016. Available from: https://ascopost.com/issues/january-25-2016/acupuncture-for-cancer-symptom-clusters
9. Maciocia G The foundations of Chinese medicine. London: Churchill Livingstone; 1989.
10. de Valois B, Degun T Using the NADA protocol to improve wellbeing of prostate cancer survivors: five case studies. Eur. J. Orient. Med. 2015;8(1):8–18.
11. Price S, Long AF, Godfrey M Exploring the needs and concerns of women with early breast cancer during chemotherapy: valued outcomes during a course of traditional acupuncture. Evid. Based. Complement. Alternat. Med. 2013;2013:165891.
12. Price S, Long A, Godfrey M What is traditional acupuncture – exploring goals and processes of treatment in the context of women with early breast cancer. BMC Complement. Altern. Med. 2014;14(1):201.
13. Walker G, de Valois B, Young T, et al. The experience of receiving traditional Chinese acupuncture. Eur. J. Orient. Med. 2004;4(5):59–65.
14. Paterson C, Britten N Acupuncture as a complex intervention: a holistic model. J. Altern. Complement. Med. 2004;10(5):791–801.
15. Rugg S, Paterson C, Britten N, et al. Traditional acupuncture for people with medically unexplained symptoms: a longitudinal qualitative study of patients' experiences. Br. J. Gen. Pract. 2011;June:306–315.
16. MacPherson H, Elliot B, Hopton A, et al. Lifestyle advice and self-care integral to acupuncture treatment for patients with chronic neck pain: secondary analysis of outcomes within a randomized controlled trial. J. Altern. Complement. Med. 2017;23(3):180–187.
17. Evans M, Paterson C, Wye L, et al. Lifestyle and self-care advice within traditional acupuncture consultations: a qualitative observational study nested in a co-operative inquiry. J. Altern. Complement. Med. 2011;17(6):519–529.
18. Deadman P Live well live long: teachings from the Chinese nourishment of life tradition. Hove: The Journal of Chinese Medicine; 2016.
19. Birch S, Lee M, Alraek T, et al. Evidence, safety and recommendations for when to use acupuncture for treating cancer related symptoms: a narrative review. Integr. Med. Res. 2019;8(3):160–166.

20. Melchart D, Weidenhammer W, Streng A, *et al.* Prospective investigation of adverse effects of acupuncture in 97 733 patients. Arch. Intern. Med. 2004;164(1):104–105.
21. Deng G, Frenkel M, Cohen L, *et al.* Evidence-based clinical practice guidelines for integrative oncology: complementary therapies and botanicals. J. Soc. Integr. Oncol. 2009;7(3 Summer):85–120.
22. Cancer Research UK Acupuncture. 2015. Available from: www.cancerresearchuk.org/about-cancer/cancers-in-general/treatment/complementary-alternative/therapies/acupuncture
23. National Cancer Institute Acupuncture (PDQ°)-Health Professional Version. National Cancer Institute; 2020. Available from: www.cancer.gov/about-cancer/treatment/cam/hp/acupuncture-pdq
24. Deng G, Rausch SM, Jones LW, *et al.* Complementary therapies and integrative medicine in lung cancer. CHEST (May 2013 Suppl.) 2013;143(5):e420s–e436S.
25. Canadian Cancer Society Acupuncture. Canadian Cancer Society; 2021. Available from: www.cancer.ca/en/cancer-information/diagnosis-and-treatment/complementary-therapies/acupuncture/?region=on
26. Deng G, Bao T, Mao JJ Understanding the benefits of acupuncture treatment for cancer pain management. Oncology (Williston Park) 2018;32(6):310–316.
27. Lu W, Doherty-Gilman A, Rosenthal DS Recent advances in oncology acupuncture and safety considerations in practice. Curr. Treat. Options Oncol. 2010;11(3–4):141–146.
28. Lee MS, Choi T-Y, Park J-E, *et al.* Moxibustion for cancer care: a systematic review. BMC Cancer 2010;10(130).
29. Xu J, Deng H, Shen X Safety of moxibustion: a systematic review of case reports. Evid. Based Complement. Alternat. Med. 2014;2014:783704.
30. de Valois B, Young T, Glynne-Jones R, *et al.* Limiting chemotherapy side effects by using moxa. Eur. J. Orient. Med. 2016;8(3):29–39.
31. Sagar SM, Wong RK Safety and side effects of acupuncture and moxibustion as a therapy for cancer. In: Cho W, editor. Acupuncture and moxibustion as an evidence-based therapy for cancer. Dordrecht: Springer; 2012. pp. 265–289.
32. de Valois B, Glynne-Jones R Acupuncture in the supportive care of colorectal cancer survivors: four case studies, Part 2. Eur. J. Orient. Med. 2018;9(1):10–22.
33. Macmillan Cancer Support The burden of cancer and other long-term health conditions. 2015. Available from: www.macmillan.org.uk/documents/press/cancerandotherlong-termconditions.pdf
34. NHS Choices Aortic valve replacement – recovery. Department of Health; 2018.
35. Maciocia G The psyche in Chinese medicine. London: Churchill Livingstone; 2009.
36. Deadman P, Al-Khafaji M, Baker K A manual of acupuncture. Hove: The Journal of Chinese Medicine; 2007.

Chapter 5

Toolkit

Introduction

The flexibility of acupuncture to address complex conditions is encapsulated in these quotations:

> Chinese medicine...is a 'tradition to think with'. (Professor Volker Scheid)[1]

> But it wasn't the same acupuncture every time anyway...every week they asked how you were in relation to different things before starting and would decide on which particular treatment would be appropriate for that week... So it wasn't like a set plan that you had to have it whether you wanted it or not, it was very flexible. (Breast cancer survivor with lymphoedema)[2]

Toolkit essentials

The importance of having a toolkit

Every practitioner has a 'toolkit'. This is the collection of tools, procedures, and approaches we acquire as our expertise develops. It may start as an 'unconscious' toolkit, comprising aspects of our training that attracted us most.

As clinical experience grows, we develop ways to deal with challenges that arise. We embark on continuing professional development (CPD), read, discuss with colleagues, and explore with our patients. Being aware of having a toolkit provides ready access to techniques to draw on when faced with clinical challenges.

Such challenges may be environmental, for example clinics that do not allow moxa, or have a treatment couch that cannot accommodate patients comfortably in a prone position. Restrictions may relate to the condition itself, such as avoiding needling in a limb affected by lymphoedema. Patients themselves may express strong opinions about how they wish to be treated, and where and how they wish to be needled. A toolbox of options provides the flexibility to meet these challenges.

A great strength of East Asian medicine (EAM) is that its diversity offers many ways to approach clinical challenges. This versatility should be celebrated by acupuncturists, as it increases our capacity to meet our patients' needs, working with them energetically and 'in the moment', whatever the context.

Every practitioner is the sum of their initial training, their subsequent CPD, and their individual clinical circumstances, as well as the personal history, experiences, and interests that enrich and influence the practitioner they become. Added to this is the practitioner's penchant for aspects of their respective style of acupuncture (theoretical framework). We grow and develop our own unique styles; 'individual practitioners and teachers practise in quite different ways from each other'.[3]

ESSENTIALS

This chapter, and the 'tools' it discusses, are not intended to be prescriptive. Rather, the tools are presented to clarify the case studies and procedures discussed throughout this book. They are also intended to stimulate practitioners' thoughts about the toolkits they might develop for themselves.

Developing a toolkit

I encourage practitioners to consciously develop their own toolkit, drawing on their respective theoretical frameworks, training, and experience, and considering the clinical context(s) in which they work.

I also recommend practitioners explore outside their own theoretical framework to acquaint themselves with the richness and versatility of acupuncture. Diversity and innovation are characteristics of the development of EAM. Continuous adaptation and transformation have made it applicable to modern health problems, and to the conditions experienced by patients in differing geographical and cultural areas of the globe.

All styles of acupuncture have much to offer both patients and practitioners. Open-minded acceptance of this enables the acupuncture profession to explore and innovate to meet the evolving healthcare needs of modern societies around the world.

The richness and diversity of EAM give us many ways to approach a clinical challenge. As Scheid says, it is a tradition to think with.

ESSENTIALS

Assembling a toolkit is a process that takes place over time. Newly qualified practitioners, or practitioners new to working with cancer survivors, might begin with a starter toolkit that contains some basic tools. As experience of working with cancer survivors grows and knowledge of these patients' requirements develops, new tools are added to create a more sophisticated toolbox for dealing with a wide range of situations.

This can be likened to starting off with the basic home toolkit for car owners and developing it to the toolboxes seen in auto repair shops, filled with specialist tools for repairing a wide range of cars.[4]

Developing treatment approaches for the individual

In clinic, I aim to develop a treatment strategy relevant to the individual, as they present at each appointment. Sometimes this will include standardised protocols when the protocol addresses the patient's need at the time. Sometimes, a protocol or point combination is the foundation for treating a patient, and over time I tailor it to the individual by adding, changing, or removing points. This process develops through applying a clearly defined treatment strategy, observing the response, and adjusting and building on the strategy. It relies on communication with and feedback from the patient. Treatment becomes a process of discovery; many of the approaches in my toolbox were discovered through this process.

Treatment principles and points

Practitioners often ask 'what point or points do you use?' A more clinically pertinent question is 'what are your treatment principles?' This shifts the focus away from points alone towards addressing the condition, expanding the range of points available for that situation. This gives flexibility, especially when conditions mean certain points cannot be used, for example in the case of lymphoedema (see Chapter 9, Cancer Treatment-Related Lymphoedema), amputation, scarring, or patient preference. Access to at least one good points compendium (see Further Information and Resources in the Appendices, online) and a good knowledge of the multiple functions of the points enable the practitioner to select alternatives with ease and confidence.

Some tools from my toolkit

I developed this toolkit over many years of research and practice. It reflects my training – the 'integrated' style taught at the College of Integrated Chinese Medicine in Reading, UK, which draws on two theoretical frameworks. These are Five Element Constitutional Acupuncture and Chinese medicine (often referred to as TCM). It also reflects what I have learned through practising, researching, and writing about acupuncture as well as sharing with colleagues and listening to feedback from my patients.

Five Element Constitutional Acupuncture approaches

Five Element Constitutional Acupuncture (referred to as Five Element acupuncture hereafter) focuses on the interaction of the five elements or phases – fire, earth, metal, water, and wood. A key characteristic is the concept of the 'constitutional imbalance' whereby an imbalance in one of the five elements may underpin symptoms of ill-health on the level of the body, mind, and/or spirit. This is the 'constitutional factor' or 'CF' (or 'causative factor'). The practitioner focuses on the patient's colour, sound, emotion, and odour (CSEO) and the pulses to diagnose the CF and monitor change.[5]

Emphasis on establishing rapport with the patient makes Five Element acupuncture appropriate for treating 'longer-term chronic problems with a mixture of physical and spirit-level issues'.[3] This is a very good approach for cancer survivors, offering elegant and often simple treatments having the potential to address complex conditions. Focusing on the CF can curb any tendencies on the part of the acupuncturist to 'get scattered' in the attempt to address multiple concurrent symptoms, such as those presented by cancer survivors with comorbidities.

From the very rich offering of Five Element acupuncture techniques, I have selected those described below as mainstays in my toolbox. This is not to say other techniques are irrelevant or less effective. These are simply the ones for which I have developed an affinity through my own study and practice; some I have used extensively in research projects, so have been able to systematically monitor their effects. More extended discussions of Five Element acupuncture can be found in the excellent textbook on the subject by Hicks *et al.*[3]

Five Element blocks to treatment

Blocks to treatment are phenomena associated with blockages in the patient's qi. These can have profound negative effects on the patient's physical and psychological health. They often underlie a patient's inability to progress during treatment, or unexplained relapse. There are four blocks:

- Aggressive Energy (AE)
- Possession: Internal Dragons (IDs) and External Dragons (EDs)
- Husband–Wife Imbalance
- Entry–Exit blocks.

While JR Worsley, founder of Leamington Acupuncture, is attributed with introducing these ideas to the practice of acupuncture in Britain and America, the concept of blocks to treatment appears to be rooted in ancient beliefs about the nature of disease.[6,7]

The blocks have their own distinct characteristics, indications, and treatment protocols; they also share common features. They may:

- pre-exist in a patient's energetic make-up, requiring the practitioner to clear them before addressing other aspects of the patient's health
- arise during acupuncture treatment, becoming apparent when a patient stops progressing or even regresses until the block is cleared
- be a *cause* of poor health, and *be caused* by poor health.

In this toolkit, I focus on Aggressive Energy (AE) and Possession, whose indications include a history of:

- life-threatening illness
- intensive drug therapy (either therapeutic or recreational)
- trauma (either physical or emotional) that affects the patient deeply on a physical, emotional, or spiritual level.

These indications suggest that clearing blocks to treatment may be particularly relevant when treating people living with and beyond cancer. Survivors will have experienced:

- the shock of a cancer diagnosis
- invasive treatments, such as surgery, radiotherapy
- intensive drug therapies, such as chemotherapy, anti-emetics, painkillers, antidepressants, hormonal treatments to prevent recurrence, medications to manage side effects
- the anxiety and deep-rooted fear associated with a life-threatening condition.

Husband–Wife Imbalance and Entry–Exit blocks are also applicable; however, as my own clinical experience of these has not been extensive, they do not feature as mainstays of my toolbox.

Aggressive Energy and the 'AE Drain'
What is it?

Aggressive Energy (AE) is described as 'contaminated' or 'unhealthy' qi, that is, qi that stagnates or accumulates and turns to toxic heat or fire in the yin organs. AE is thought to underlie serious physical illness and emotional instability including emotional states such as despair and depression. Its aetiologies are:

- internal causes, such as emotional trauma
- external pathogenic factors (wind, cold, damp, dryness, fire, or heat) invading the body or arising internally.

When the body's qi is strong, it can recover from these events, whether internal or external. However, AE may develop if an emotional state or pathogen lingers in the body over time.

How do we identify Aggressive Energy?

Of the predisposing circumstances stated by Hicks *et al.*[3] that indicate the presence of AE, the most relevant to cancer survivors are:

- **Physical illness that is serious or life-threatening** – cancer is of course one of these. In addition, cancer survivors may also have other long-term chronic illnesses (comorbidities), such as hypertension, obesity, mental health problems, chronic heart disease, chronic kidney disease.[8]
- **A history of intensive drug therapy** – as well as systemic anti-cancer treatments, cancer survivors may have taken or continue to take prescribed medicines for cancer-related issues (such as adjuvant hormonal treatments) as well as for comorbidities.
- **Severe mental or spiritual problems** – cancer survivors may experience chronic or intermittent feelings of despair, hopelessness, and resignation, while many survivors talk about feeling 'out of balance' and 'out of control'.

How do we treat it?

AE is both diagnosed and treated with an AE Drain. This is administered routinely as a first treatment by many Five Element practitioners (unless Possession is suspected, see later in this chapter).

It should also be considered during a course of treatment when a patient fails to respond to treatment, or their health unexpectedly declines. In these circumstances, it is also advisable to check whether cancer recurrence is a possibility.

How do we do an AE Drain?

The patient may be sitting up, and if so they should be well supported in case needle shock causes fainting. In my experience, this is rare but possible. To avoid this possibility, the patient may be positioned lying prone.

Procedure (Table 5.1 and Figure 5.1):

- Insert needles **superficially** (0.1 cun is recommended) into the back shu points of the yin organs. Do not aim to obtain needle sensation (deqi).
- Insert a 'check' needle at each of three points in the muscle, about 2 centimetres lateral to the inner Bladder line. Check needles should be positioned in the muscle adjacent to each grouping of points.

An AE Drain combines both diagnosis and treatment:

- **Diagnosis** – AE is present if erythema (redness) develops around any of the needles in the back shu points, but not if redness also develops around the check needles.
- **Treatment** – if erythema is present, retain the needles until the redness disappears. This often occurs within 10–20 minutes; sometimes, erythema may take longer to drain. If this exceeds available clinic time, remove the needles, and repeat the treatment at the next session.

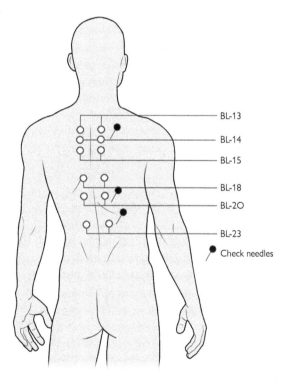

FIGURE 5.1: POINTS FOR THE AE DRAIN

Table 5.1: Points for the AE Drain

Yin organ	Back shu point	Check needles
Lung	BL-13 *Feishu*	
Pericardium	BL-14 *Jueyinshu*	Check needle
Heart*	BL-15 *Xinshu*	
Liver	BL-18 *Ganshu*	Check needle
Spleen	BL-20 *Pishu*	
Kidney	BL-23 *Shenshu*	Check needle

*Some Five Element schools advise against placing needles in the back shu point of the Heart unless Aggressive Energy is detected in the Pericardium or if it is present in both the Kidney and Lung but not in the Pericardium. In discussions with many Five Element practitioners, I have found it is common practice to include the Heart at the beginning of the procedure.

What reaction might we expect?

Reactions vary according to the individual; most people report feeling different after AE is cleared. They may say they are feeling better in themselves and report improvements in symptoms at their next treatment. Feeling very tired is common after this treatment, after which they begin to feel energised. Sometimes, reactions may be dramatic, as shown in Poppy's vignette below.

Tips from my clinical experience

- This is a useful first treatment when people are anxious about having acupuncture. I find it particularly useful for individuals referred for acupuncture by a biomedical healthcare professional. These patients may expect acupuncture to be painful; they are pleasantly surprised to find it pain free, and they have had up to 15 needles inserted! This can be a great psychological boost for such patients.
- I was taught to administer AE Drains with the person sitting upright and have not had problems with patients fainting. Many schools now recommend the patient lying in the prone position to ensure safety should they faint. This can be uncomfortable for patients if there is no face hole in the treatment table, and for patients who experience claustrophobia, have breast pain, scarring on the torso, or have a stoma.
- Over many years, I have experimented with how to introduce this to patients. I do not refer to it as 'aggressive energy'; in general, I say it is preparation for future acupuncture treatment. If possible, I match this to a patient's interests; for example, for a patient interested in gardening, I say this is like preparing the soil to receive seeds; for one who does DIY, I liken it to preparing wood to receive paint. Sometimes, I say it is like a gentle detox treatment.
- I have observed, and many patients have reported, changes even when there is no sign of erythema.
- Although needles are usually inserted bilaterally, good results can be obtained with unilateral insertion for cancer survivors at risk of lymphoedema[9] (see Chapter 9, Cancer Treatment-Related Lymphoedema).

- Many women report alleviation of hot flushes and night sweats (HFNS) following an AE Drain (see Chapter 8, Cancer Treatment-Related Hot Flushes and Night Sweats).

VIGNETTE: POPPY AND THE POWER OF THE AE DRAIN[10]

Background

Poppy, aged 44, completed breast cancer treatment (surgery, chemotherapy, and radiotherapy) ten months prior to joining a study of using acupuncture to manage tamoxifen-related HFNS.

During the initial consultation, Poppy discussed the aches and pains her GP attributed to tamoxifen. She said these aches, which occurred under both armpits and around her back, felt as if someone was 'squeezing' or 'gripping' her. They were worse on getting out of bed in the morning, or rising from a sitting position, when they were accompanied by a sharp spasm of pain. Numerous investigations had not identified a cause. Although her doctor was unconcerned, Poppy found these more uncomfortable and distressing than her copious HFNS.

The first treatment

Following standard procedure in this research, Poppy's first treatment was an AE Drain. Considerable erythema appeared around the needles in the Bladder points, which diminished over the 25 minutes the needles were retained.

Progress through treatment

At her next treatment a week later, Poppy delightedly reported she had been pain-free on waking the day after treatment, and the pain had not returned until four to five days later. Even then, the discomfort was tolerable. This did not need attention until her seventh treatment, when Poppy specifically asked for 'that back treatment' to be repeated.

In all her written feedback about the benefits of having acupuncture treatment for HFNS, Poppy stressed that acupuncture had 'instantly unblocked the awful aches and pains I'd been suffering from since chemo and radiotherapy' the previous year.

Summary

Poppy's case illustrates how Aggressive Energy can manifest in an individual, and shows how effective an AE Drain can be in clearing troublesome symptoms.

Possession (or Seven Dragons, Internal Dragons and External Dragons)
What is it?

In Five Element acupuncture, 'Possession' refers to a state where a person may be out of control of their mind and spirit. It may manifest along a spectrum from obsessive thoughts to being invaded and controlled by unhelpful spirits.[3]

Its aetiologies may be from external or internal causes, and may be the result of physical, mental, or spiritual influences. When a person is in good overall health, their resilience will deal with the disturbance. Vulnerability to Possession is increased by several factors, of which those generally pertaining to cancer survivors include:

- **Underlying poor physical or psychological health** – cancer and its treatments are a factor here.
- **Emotional shocks** – these scatter the qi and may leave people feeling traumatised and temporarily out of control. When the qi is strong, individuals can recover their equilibrium; however, when the qi is not strong, the intensity of the emotional experience may become overwhelming. A diagnosis of cancer is almost certainly an emotional shock, and other emotional shocks may occur at any stage during and beyond cancer treatment. Thus, we can presume that this will be common factor in cancer survivorship.
- **Physical shocks** – surgery is key. In the UK, 68% of people undergo surgery as part of their primary cancer treatment;[11] many have subsequent surgeries as part of their ongoing cancer treatment, in addition to surgeries that are common in the usual course of healthcare. Surgery can affect the shen, leaving it temporarily separated from the body, so it is no longer housed in the Heart. This increases vulnerability to Possession.
- **Drug 'abuse'** – while Hicks *et al.* specifically refer to drug 'abuse', I also include prescribed medicines used in cancer treatment, for example long-term use of opioids for chronic post-cancer pain.

How do we identify Possession?
While the aetiologies may alert us to the possibility of Possession, diagnosis is more commonly based on the patient's presentation: 'one key sign is that something about the patient is extremely unusual'.[3] Examples include:

- 'Veiled' eyes – it is difficult to make a connection with the patient.
- Unusual speech or behaviour – for example, it is not possible to establish rapport or take a case history.
- Intense dream life, recurrent terrifying or evil dreams; also, images that haunt a patient in their waking life.
- Obsessions or addictive behaviour or voices in the mind – see Heather's vignette below.
- Patient says they 'feel' possessed or out of control.
- Acupuncture treatment doesn't progress, or the treatment has some effect but the patient relapses.

VIGNETTE: HEATHER – POSSESSION, OBSESSIVE BEHAVIOURS, AND A CASE OF LEARNING FROM A PATIENT[10]

Background

Heather, aged 46, completed breast cancer treatment (surgery, chemotherapy, and radiotherapy) 16 months prior to joining a study of using acupuncture to manage tamoxifen-related HFNS.

During the initial consultation, Heather explained that with regard to her cancer, she was afraid to say she was feeling well 'in case it all goes wrong'. This would be 'tempting fate'.

Progress through treatment

Heather attended for three treatments before withdrawing from the study. She responded well to the AE Drain at her first treatment, reporting that she felt 'really a lot calmer, not so wound up…or fidgety' afterwards. Her family and friends also noticed she was not so 'uptight'. After the second treatment (Table 5.4), she reported that HFNS had reduced, and she was still feeling relaxed.

During these treatments, Heather disclosed her fear of change. She was locked into a belief system that dictated her cancer would return if she changed anything in her daily life. This was clearly debilitating and was causing tensions at home.

This was my signal to treat Possession. However, at her third treatment, Heather said she was feeling more positive about change and she was talking to her partner about moving house. From this, I judged that the treatment was influencing her belief system about change and I did not treat Possession.

I was therefore surprised to receive a letter from Heather saying she was unable to attend further sessions due to 'transportation problems'; she regretted this, as she found treatment 'valuable and most effective with my hot flushes and sweats'.

Heather had not previously mentioned transportation as a potential issue; she declined to discuss her decision to leave the study with me over the phone. From this, I suspected Heather may have retreated to her obsession about change. Improvements in her HFNS may have triggered concerns that this change would cause the cancer to return, so it was safer to discontinue treatment.

Learning from the patient

Of course, I will never know her true reasons. However, my assessment of Heather's response and her possible motives was a powerful influence on my approach to future study participants. It convinced me it was necessary to adapt the study protocol to address blocks to treatment where appropriate.

Summary

Heather's need to maintain the status quo to keep the cancer at bay was clearly an obsession and an indication for treating Possession.

How do we treat it?

Possession is treated by using Internal Dragons (IDs) and/or External Dragons (EDs), approaches also known as Seven Dragons. There are general rules for choosing which to use:

- **Internal Dragons** are indicated if the patient's problem is from an internal cause, such as emotional shocks, instability, or poor psychological health.
- **External Dragons** are indicated if the problem appears to be from external causes, such as surgery or drugs.

It may be difficult to discern whether the cause is internal or external, and many cancer survivors will have experienced both internal and external causes. For example, as discussed above, they will have experienced the shock of diagnosis, and may have experienced surgery and possible use of prescription drugs that are powerful or potentially addictive. In such cases, Hicks *et al.* recommend using Internal Dragons first, and if this does not make a change, to then use External Dragons.

However, the choice of which of these treatments to use may be influenced by purely practical factors, such as limited access to the points. For example, I have used External Dragons in lieu of Internal Dragons on patients for whom recent surgery made it inappropriate to needle on the front of the torso (see Lily's vignette below).

How do we do Seven Dragons treatments?

These treatments are sometimes called 'Seven Dragons' as they each use seven acupuncture points (Table 5.2, Figure 5.2, and Figure 5.3).

Table 5.2: Points for Seven Dragons treatments

	Internal Dragons (IDs)	External Dragons (EDs)
Position	Patient lying on back, arms at sides, legs extended.	Patient seated on chair facing treatment table with feet on the floor and able to support themselves by folding arms on the table and leaning forward.
Points used (bilateral needling)	Extra point 0.25 cun below REN-15 *Jiuwei* ST-25 *Tianshu* ST-32 *Futu* ST-41 *Jiexi*	DU-20 *Baihui* BL-11 *Dazhu* BL-23 *Shenshu* BL-61 *Pucan*
Procedure	For both procedures: • Needle points from top to bottom, using even or sedation technique. • Work from right to left. • After inserting all needles, turn each needle 180° counterclockwise. • Leave needles in place for 20 minutes or until changes in the patient have occurred. • Remove needles from top to bottom, working from right to left.	

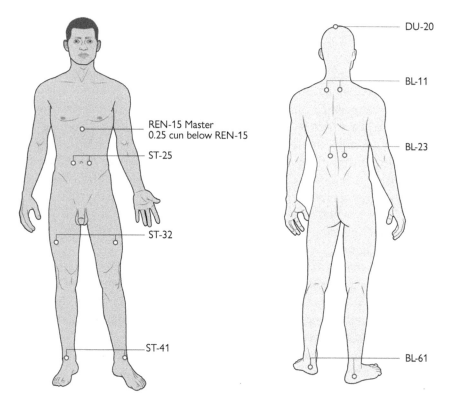

FIGURE 5.2: POINTS FOR INTERNAL DRAGONS   FIGURE 5.3: POINTS FOR EXTERNAL DRAGONS

What reactions might we expect?

Reactions vary according to the individual, and may occur at any time – during treatment, soon afterwards, or some time afterwards. During treatment, they may range from no apparent reaction to very noticeable visual and audible reactions that may include shaking, strange noises, feeling ill. While there are some anecdotal accounts of extremely dramatic reactions, patients may simply feel relaxed during the treatment (my patients often fall asleep).

Feeling tired or feeling energised after the treatment are common. Individuals may experience a fundamental transformation, with the signs of Possession disappearing. They may report feeling lighter, freer, or more in control of life, or they may be aware of feeling better in themselves while being unable to describe the changes.

Tips from my clinical experience

- Five Element acupuncturists are often trained to clear Possession at the first treatment if it is suspected, addressing this block before clearing Aggressive Energy. I find this can be clinically challenging, especially with acupuncture-naive patients, who may be anxious about having acupuncture for the first time and who are unfamiliar with needle sensation. Some patients, particularly those with body image issues, may feel very vulnerable exposing the yin side of their torso at the first treatment. I choose to clear Dragons when I am confident that I have gained the patient's trust.

- In general, I aim to administer External Dragons as soon as possible after any surgical intervention (whether cancer related or not).
- There are many variations to the method for administering Seven Dragons treatments. I have been taught to insert and remove the needles working from top to bottom and from right to left.
- Many cancer survivors say the experience of having cancer has made them feel they have lost control of their lives. To ground the treatment and help the patient regain a sense of control, I needle any of the following after removing the needles for the Seven Dragons treatment:
  - the yuan source points of the Small Intestine and Heart, SI-4 *Wangu* and HE-7 *Shenmen*
  - ST-36 *Zusanli*
  - the yuan source points of the patient's constitutional factor (CF) if known.[12]
- I don't administer IDs and EDs in the same session, nor do I combine them with an AE Drain in the same session. Each of these are strong interventions, which in combination may overwhelm the patient.
- When discussing this treatment with patients, I do not use the word 'Possession' which may be perceived negatively or as a judgement. I sometimes refer to it as 'the Seven Dragons', but mostly talk about it as a treatment intended to clear any blocks to their energy that may have arisen because of cancer treatment.
- Indicated for nightmares and distressing dreams, Seven Dragons can also restore a healthy dream life. Many survivors report that their dream life ceased at the time of their diagnosis and they 'recovered' their ability to dream after this treatment.
- 'Possession' has historically been taught with an aura of mystique and drama; 'Possession' is, after all, quite a powerful and potentially frightening term. I personally feel this approach disempowers practitioners. Generally, I call on these treatments when:
  - things don't make sense
  - I cannot put my finger on what is amiss in what the patient is telling me (or not telling me)
  - my diagnosis doesn't add up.

Administering a Seven Dragons treatment is unlikely to do harm. Even if Possession is not present, the treatments are very good for stabilising the patient and can be beneficial.

VIGNETTE: LILY AND A CASE OF USING EXTERNAL DRAGONS WHEN INTERNAL DRAGONS ARE NOT POSSIBLE[10]

Background

Lily, aged 51, completed breast cancer treatment (surgery, chemotherapy, and radio-therapy) seven months prior to joining a study of using acupuncture to manage tamoxifen-related HFNS.

During the initial consultation, Lily reported poor quality sleep; she slept only two hours. This started 16 years previously, when fire destroyed her property. Since the blaze, she habitually wakened at 2.30am (the time the fire started) to 'go on patrol' and check the whole house. She also experienced nightmares, horrid dreams, and was 'frightened to relax and go into a deep sleep'. Consequently, Lily had become accustomed to going without sleep.

Initial progress through treatment

While this obsessive need to check the house every night suggested Possession, Lily initially did well on the standard protocol for the study (Table 5.4). HFNS reduced in frequency and intensity and her sleep began to improve. However, she was still waking at 2.30am to 'go on patrol', and her dreams were still disturbing.

After her fourth treatment, she seemed to get worse: HFNS became more severe and nosebleeds (which had plagued her for most of her life, but which had not occurred during the previous year) returned. I decided to treat Possession at the next treatment if there was no improvement in the intervening week.

Internal or External Dragons?

Given the obsessive nature of Lily's night-time behaviour and the nature of her dreams, IDs seemed the relevant treatment. However, she had recently undergone breast recon-struction, and it seemed inappropriate to needle into the tender scarred area on the front of her torso. Thus, I opted to administer EDs.

Lily relaxed visibly during the treatment, although at the end she felt 'absolutely wiped out'. The next week, she was in good spirits: HFNS had reduced again, and she was 'definitely sleeping better'. She was now going to sleep at 10pm, waking at 3am but staying in bed, and dozing until 5am. The nose bleeds ceased.

Short- and long-term feedback

At her next and final (eighth) treatment, Lily delightedly reported she'd had the best week ever, with only four HFNS all week. She was sleeping five hours at a stretch, hadn't patrolled the house for two weeks, and her energy had improved remarkably.

When asked if she found being in the study beneficial, she replied that during the first weeks, she hadn't been sure. However, since the 'treatment on her back' (EDs) she was feeling 'remarkably different and much better… I feel alive now!'

Summary

Lily's case illustrates many of the aspects of Possession discussed above. There are multiple factors leading to the possibility of Possession, including emotional shocks (the fire, cancer diagnosis) and physical shocks (surgeries), plus intense medication (chemotherapy). Signs and symptoms of Possession include the obsessive behaviour (going on patrol every night), intense dreams, and the relapse midway through her course of acupuncture treatment.

This case also illustrates that it is effective to use EDs when IDs are indicated but not possible because of recent surgery.

Treating the spirit

Treating the spirit is fundamental to Five Element acupuncture, to 'initiate deep and fundamental changes [to affect] how patients feel in themselves'.[3] This approach is particularly useful when treating cancer survivors who are anxious, and particularly those who are experiencing fear of recurrence.

This approach draws on a wide range of points too numerous to list here; in fact, Hicks *et al.* specify 72 points in their list of points used specifically to treat the spirit.[3] Of these, I find Kidney chest points between KID-22 *Bulang* to KID-27 *Shufu* especially helpful when working with cancer survivors. Using these points, particularly with moxibustion, helps to strengthen the qi of the Kidney, Heart, Pericardium and Lung when it 'has been depleted through grief, fear and shock', and they are indicated for people who are 'struggling to cope with...daily life'.[3]

When working with my preferred spirit points (Table 5.3 and Figure 5.4) I use direct moxa (three to five cones) on selected points and usually I do not needle. As a rule, I use these points unilaterally on breast cancer patients who have or are at risk of lymphoedema (see also Chapter 9, Cancer Treatment-Related Lymphoedema). Patients (and some practitioners) may be sceptical that such a minimal intervention will have an effect; however, as shown by the experience of Ann (see Chapter 14), three to five small cones on these points – even unilaterally – can profoundly affect how someone feels.

Table 5.3: Selected spirit points

Points	Indications[13]
KID-24 *Lingxu*	Revives the spirit and calms the mind; useful for patients experiencing profound depletion of body, mind, and spirit.
KID-25 *Shencang* and KID-27 *Shufu* in combination	Strengthens and nourishes body, mind, and spirit; reinvigorates qi; and supports the person in building their own reserves.
REN-17 *Shanzhong*	The front mu point of the Pericardium is indicated for despondence, sadness, and feeling disconnected from inspiration.

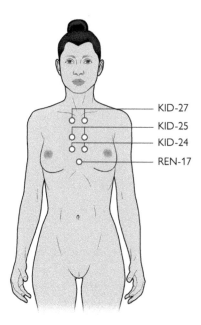

FIGURE 5.4: SELECTED SPIRIT POINTS

Treating the constitutional factor

Diagnosing and treating the constitutional factor (CF, also referred to as the causative factor) is fundamental to Five Element acupuncture. A full discussion of its theory and practice falls outside the purpose of this book.

However, I have had much clinical success treating cancer survivors by addressing the CF – either exclusively, or in combination with other approaches. The case study of Alauda illustrates how adjusting the treatment strategy to treating the CF helped to shift a deep emotional issue (see Chapter 8, 'Case study: Alauda and long-term management of HFNS'). Similarly, Claire experienced a significant shift when treatment focused on the CF (see Claire's case study in Chapter 11, Survivorship: Navigating the Milestones).

Summary of benefits of Five Element acupuncture for cancer survivors

Five Element acupuncture is suitable for supporting cancer survivors. Focus on the CF can address the often-complex presentations of these patients. This focus can also restrain any temptation on the part of the practitioner to attempt to treat every symptom, while the capacity to address the levels of body, mind, and spirit has the potential to comprehensively address the complexities of survivorship.

In general, Five Element acupuncture uses relatively few needles, often two to four points in a treatment.[2] This can be appealing to cancer survivors, who may be anxious about needles, especially after their experience of chemotherapy.

Finally, the capacity of Five Element acupuncture to deal with blocks to treatment can play a valuable role in improving the overall health of cancer survivors.

The extraordinary vessels
What are they?
The eight extraordinary vessels are the:

- Directing (or Conception or *Ren Mai*)
- Governing (*Du Mai*)
- Penetrating (*Chong Mai*)
- Girdle (*Dai Mai*)
- Yin Motility (or Yin Stepping or *Yin Qiao Mai*)
- Yang Motility (or Yang Stepping or *Yang Qiao Mai*)
- Yin Linking (*Yin Wei Mai*)
- Yang Linking (*Yang Wei Mai*).

Together these extraordinary vessels present 'a complex and important regulatory, balancing and integrating system that complements the main and connecting channels'.[14] In addition to circulating Kidney essence, these vessels enable a deeper level of treatment that functions as a way to address the patient's constitution.

Each extraordinary vessel has its own range of influence through the body and its own functions. A detailed discussion of the particulars of each of the eight extraordinary vessels is outside the range of this toolkit, and I refer readers to other texts for in-depth discussion (see Further Information and Resources in the Appendices, online). In this toolkit, I discuss the two most useful extraordinary vessels in my work with cancer survivors – the Directing Vessel and the Yang Linking Vessel.

Why do we use them?
Each extraordinary vessel has a 'confluent' or 'opening' point and a 'coupled' point. Needling the opening and coupled points together influences the area of the body covered by that extraordinary vessel, enabling treatment of symptoms to occur along the vessel's pathway.[14]

For example, the Directing Vessel originates between the kidneys, flows down to the perineum at REN-1 *Huiyin*, rises on the midline to the abdomen before travelling up the centre of the chest, throat, chin and face, circles around the lips and inside the mouth, then divides and enters the eyes, ending at ST-1 *Chengqi* (Figure 5.5). Thus, the Directing Vessel influences the abdomen, chest, lungs, throat, and face.[15] This access facilitates a generous scope for influencing the body – and for treating complex presentations of symptoms – by needling two points. This is useful clinically, especially for cancer survivors who may have 'had enough of needles' during cancer treatment.

Furthermore, the extraordinary vessels are indicated for 'complicated' presentations, that is, conditions that are chronic with 'multiple, confusing patterns and many different symptoms in different body systems'.[14] These are presentations we expect to find when working with cancer survivors.

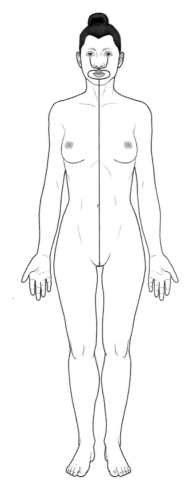

FIGURE 5.5: PATHWAY OF THE DIRECTING VESSEL

How do we use them?

My preferred method for using the extraordinary vessels is Maciocia's gender-based host–guest style.[14] For this method:

- Needle both the opening (host) and coupled (guest) point of the chosen extraordinary vessel.
- Needle the opening point first, followed by the coupled point. The two points are needled unilaterally and contralaterally. For women, the opening point is on the right side and the coupled point is on the left side; for men, the opening point is on the left side and the coupled point is on the right side (however, see the Notes below for modifications to this).
- Needle to obtain needle sensation (deqi); no further needle stimulation is necessary.
- When using additional points, needle these after needling the coupled point, starting from the top of the body and working downwards.

- Retain the needles for about 20 minutes.
- Remove the needles in reverse order, that is, starting with any additional points working from the bottom up, followed by the coupled point and ending with the opening point.

Notes
It is advisable to use:

- no more than four to five points in addition to the opening and coupled points
- only one extraordinary vessel in a treatment.

When working with cancer survivors, adopt a pragmatic approach to the gender-based needling and switch the sides if necessary. For example, if a woman had breast cancer on her right side, then use the opening point on the left side and the coupled point on the right, to avoid needling in the arm with or at risk of lymphoedema.

Working with the Directing Vessel
What is it?

Opening point:	LU-7 *Lieque*	Needle right side for women, left side for men
Coupled point:	KID-6 *Zhaohai*	Needle left side for women, right side for men

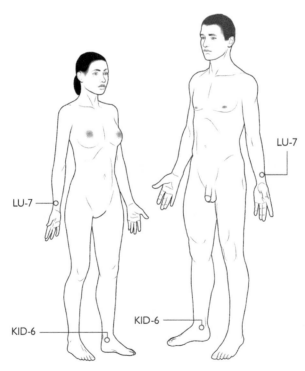

FIGURE 5.6: OPENING AND COUPLED POINTS OF THE DIRECTING VESSEL (GENDER-BASED)

Why do we use it?

The Directing Vessel is the extraordinary vessel I draw on most for working with cancer survivors. Of its many functions, I use it primarily for the purposes set out below.

Nourish yin

The Directing Vessel, also known as the Sea of the Yin channel, helps regulate the qi of all the yin channels.[16] As such, it can be used to nourish yin, especially for menopausal and post-menopausal women, when it can be used to tonify Blood and yin and reduce empty heat symptoms from yin deficiency.

This makes it useful for addressing hot flushes, night sweats, feelings of heat, dry mouth at night, dizziness, and insomnia, symptoms associated with cancer treatment-related menopausal symptoms (and natural menopause). To address these, combine the opening and coupled points with REN-4 *Guanyuan* and SP-6 *Sanyinjiao* (Table 5.4).

Promote transformation, transportation, and excretion of fluids

The Directing Vessel functions to distribute fluids correctly in the abdomen, and for this reason Maciocia recommends it for treating oedema[14] and thus, lymphoedema. This may be most effective in early stages when lymphoedema is still an accumulation of protein-rich fluid and before tissue changes cause fibrosis and build-up of adipose tissue (see Chapter 9, Cancer Treatment-Related Lymphoedema).

To use, needle the opening and coupled points (observing the Notes above) and combine with points on the Directing Vessel that stimulate metabolism of fluids by the Triple Burner. These include:

- REN-17 *Shanzhong* to influence the upper burner
- REN-12 *Zhongwan*
- REN-9 *Shuifen* to influence the middle burner
- REN-5 *Shimen* to influence the lower burner.

When using these REN points, I may choose to use needles only, moxa only, or combine moxa and needling, depending on the aims for treatment for the individual.

Activate the Triple Burner

In addition to controlling the water passages and excretion of fluids, the Triple Burner controls the transportation and penetration of qi in all parts of the body.[14] These functions are closely intertwined – the Triple Burner ensures that fluids flow freely and correctly through the body. This is made possible by its control of the flow and penetration of qi, which essentially also controls the transformation and movement of fluids.

These functions may be integral in the management of lymphoedema. To enable this, the opening and coupled points are combined with points on the Directing Vessel as discussed above.

Working with the Yang Linking Vessel
What is it?

Opening point:	TB-5 *Waiguan*	Needle right side for women, left side for men
Coupled point:	GB-41 *Zulinqi*	Needle left side for women, right side for men

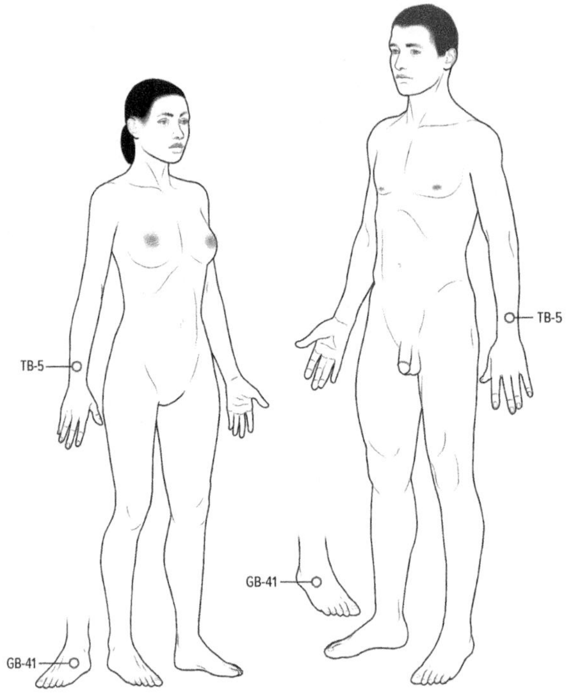

FIGURE 5.7: OPENING AND COUPLED POINTS OF THE YANG LINKING VESSEL (GENDER-BASED)

Why do we use it?

I also use the Yang Linking Vessel when working with cancer survivors, particularly those treated for head and neck cancers.

The Yang Linking Vessel connects all the yang channels and is said to dominate the exterior of the entire body.[14,16] Tracing a route along the lateral aspect of the body, it influences the leg, sides of the body, lateral aspect of neck and head, and the ears (Figure 5.8). It is used for symptoms such as pain in the lateral aspect of the leg and pain in the lateral side of the neck.

This makes it especially useful when addressing the consequences of head and neck surgery. These survivors may present with symptoms on the lateral leg from graft surgery, lateral neck and shoulder pain from interventions local to the tumour, and hearing and other ear problems resulting from radiotherapy.

To use, combine the opening and coupled points with points relevant to the patient's presentation.

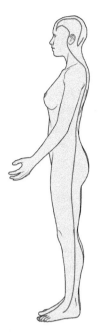

FIGURE 5.8: PATHWAY OF THE YANG LINKING VESSEL

VIGNETTE: JR AND THE YANG LINKING VESSEL

Background

JR, aged 65, completed treatment for cancer of the right tonsil (surgery, chemotherapy, and radiotherapy) 16 months prior to joining a study of using acupuncture to improve wellbeing for people with cancer treatment-related lymphoedema (see Chapter 9, Cancer Treatment-Related Lymphoedema).

His main complaints were pain in the right neck and shoulder and an awful taste in the mouth. On the study questionnaire – the Measure Yourself Medical Outcome Profile (MYMOP) – he rated these as 5/6 and 6/6 points respectively on a 7-point scale where '0' is as good as it can be and '6' is as bad as it can be. Doing daily exercises using his right arm was the activity he wished to be able to do, and which he rated at 5/6. He was taking codeine and ibuprofen daily every four hours to manage the pain.

Initial progress through treatment

JR attended for 13 acupuncture treatments over three months. At his first treatment, I administered an AE Drain, and I cleared Internal Dragons at the second.

The remaining 11 treatments were all built on the foundation of opening the Yang Linking Vessel to help relieve the pain and stiffness in the shoulder and side of his neck. For treatments 3–7, I opened the Yang Linking Vessel, and then focused on:

- addressing the bad taste in his mouth by resolving phlegm (ST-40 *Fenglong*)
- clearing the sinuses (LI-4 *Hegu*, LI-20 *Yingxiang*, M-HN-3 *Yintang*)
- regulating the fluids in the mouth (REN-24 *Chengjiang*).

I also treated his CF, which I assessed as fire, mostly using the yuan source points of the Heart and Small Intestine channels (HE-7 *Shenmen* and SI-4 *Wangu*).

At the end of these seven treatments, JR reported alleviation of the pain in his shoulder and neck, to the extent that he had not taken any pain medication during the previous two weeks. The bad taste had improved, and he was comfortable with it, changing his desired treatment outcome to improving discomfort behind the ear and along the jawline.

Continued progress
Over the next six treatments, I began each treatment by opening the Yang Linking Vessel, as this runs through the area that was troubling JR. I supplemented this with local points for the shoulder. As this was a study in which needling the affected side was contraindicated, I needled points on the opposite side (e.g. GB-21 *Jianjing*, TB-15 *Tianliao*, SI-10 *Naoshu*, SI-11 *Tianzong*, SI-12 *Bingfeng*, and M-BW-35 *Huatuojiaji* points). However, I used stick moxa on the affected side to relieve the stiffness and discomfort in the shoulder and neck. At his ninth treatment, JR said his right arm was 'working like magic'.

Short- and long-term feedback
At the end of 13 treatments, JR's scores showed noticeable reductions. He rated his symptoms and activity at 2/6, a reduction from the 5/6 and 6/6 at the beginning of treatment. He reported reduction in pain and improvements in overall quality of life, as well as being able to do his daily exercises. Writing at the end of treatment he said:

> I found it [acupuncture] gave me more energy at the beginning of the week but by the end I felt I needed topping up. It also made me more relax [sic] to do my exercises, and more freedom of arm and shoulder movement. I felt that every time I came each week I felt better. It's been a great improvement in my life and wellbeing.

Participating in a research-related activity some months later, JR expressed how he felt about having acupuncture:

> Well I looked forward to going to acupuncture. I mean, most things you have to go through I don't look forward to going to! I've got to go in tomorrow, with a camera down the throat, I'm not looking forward to that, but with the acupuncture I felt better every time I went, so…oh yeah! I felt better going and even better when I left.

His long-term feedback suggests continuation of treatment would have been beneficial:

> Yes, as I said, when I was having acupuncture, I could move my arm and my shoulders, and then when it seized up again I had to go back to the tablets to be able to do it…it gradually wore away.[2]

Summary
It is challenging to assess the effects of specific acupuncture points when used in combinations of multiple points. However, the Yang Linking Vessel may have played an important

role in JR's progress. This is supported by the improvements in the first phase of treatment, as during this time, I used only the two points of the Yang Linking Vessel to address the shoulder and neck problems and I focused on treating the foul taste. Nevertheless, he reported great improvements in the shoulder and arm movement and reduction of pain, to the extent that he greatly reduced his pain medication. An important feature of JR's long-term feedback highlights the need for ongoing treatment for these chronic conditions.

A protocol for addressing cancer treatment-related hot flushes and night sweats

I developed this approach when designing research into using traditional acupuncture to manage breast cancer treatment-related HFNS for women taking tamoxifen (discussed in Chapter 8, Cancer Treatment-Related Hot Flushes and Night Sweats).[17]

Table 5.4: A protocol for addressing HFNS

Treatment principles	Points	Method Insert all needles using even technique and obtain deqi. All points are used unilaterally, avoiding needling on the arm on the side of the affected breast.
Nourish Kidney yin	Open the Directing Vessel: LU-7 *Lieque* KID- 6 *Zhaohai*	To open the Directing Vessel: Insert needle into LU-7 first (on the side not affected by breast cancer) then KID-6 on the opposite side. Retain for at least 20 minutes.
	REN-4 *Guanyuan* SP-6 *Sanyinjiao*	Once LU-7 and KID-6 are inserted, needle the remaining points. Do not manipulate the needles. After the 20 minutes, remove all needles. KID-6 is penultimate needle removed, and LU-7 the last.
Stop night sweats	HE-6 *Yinxi* KID-7 *Fuliu*	
Clear heat	LI-11 *Quchi*	
Resolve damp*	SP-6 *Sanyinjiao* LU-7 *Lieque*** LI-11 *Quchi*	

*This illustrates drawing on the multiple functions of a point to address multiple conditions. For example, SP-6 *Sanyinjiao* functions to both nourish Kidney yin and resolve damp.
**As a function of regulating the water passages.

The protocol (Table 5.4 and Figure 5.9) assumes Kidney yin deficiency as the root of hot flushes and incorporates strategies for managing night sweats and for clearing heat and damp, which colleagues I consulted at the time observed to be associated with tamoxifen.[17]

It is built on the foundation of opening the extraordinary vessel, the Directing Vessel, as discussed above. I adapt the gender-based approach to needling to take account of limbs with or at risk of lymphoedema. Thus, if it is not possible to use a point because of lymphoedema-related contraindications, I reverse the points as necessary, needling LU-7 on the left and KID-6 on the right for women (or LU-7 on the right and KID-6 on the left for the rarer instances of male breast cancer) (see Chapter 9, Cancer Treatment-Related Lymphoedema).

In the study, the first treatment was an Aggressive Energy Drain; in the remaining seven treatments of the study, I supplemented the 'core protocol' (Table 5.4) with 'points for the patient' to provide semi-individualised treatment. In routine clinical practice, I also adapt this core protocol as appropriate, adding points for the patient or reducing the number of points for patients who are sensitive to needling.

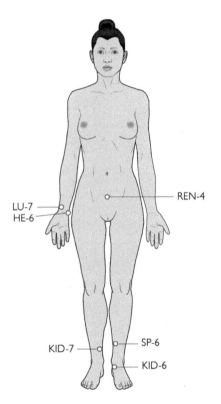

FIGURE 5.9: A PROTOCOL FOR ADDRESSING HFNS

Protocol for addressing cancer treatment-related lymphoedema

This protocol (Table 5.5 and Figure 5.10) is adapted from Maciocia's protocol for oedema.[14] I have used it clinically, but not extensively under research conditions.[9] However, my observation and patient feedback suggest beneficial effects as evidenced by the case study of Ann (see Chapter 14).

Table 5.5: A protocol for addressing cancer treatment-related lymphoedema

Treatment principles	Points	Method
		Insert all needles using even technique and obtain deqi. All points are used unilaterally, avoiding needling on the limb affected by or at risk of lymphoedema.
Promote transformation, transportation, and excretion of fluids	Open the Directing Vessel: LU-7 *Lieque* KID- 6 *Zhaohai*	To open the Directing Vessel: Insert needle into LU-7 *Lieque* first (avoiding the side affected by lymphoedema) then KID-6 *Zhaohai* on the opposite side. Retain for at least 20 minutes. Once LU-7 *Lieque* and KID-6 *Zhaohai* are inserted, needle the remaining points. Do not manipulate the needles. After the 20 minutes, remove all needles. KID-6 is penultimate needle removed, and LU-7 the last.
Stimulate the metabolism of fluids by the Triple Burner	REN-17 *Shanzhong*[*] REN-12 *Zhongwan*[**] REN-9 *Shuifen*[**] REN-5 *Shimen*[***]	When designing a treatment for a particular patient: • I choose from the points in these two sections, taking account of the location of the swelling as well as the patient's other presenting conditions. • I then select the point(s) that will address these best. I would not use all these points but would select those that would give me the widest and most appropriate treatment effect within the context of the individual patient. • I also select one point on the Triple Burner itself, from those listed.
Activate the Triple Burner. The main points to activate the Triple Burner are on the Directing (Ren) channel, rather than on the TB channel; however, points on the TB channel can also be used	REN-17 *Shanzhong*[*] REN-12 *Zhongwan*[**] REN-9 *Shuifen*[**] REN-6 *Qihai*[***] REN-5 *Shimen*[***] REN-3 *Zhongji*[***] TB-4 *Yangchi* TB-5 *Waiguan* TB-6 *Zhigou*	

[*] These points act on the upper burner.

[**] These points act on the middle burner.

[***] These points act on the lower burner.

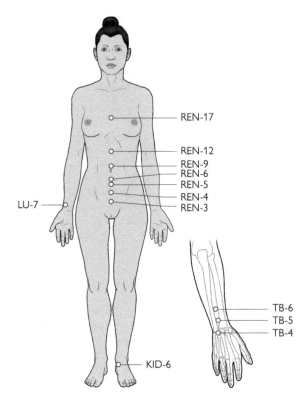

FIGURE 5.10: A PROTOCOL FOR ADDRESSING CANCER TREATMENT-RELATED LYMPHOEDEMA

Using microsystems

Microsystems can be invaluable when working with cancer survivors. Like distal points, they can be used to treat an area of the body that may not be accessible to local body acupuncture.

Microsystems are based on the idea of a *somatotopy*, that is, the projection of the whole of the body in a particular part of the body. This idea underpins many micro-systems used within acupuncture, examples of which include:

- auriculotherapy
- scalp acupuncture
- Korean hand therapy
- wrist, ankle, or tongue acupuncture.

These concepts are found in other systems of diagnosis and treatment, such as reflex-ology and iridology.

My preferred microsystem when working with cancer survivors is ear acupuncture or auriculotherapy, a therapeutic intervention using stimulation of the external ear to alleviate health problems elsewhere the body.[18] It is based on the concept that for every part of the body, there is a corresponding reflex point on the external ear that can be used for both diagnosis and treatment.[19] The reflex point, which is an area rather than a precise point, can be stimulated in a range of ways including needles, electrostimulation, press needles, ear seeds, and magnets. Ear acupuncture can be used on its own as a form of treatment or combined with body acupuncture.

The tools discussed below can easily be incorporated into the practitioner's toolkit. For a full understanding of auriculotherapy (or other microsystems), training and access to the many excellent books available are recommended.

The NADA protocol
What is it?
The NADA protocol uses five points on the surface of the ear. Developed in the 1970s by the National Acupuncture Detoxification Association (NADA) for use in substance detoxification, it is now used for a variety of conditions in healthcare settings around the world, as well as for major emergencies where trauma and post-traumatic stress disorder are present.[20] Anecdotal evidence that NADA relieved HFNS accompanying substance detoxification led to my investigation of its usefulness in managing cancer treatment-related vasomotor symptoms.[21]

Why use it?
The NADA protocol is useful in institutional settings, especially where cost of service delivery is a consideration. Its many distinctive features include these advantages:

- No diagnosis is required.
- It is quick and easy to administer.
- There is no need for patients to remove clothing, thus minimising problems for patients with body image issues. It is also useful in clinics where privacy may not be possible.
- Working with the ears avoids the issues of contraindications to needling areas of the body with or at risk of lymphoedema.
- It can be delivered in a group setting, with the potential for one practitioner to treat up to 20 patients in an hour and a half.[22]

In some countries or regions, non-acupuncturists can be trained as NADA specialists to deliver it (practitioners are advised to check their local or national regulations regarding acupuncture practice).

NADA has been researched for managing cancer treatment-related HFNS in breast and prostate cancer patients[23,24] (see Chapter 8 Cancer Treatment-Related Hot Flushes and Night Sweats, and Stan's vignette below).

ESSENTIALS

The spirit of NADA

When using NADA, one should be aware of the 'spirit of NADA', its underpinning philosophy. Dr Michael Smith, the main pioneer of this treatment, emphasised that NADA 'creates a zone of peace within so patients can begin to experience their own inner strengths'.[25] To this end, he discouraged mapping the earpoints to their functions, and encouraged explaining them in terms of what they give the recipient: 'serenity, patience, wisdom, courage and acceptance'.[26]

NADA enables the patient to feel safe, to open to themselves, and to allow healing to take place in the person's own time and space, to recover their essential self. As we shall see, this treatment can play a vital role in supporting cancer survivors.

How do we do NADA treatment?

The patient may be sitting or lying down. Needles are inserted into the five auricular acupuncture points specified for each ear (Table 5.6 and Figure 5.11). Insertion should use a rapid, single-handed motion with 180° rotation, to a shallow depth that supports the needle tip in the cartilage. No further stimulation is required. The needles are retained for 30–40 minutes.

Special detox acupuncture needles are recommended. These are single-use, sterile, stainless steel 0.20mm diameter and 7mm long; those with brightly coloured plastic handles are preferred for group delivery for ease of finding if needles fall from the ears.

The ears points are slightly more prone to bleeding than body points when the needles are removed, so guidelines for dealing with and disposing of blood should be followed.

Table 5.6: NADA protocol points

Left ear	Right ear
Auricular Sympathetic	Auricular Sympathetic
Shenmen	*Shenmen*
Kidney	Kidney
Liver	Liver
Lower Lung	Upper Lung

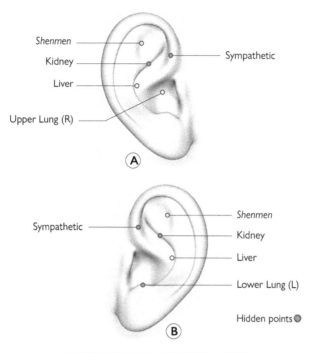

FIGURE 5.11: NADA PROTOCOL POINTS

Notes on group treatment

NADA was designed to be given in a group setting. Feeling isolated is a known consequence of cancer survivorship, thus the group setting can be helpful for survivors. In the cancer centre where I work, many of the individuals attending for NADA treatment formed strong social bonds. One group of prostate cancer survivors actively used their NADA morning as a social event, arranging to have cakes and tea together after treatment.

May's vignette (below) illustrates how this group setting can also be helpful for individuals who feel they are the only person experiencing symptoms.

VIGNETTE: MAY AND THE BENEFITS OF THE NADA GROUP SETTING

May, a breast cancer survivor, found the group setting the most beneficial aspect of her eight-week course of NADA treatments. These helped her realise she wasn't the only woman experiencing frequent and distressing HFNS.

At her four-week follow-up after NADA treatment ended, she wrote 'It was helpful to meet other women with similarly severe symptoms.' Until attending for NADA sessions, she felt 'isolated' and 'alone', saying she was 'totally unprepared for the huge and unpleasant side effects tamoxifen has had on me'.

At her 18-week follow-up, she said that prior to the NADA treatment, she felt 'isolated and that nobody cared. I don't feel like that now.'[26]

Being in a group with others having similar experiences can be beneficial in helping survivors to come to terms with the new normal. However, it is astute to be aware that sometimes it can be unhelpful.

On occasion, I have observed groups where there has been a disruptive element – a survivor who feels a need to play to an audience, or who spreads erroneous, frightening information about cancer. This can be managed by encouraging the groups to enjoy NADA treatment in silence.

It is also particularly difficult for a group if one of their members has a cancer recurrence, a situation which may occur and is unavoidable. Finally, June's vignette illustrates how, for some, the idea of group treatment is simply overwhelming.

VIGNETTE: JUNE AND AN AVERSION TO GROUP TREATMENT

June read and understood that NADA treatment would be delivered in a group when she joined a study of NADA for breast cancer treatment-related HFNS. However, at her first treatment she declared she would not participate if she had to be in a group. I offered to treat her separately if a treatment room was available.

At her third treatment, June reported she had discovered a new lump and broke down completely. She was so distressed, I called in a nurse for assistance. The nurse gave June information about any potential lump, assessed her to make sure she was not a danger to herself, and organised an emergency appointment with the psychiatrist. I treated June using earpoints *Shenmen* and Kidney, making sure she could get home after this dramatic episode.

I was surprised that June attended for her next (fourth) treatment. In fact, she was now feeling much better – she had confirmation that the lump was not a recurrence, her HFNS were reducing and her sleep improving. She was reluctant to take the venlafaxine prescribed by the psychiatrist. Over the next two weeks, her symptoms continued to improve, and she also asked to join the group for treatment!

June continued to do well, and when her NADA treatment ended, she chose to have acupuncture treatment regularly to 'continue to recover health and energy'.[26]

Tips from my clinical experience

- As well as using NADA in group settings, I use it when treating patients individually. Then, I may use it on its own or in combination with body acupuncture.
- For breast cancer survivors with bilateral risk of lymphoedema, I often combine NADA points with points on the lower body.
- NADA is especially useful when patients experience extreme anxiety or agitation,

as it calms and grounds strong emotions. In such circumstances, I may use it on its own or in combination with body points.

- NADA is very flexible. Although the protocol is five points in each ear, it is easily adapted to an individual's needs and tolerance. Depending on the patient, I might needle five points in one ear only, or I might needle *Shenmen* only.
- Patients may notice changes immediately during or after treatment, or it may take several treatments before benefits become apparent.
- Ear seeds or magnets can be applied to the earpoints in addition to or instead of needles. I offer this to patients for continued stimulation of the points as a means of symptom control between acupuncture treatments. My favourite point for this is *Reverse Shenmen*, discussed below.

VIGNETTE: STAN AND USING NADA TO IMPROVE WELLBEING FOR PROSTATE CANCER SURVIVORS[27]

Prostate cancer history

Stan, aged 74, was a retired businessman, diagnosed with early stage prostate cancer 11 years before having NADA treatment. Initial cancer treatment included external beam radiotherapy and low-dose brachytherapy, followed by a three-year course of the pituitary down-regulator goserelin (Zoladex®). Later, rising PSA levels led to further Zoladex® treatment, later changed to three-monthly injections of triptorelin (Decapeptyl IM®). While this successfully controlled the prostate cancer, he was troubled by many consequences of cancer treatment.

General health history

Stan was referred to the NADA prostate service by the urology research nurse. His main troublesome symptoms were HFNS and hip pain.

He experienced six to seven daytime flushes, and three night sweats interrupted his sleep. These incidents were accompanied by anxiety, a tingling sensation, and cold shivering. Constant pain in his hips, diagnosed as osteoarthritis, was managed with tramadol hydrochloride and ibuprofen. Nausea, a side effect of this medication, was controlled with prochlorperazine maleate.

Bladder frequency and urgency meant Stan urinated six to seven times during the day, and that many times again during the night. Oxybutynin was helpful in managing this. Constipation was a long-term issue, although he was managing some movement once a day. In addition, erectile dysfunction was a consequence he had come to terms with, especially as the cancer treatment appeared to be working. Comorbidities included asthma and allergies to certain medications and foods.

Progress through treatment

Stan did not report significant changes until his fourth NADA treatment, when HFNS reduced in frequency and the accompanying sensations started to change: 'tingles' disappeared, flushes were now a 'slow hotness', and he had more bladder control. Mood and energy levels were 'very good'; he felt more relaxed and clear-minded. His wife remarked that Stan was more focused and positive.

At his fifth treatment, he reported further improvements in HFNS, good energy levels, and 'very much improved' bladder function, with only one to two incidents at night. Symptoms continued to improve and at his eighth and final treatment, Stan summarised the benefits he experienced. HFNS were now moderate and no longer accompanied by anxiety. Bladder urgency had disappeared, and he no longer needed to use Senokot® to encourage bowel movements. Sleep was better and he could easily get back to sleep if wakened by a flush. Hip pain was 'reduced by 80%'; he was no longer taking tramadol or ibuprofen.

Long-term feedback
At his 18-week follow-up, Stan wrote:

> I feel much more relaxed and not much anxiety and stress pre and post hot flush. Still have hot flushes but without attending embarrassment. Acupuncture was [a] great experience – emotionally and psychologically.

Summary
Stan provides a study of a survivor who has survived his diagnosis by over ten years, and whose presentation is complicated by comorbidities, the problems of ageing, and the cocktail of medications prescribed to manage these health issues. NADA treatment appears to have been beneficial for addressing the consequences of cancer treatment (hormone therapy-related HFNS), as well as symptoms of ageing (osteoarthritis). It may be that bowel performance improved because Stan was able to reduce the pain medication, of which constipation is a side effect.

This study illustrates the potential benefits of NADA for emotional, as well as physical, wellbeing. It also demonstrates the power of a relatively simple form of acupuncture treatment to impact a wide range of health issues.

Shenmen and Reverse Shenmen
As an adjunct to treatment, I offer patients seeds, beads, or magnets on earpoints. While I might use some or all the points of a treatment protocol, I usually use a single earpoint.

My favourite point to use is *Reverse Shenmen*, used widely by NADA specialists especially to address trauma-related issues.[28] Its location on the back of the external ear gives it the advantage of being virtually invisible to others. This may be less irritating when sleeping or using phones than points on the front of the ear. I use it primarily as a support tool for patients to self-manage between treatments.

The location
To find *Reverse Shenmen*, first locate earpoint *Shenmen* in the triangular depression at the top of the ear. Place a thumb on *Shenmen* and a forefinger on the back of the ear opposite

your thumb. This position on the back of the ear is *Reverse Shenmen* (Figure 5.12). Veins or colour changes may also indicate the location of this point.

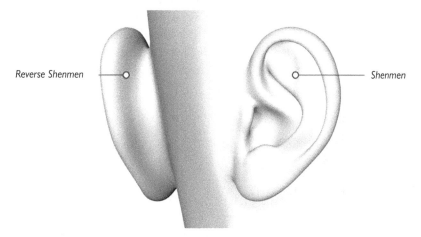

Reverse Shenmen   Shenmen

FIGURE 5.12: *REVERSE SHENMEN* AND *SHENMEN*

The materials
A variety of options are suitable, including vaccaria seeds, gold magnetic beads, or tourmaline ear stones. These are secured to the ear using a small piece of tape.

The method
Clean the area with a disinfectant wipe to improve the adherence of the tape. Position the seed/bead/stone over the point; press lightly to secure the tape.

The recipient can be instructed to:

- press the seed gently as needed or leave it in place without touching
- leave the seed/bead/stone in place until it falls off (can be a week or longer) or they can remove and discard it.

Cautions

- Occasionally, there may be an allergic reaction to the tape, in which case a different type of tape should be tried. Alauda could not tolerate the tape on the ear seeds I usually use; we found she could tolerate the tape on tourmaline ear stones (see Alauda's case study in Chapter 8, Cancer Treatment-Related Hot Flushes and Night Sweats).
- Remove the seed/bead/stone if it irritates the ear.
- Patients may need reassurance that the bead/seed/stone will not fall into their inner ear.

Four Gates and Three Gates
What is it?

I often use Four Gates, bilateral LIV-3 *Taichong* and LI-4 *Hegu* (Figure 5.13), as a first treatment. It introduces patients who have never had acupuncture to needle sensation, giving them a good sense of what treatment feels like. From my perspective, is easy to obtain needle sensation and the combination gives me valuable information about the patient's response to acupuncture, both during and following the session.

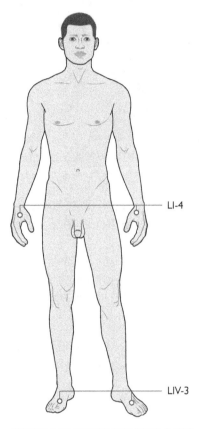

LI-4

LIV-3

FIGURE 5.13: POINTS FOR FOUR GATES

Why use it?

For the patient, and especially for acupuncture-naive patients, it can be relaxing. It is also indicated for anxiety and LIV-3 *Taichong*, the main point on the Liver channel to calm the mind, combines well with the strong calming effect of LI-4 *Hegu*, which soothes the mind and allays anxiety.[29]

VIGNETTE: DEE AND USING FOUR GATES TO OVERCOME FEAR AND ANXIETY[30]

Dee, aged 57, was a colorectal cancer survivor referred to the hospital outpatient acupuncture service by her oncologist for 'a number of vague symptoms including anxiety, poor sleep, and abdominal discomfort'. At her first appointment, Dee was positive and forthcoming; however, her anxiety about having acupuncture was apparent. She especially feared needles. My priority at that treatment was to have her experience needling so she could decide whether to continue treatment.

I chose Four Gates for its relaxing and calming effects. It had the desired effect. On inserting the first needle (LI-4 *Hegu* in her left hand), Dee visibly relaxed. After I inserted all four needles, she said she was experiencing a 'floating sensation' that was pleasant and relaxing. She chose to continue treatment.

Simple and elegant, Four Gates has wide-ranging effects that may be appropriate for patients presenting with complex symptom patterns including pain, anxiety, HFNS, and bowel disorders. On an emotional level, Four Gates soothes the mind, calms anxiety, and addresses general nervous tension.[15] It can support the process of 'letting go' and is indicated for deep frustration and suppressed anger.[3] I often add extra point M-HN-3 *Yintang*, for its potential to calm the mind, alleviate anxiety, and promote sleep in insomnia.[15]

If the patient experiences strong beneficial effects from this treatment, it may remain the basis of the treatment I use. I add points to it gradually, tailoring it to the individual's needs and responses, as illustrated by Rosa's vignette.

VIGNETTE: ROSA AND USING FOUR GATES TO ADDRESS COMPLEX PHYSICAL AND EMOTIONAL SYMPTOMS[12]

We met Rosa, aged 63, in Chapter 4. Surgery for Stage II sigmoid colorectal cancer nearly two years previously left her with 'increasing problems with her bowels', and her consultant referred Rosa to the hospital outpatient acupuncture clinic. Presenting with complex physical and emotional symptoms, Rosa's priorities for acupuncture treatment were to improve bowel movements (constipation) and relieve anxiety.

Four Gates was an elegant way to address Rosa's priorities, as it is effective for both constipation and anxiety. The strong downward movement of LI-4 *Hegu* acts to move the stools and LIV-3 *Taichong* is indicated for constipation when 'failure of qi to flow freely binds the stool'.[16] The synergistic action of the two points enhances the power of LI-4 *Hegu* to soothe the mind and calm anxiety and LIV-3 *Taichong* to address general nervous tension from stress.[15]

Four Gates also was indicated for several other of Rosa's symptoms, relieving the abdominal pain and spasm[16] she was experiencing while also addressing the complex emotions relating to her cancer experience. For this, LI-4 *Hegu* supports the process of 'letting go' while LIV-3 *Taichong* is indicated for deep frustration and suppressed anger.[3]

Four Gates was the foundation for Rosa's treatment. I gradually supplemented it with additional points that supported my treatment principles (such as ST-25 *Tianshu*,

SP-15 *Daheng*, ST-37 *Shangjuxu* to regulate the bowels and HE-7 *Shenmen*, P-3 *Quze*, and extra point M-HN-3 *Yintang* to regulate and calm the spirit). At her eighth treatment, Rosa said her bowel performance was 'as good as it could be' and reported that her anxiety had reduced.

Adapting Four Gates – 'Three Gates'

I adapt Four Gates for cancer patients with or at risk of lymphoedema, avoiding needling in the affected or 'at-risk' limb, thus making it 'Three Gates'. Obviously, this is not suitable for patients who have, or are at risk of, bilateral lymphoedema, for whom other approaches may be found (see Chapter 9, Cancer Treatment-Related Lymphoedema).

Shen disturbance, Mind Unsettled and Unsettled Ethereal and Corporeal Soul

Cancer survivors often present with restlessness, insomnia, irritability, anxiety, and poor memory. These signs correspond to shen disturbance, or Mind Unsettled (anxiety, mental restlessness, insomnia, and agitation) accompanied by Unsettled Ethereal Soul (nightmares, irritability, and absent-mindedness). Unsettled Corporeal Soul may also be present, manifesting with anxiety with breathlessness and a feeling of tightness of the chest, worrying a lot, and somatisation of the emotions on the skin (e.g. itchy rashes).[29]

While these symptoms often accompany HFNS, they are experienced by many cancer survivors. I address these either by focusing solely on the disharmony or addressing it as part of the overall treatment strategy. To calm the shen, I select points on the Pericardium and Heart channels, favouring:

- HE-7 *Shenmen*, P-3 *Quze*, P-6 *Neiguan*, P-7 *Daling*
- the associated back shu points, BL-14 *Jueyinshu*, BL-15 *Xinshu*
- the associated front mu points, REN-17 *Shanzhong*, REN-14 *Juque*
- associated points from the outer Bladder line, BL-43 *Gaohuangshu*, BL-44 *Shentang*.

There are many others to choose from.

For patients presenting with dream-disturbed sleep, Pericardium points are useful, especially REN-15 *Jiuwei* in combination with moxa on REN-17 *Shanzhong*. When dreams are distressing or develop into nightmares, I consider:

- clearing Internal (or External) Dragons (see Possession above)
- using moxa on BL43 *Gaohuanshgu* and Ren17 *Shanzhong* (see 'Toasted Pericardium Sandwich' below).

Moxibustion (moxa)
Why do I use it?
I use moxa for many purposes, including to:

- nourish Blood and qi
- warm yang
- nourish yin
- nourish the body fluids.

Another reason to use moxa is to engender a state of deep relaxation for the patient. Many people enjoy moxa, taking pleasure in both the aroma and warmth. In such cases, I may use it liberally.

When using moxa, I am guided by the patient's responses, including whether they like the treatment, whether it facilitates a state of deep relaxation, and providing it does not exacerbate any symptoms, such as HFNS. I don't use it for patients who are sensitive to the smell or to smoke, or those who are sceptical or fearful about the process.

For patients who are sensitive to, or actively dislike, needling, moxa can be a useful alternative. In such cases, I substitute moxibustion partially or wholly for needling (see Claire's case study in Chapter 11, Survivorship: Navigating the Milestones).

How do I use it?
I draw on a range of methods for applying moxa, including:

- indirect stick moxa (using either herb or compressed smokeless moxa sticks)
- moxa on the needle (warm needle)
- direct moxa using cones of moxa punk
- electronic moxa device (e.g. Premio-10 moxa pen).

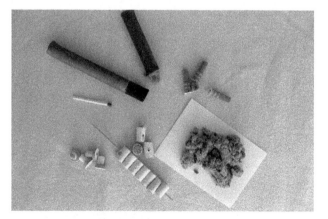

FIGURE 5.14: VARIOUS STYLES OF MOXA

Both context and patient preference influence the type of moxa I choose. I happily use smokeless moxa in clinics fitted with smoke alarms and when patients dislike or are sensitive to moxa smoke. I do not use techniques that burn or scar the skin; these methods might be difficult to use in some institutional settings or for some patients.

Introducing moxa into institutional settings can be challenging – its aroma may be unacceptable and there are considerable safety issues. This is the case in medical settings, where flammable materials such as medical gases may be present in the treatment room. Patients on oxygen should not use moxa in proximity to the oxygen source. In addition, cancer survivors who have a breathing stoma may experience irritation from smokeless moxa as well as moxa smoke.[9]

Explaining the concept of moxa to non-acupuncturists can be challenging, especially to medical professionals. However, in situations where it is possible to use moxa, it can have many applications for cancer survivors including the management of HFNS. Of the many possible ways to use moxa, three that I find particularly useful are discussed below.

Treating the spirit
Using moxa on the spirit points is discussed earlier.

'Toasted Pericardium Sandwich'
This is helpful for anxious patients, and I also include it in strategies to manage HFNS. I have nicknamed it the 'Toasted Pericardium Sandwich' as it uses moxa on points on the posterior and anterior of the body at the level of the pericardium (Figure 5.15). I apply moxa cones (and do not needle) to:

- BL-43 *Gaohuangshu* (usually 15 cones, bilateral)
- REN-17 *Shanzhong* (three to five cones).

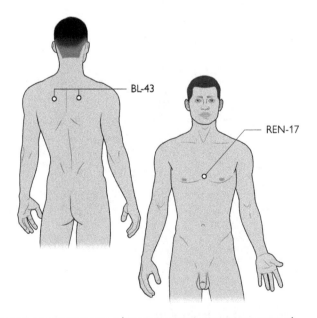

FIGURE 5.15: POINTS FOR A 'TOASTED PERICARDIUM SANDWICH'

According to several classical texts, BL-43 and Ren-17 are contraindicated to needling and I choose to follow these recommendations in clinical practice.[16]

On completing the moxa, I ask the patient to take three deep slow breaths in their own time, focusing on the warmth generated by the treatment. Many patients find this deeply relaxing. I discovered its usefulness for anxiety and dream-disturbed sleep when working with Rose (see Chapter 11, Survivorship: Navigating the Milestones).

I also like the elegance of using the deep nourishing properties of BL-43 *Gaohuangshu* when working with cancer survivors. Indicated for all kinds of deficiency, including that of the Lung, Heart, Kidney, Spleen, and Stomach, its tonifying effect is said to 'strengthen the original qi and treat every kind of deficiency'.[16] It nourishes and calms the Heart, improving poor memory and insomnia, nourishes yin, and is indicated for spontaneous sweating – all symptoms commonly associated with shen disturbance and frequently reported by survivors experiencing cancer treatment-related HFNS.

Classical texts favoured treating BL-43 *Gaohuangshu* using moxa, often in large amounts (300 cones), following this with moxa on points below the umbilicus to draw the heat downwards.[16] However, my clinical experience suggests this last stage may not be necessary.

Combining BL-43 *Gaohuangshu* with REN-17 *Shanzhong,* the front mu point of the Pericardium, functions to enhance the therapeutic effects and is especially helpful for calming the shen. In addition, the 'Toasted Pericardium Sandwich' helps to open the chest, useful for patients who may be grieving or for those who present with signs of constriction in the upper jiao.

Moxa on ST-36 Zusanli

ST-36 *Zusanli* has been used for centuries in East Asian medicine for strengthening the body, improving health, and supporting the immune system. Qin Cheng-Zu (Song dynasty) stated that 'all diseases can be treated' using this point, and Sun Si-miao advised using regular moxibustion on ST-36 to preserve and maintain health.[16] In modern clinical use and in research, it is the most commonly used acupuncture point for immune strengthening and regulation.[31–33]

Teaching patients to self-moxa

ST-36 *Zusanli* also has the advantage that it can be accessed easily by the patient (Figure 5.16). Thus, patients can be taught to self-moxa ST-36, to:

- tonify qi and Blood
- calm the spirit
- address emotional disorders that have their roots in Heart Blood deficiency.[16]

When teaching patients to self-moxa, I demonstrate the technique to them, including how to light and safely extinguish the moxa. I then have them demonstrate those techniques to me to ensure they have understood the procedure. At the next appointment, I follow up to answer any questions arising and to confirm that they are administering the moxa safely and correctly.

I recommend the amount of time to apply the moxa on each point – usually three to five minutes per side. I also allow patients to sample smokeless or herbal moxa so they can choose which they prefer to use. Issues to consider include whether they are likely to set off a smoke alarm, and the aroma they (and their cohabitees) prefer.

I also give written instructions, shown below.

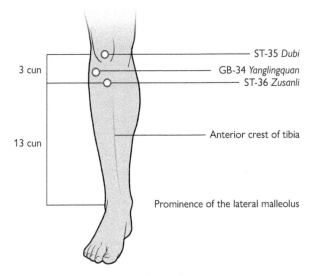

FIGURE 5.16: ST-36 *ZUSANLI*

ESSENTIALS

Information for patients: how to locate ST-36 *Zusanli*

Moxa is used over an acupuncture point on each leg, just below the knee (Figure 5.16). You will need to find these points. Make sure you have a marker pen ready.

To find this point, you will need to find your kneecap and shinbone. Your kneecap is a bone at the top of your knee. It is about two inches in diameter. Your shin bone is the long bone on the front of your leg below your knee.

To find the point on your right leg, use your right hand:

- Sit with your feet on the floor.
- Your kneecap is the area on your knee that sticks out. Feel down this to the place where it ends. This is the bottom of the kneecap and below it there is a slight indentation.
- Hold your four fingers firmly together and place your index finger horizontally across the bottom of your kneecap.
- Use your marker pen to make a small horizontal mark on your leg along the edge of where your little finger now sits.
- Use your index finger to run down the shinbone to the level you have just marked. Roll this finger to the right and use your marker pen to make a vertical line on your leg down the outside of your finger.

The point for your moxa treatment is where these two lines meet. Mark this point with your marker pen.

Repeat these steps to find the acupuncture point on your left leg, rolling your left finger to the left in the final step.

Remember the acupuncture point on each leg is on the same side as your little toe.

Many patients opt to have this point marked up for them in clinic, keeping it marked with a pen of their choosing. They may ask to have it checked at each appointment. Others, however, may feel confident to locate the point after one or two demonstrations.

To apply moxa to the point, I give the instructions below.

ESSENTIALS

Information for patients: how to moxa ST-36 *Zusanli*
Before using moxa, you will need to have the following items to hand:

- moxa stick
- moxa extinguisher
- moxa lighter
- timer.

Light one end of the moxa stick with the lighter. It may take a few seconds or a minute to build up a good heat. When the stick is correctly lit, you will be able to hold the lit end about 2–3cm from your hand. You will feel a pleasant radiating warmth. The moxa is ready to use.

Never allow there to be direct contact between your skin and the lit end of the moxa stick.

How to carry out the procedure
Find a space where you can be comfortable and will not be disturbed.

Locate the acupuncture point on each leg. You can mark these with your pen. The marks may remain visible for several days. You can refresh the marking with the pen at intervals to keep the marks visible.

Light the moxa stick. Test it, and when it is warm enough, set your timer for the time recommended by your practitioner. Then:

- hold the moxa stick over the mark on one leg – about 2–3cm away from your skin
- apply for the recommended time (use your timer for this).

Adjust the temperature:

- If it feels too hot, move the moxa stick further from your skin.
- If it feels too cool, move it closer to the skin.

Check that the moxa stick is giving off enough heat. If not, apply the lighter to it for a few seconds.

From time to time, brush off any ash that forms on the end of the stick. Do this by gently brushing the tip against the moxa extinguisher. This helps the moxa stick stay hot. The ash will drop into the bowl-shaped cup of the extinguisher. The sensation should always be one of a pleasant, radiating warmth.

After the recommended time, the skin should redden slightly. This redness will go away shortly after the treatment has finished.

Repeat this procedure on the other leg.

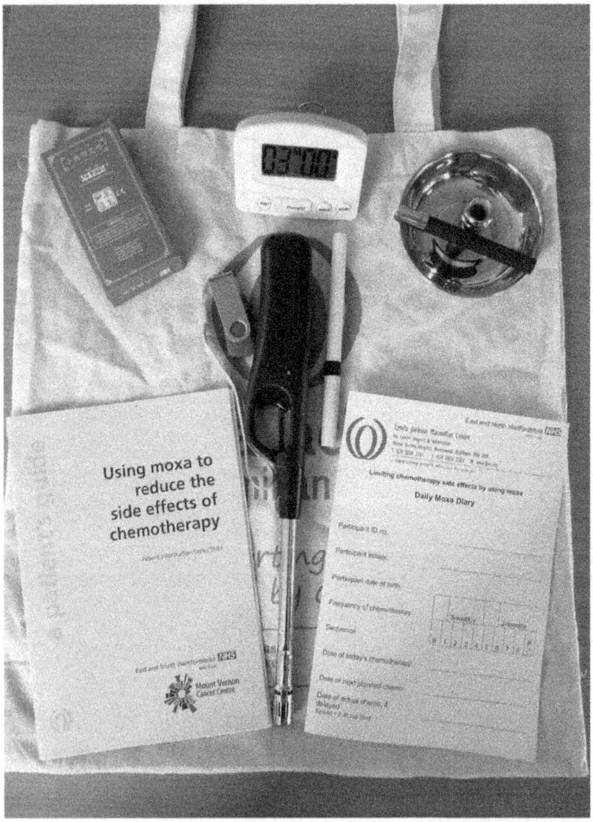

FIGURE 5.17: ITEMS IN A 'HOME' MOXA KIT. KIT CONTAINS (CLOCKWISE FROM TOP LEFT): MOXA, TIMER, MOXA EXTINGUISHER, MOXA DIARY, WRITTEN INSTRUCTIONS FOR USING MOXA, LIGHTER FOR MOXA (CENTRE)

These materials were produced for teaching chemotherapy patients to self-moxa ST-36.[*]

- Moxa leaflet: www.ljmc.org/pi_series/pi81_moxa.pdf

---

[*] A study using moxibustion to reduce side effects of chemotherapy; 2020. Available from: https://www.cancerresearchuk.org/about-cancer/find-a-clinical-trial/a-study-using-moxibustion-to-reduce-side-effects-of-chemotherapy

- Moxa video: www.youtube.com/watch?v=KKtTvHPGzyY

Exploring some myths about moxa and cancer treatment

In EAM, biomedical treatments for cancer are generally regarded as heating and the advice is to avoid using moxa. Similarly, the dominant association of menopausal and cancer treatment-related hot flushes with Kidney yin deficiency has led to moxibustion being widely contraindicated as a treatment approach (discussed in Chapter 8, Cancer Treatment-Related Hot Flushes and Night Sweats). In addition, a common perception is that moxibustion is indicated only for conditions of damp, cold, and yang deficiency.

A growing body of literature in the English language explores the use of moxa classical texts and descriptions of clinical practice and challenges these beliefs. In her book *Moxibustion: The Power of Mugwort Fire*, Lorraine Wilcox discusses the two historical opposing schools of thought about whether moxibustion can be used in heat patterns.[34] Among the many classical arguments on either side are the theories of Zhu Danxi (Yuan Dynasty) who 'perfected the theory that moxibustion can be used in heat patterns' and who developed a theory of using moxibustion to nourish yin by supplementing yang to generate yin.

Skya Abbate notes that moxibustion is used in Japanese acupuncture to tonify yin. She also describes instances in Chinese medicine where it is indicated for yin deficiency and quotes Chapter 73 of the *Ling Shu* (the *Spiritual Pivot*), which says 'deficiency of both *yin* and *yang* should be treated by *moxibustion*'.[35] Xiaorong *et al.* give guidance for the clinical application in menopausal syndrome, recommending gentle moxa on KID-3 *Taixi* and KID-2 *Rangu* (6–20 minutes each point daily, for ten treatments) for 'vexing heat in the chest, palms and soles'.[36]

My clinical observation of pale, swollen tongues in breast cancer survivors suggested to me that moxa was appropriate for managing HFNS for some patients. The positive response of the first patient with HFNS to whom I applied moxa encouraged me to continue to explore this approach. (I didn't sleep for a week after administering this for the first time; my patient, on the other hand, reported she had slept better than ever after the moxa treatment!)

Contemporary research in the West has also begun to use moxa in protocols for treating HFNS. Lesi *et al.* used moxibustion in addition to needling[37] (see Chapter 8, Cancer Treatment-Related Hot Flushes and Night Sweats), while Park *et al.* found moxibustion alone reduced frequency and severity of HFNS in women undergoing natural menopause.[38]

Prescription for rest

The balance between activity and rest is important for everyone; for cancer survivors, the impetus to get back to normal activities may mean they undervalue the importance of rest. I encourage my patients to take an afternoon rest, advising them as shown below.

ESSENTIALS

Prescription for rest

Each day (or as many days as possible), ideally between 1pm and 3pm:

- Lie down for 10–20 minutes.
- Close your eyes.
- Imagine you are recharging your batteries.
- You may or may not fall asleep, as you choose, or as you need to.
- Avoid reading or watching TV.
- Avoid feeling guilty!
- Do this as often as possible. If you miss a day or two, get back into the swing of it.

Notice how your energy changes when you adhere to this practice, and what happens on the days you miss.

Tips from my clinical experience

- I was taught the importance of rest in my acupuncture training; however, it was through my own experience of trauma and surgery that I learned the real value of this practice in aiding recovery, building strength, and overcoming consequences of illness. Patients who do this regularly soon notice they have more energy. In my work with patients experiencing HFNS, those who take a midday rest often report a reduction in flushing incidents.
- Some patients are resistant to the idea of resting or taking a nap during the day, equating it with laziness. I encourage them by emphasising that this is an activity that actively contributes to their recovery. I also encourage them to think about this as 'recharging their batteries'.

Getting active

Encouraging cancer survivors to be physically active is integral to their ongoing healthcare. Physical activity also contributes to managing many consequences of cancer treatment, as well as other chronic conditions (see Chapter 13, Reducing Risk of Recurrence and Subsequent Primary Cancers).

Using diaries

Having the patient keep a diary of their most troublesome symptom can be beneficial to both practitioner and patient. In research and clinical practice, I regularly use:

- the Hot Flush and Night Sweats Diary to monitor hot flushes and night sweats (see Appendices, online)
- the Bowel Diary to monitor bowel movements in the case of colorectal cancer

survivors (many examples are available online; search for Bowel Diary and/or Bristol Stool Scale).

In addition to benefits of keeping a Hot Flush and Night Sweats Diary (as discussed in Chapter 8, Cancer Treatment-Related Hot Flushes and Night Sweats), diaries can be useful for identifying sudden traumatic events that the patient might perceive to be unrelated to their symptom, or that they may not wish to disclose. Elizabeth's vignette (below) illustrates how changes recorded in her Bowel Diary* uncovered important information about stresses in her life.

Attitudes to keeping diaries

Patients have a variety of attitudes to keeping diaries. Elizabeth was a diligent diary keeper. For Alauda (see Alauda's case study in in Chapter 8, Cancer Treatment-Related Hot Flushes and Night Sweats), recording bordered on 'the obsessive' (her own description). She has kept her hot flush diary faithfully for years, lately using it mainly for her own information to monitor how her habit of 'burning the candle at both ends' affects her HFNS. Other patients may abandon keeping the diaries after an initial effort, either deciding they are too bothersome to keep, or that they only serve to emphasise their symptoms. While I do point out the potential value of keeping diaries, I never insist that patients keep them.

VIGNETTE: ELIZABETH AND BOWEL DIARIES

Background

Elizabeth, aged 50, was referred for acupuncture for 'pain and troublesome bowels'. Her oncologist thought pain in the back and groin were the consequence of chemoradiation to treat squamous cell cancer of the anal verge, diagnosed eight years previously.

Disabling pain restricted Elizabeth's activities and disrupted her sleep. She also experienced frequent, uncontrollable, and urgent bowel movements, reporting five to seven movements per day with frequent accidents, wind, and bloating. This seriously affected her quality of life; shopping and housework were challenging, and she was reluctant to leave the house for fear of embarrassing accidents.

Progress through treatment

Elizabeth attended for acupuncture weekly and was a dedicated keeper of the bowel diaries I gave her every week. One day she said, 'I think of you every time I have a bowel movement.' When I expressed surprise, she explained, 'I go to the toilet, I wash my hands, and I fill in my diary.'

Elizabeth's diaries were invaluable records of her progress, which seemed imperceptible. By referring to previous diaries, we could review the progress she was making. This reassured both of us. Eventually we reached a stage when her bowel movements became regular and predictable, and accidents became infrequent. Elizabeth regained her confidence and registered for a college course, a dream she had long cherished.

---

*   Many examples of bowel diaries are available online; search for Bowel Diary and/or Bristol Stool Scale.

The importance of the diaries in highlighting hidden factors

It was perplexing when she came for treatment one day and reported an unusual spike in bowel activity, increasing from an average of four per day to almost hourly over a period of three days. I asked my usual questions about changes in diet, activity, how she was feeling. However, she maintained that none of these things had changed. I puzzled over her diary, noting that her bowels had been performing regularly for a considerable period, and that this spike was most unusual.

Then it came tumbling out. Although I was aware of tensions at home, a significant crisis occurred with intense emotional fallout. This precipitated the severe increase in her bowel activity. Ashamed of this situation, Elizabeth had not revealed it to any of her healthcare professionals. Although we had established very good rapport over our many months of working together, I doubt Elizabeth would have revealed these circumstances if I hadn't puzzled over her diaries.

Summary

Elizabeth's diligent diary keeping provided valuable information for charting slow progress. More importantly, the diaries were a key to revealing her carefully guarded circumstance. This allowed me to understand why progress had been slow, as she was living with emotional strain. It also highlighted the significance of the relationship between the emotions and gut performance. With colorectal cancer survivors, it is easy to focus on physical causes of gut irregularities without considering the powerful impact of the emotions on bowel performance.

Other practitioners, supervision, and reflective practice

These are indispensable tools in my toolkit, so second nature to my professional life that I nearly forgot to mention them.

Other practitioners have been essential to my development as a practitioner. Through networks, teaching, CPD, and supervision, I have learned much from the experiences and insights of my colleagues. My ideas and practice have been enriched through this exposure. (In fact, developing the concept of a toolkit was inspired by the work of my friend and colleague, Dr Claudia Citkovitz.)

Since before qualifying, I have participated in regular supervision, and this is my most valued CPD activity. To travel the journey of being an acupuncturist alongside peers, to share clinical challenges and solutions, and to do this in a safe, confidential space consistently and over many years has helped to shape my ideas, my practice, and my own toolkit.

Allied with this is reflective practice, taught at many acupuncture training institutions. It is important to consciously examine the process of planning a strategy, observing the result, and adjusting, while asking questions at all stages. For me, reflective practice can be as formal as writing a case study for publication or it may be an activity that I carry out in my supervision group. Without it, I would never have been able to write this book.

CHAPTER SUMMARY

- A toolkit provides a rich resource of interventions that help to meet a variety of clinical challenges.
- A toolkit facilitates flexibility to meet constraints that may be environmental or condition-related.
- The tools discussed in this chapter are not prescriptive; they are intended to illustrate how I work and shed light on the case studies presented throughout this book.
- Practitioners are encouraged to develop their own toolkits, relevant to their training, the type of patients they see, and the contexts in which they work.
- Acupuncture is part of 'a tradition to think with'.

References

1. Scheid V Traditional Chinese medicine: What are we investigating? The case of menopause. Complement. Ther. Med. 2007;15:54–68.
2. de Valois B, Asprey A, Young T 'The monkey on your shoulder': a qualitative study of lymphoedema patients' attitudes to and experiences of acupuncture and moxibustion. Evid. Based Complement. Alternat. Med. 2016;Article ID 4298420.
3. Hicks A, Hicks J, Mole P Five element constitutional acupuncture. Edinburgh: Churchill Livingstone; 2004.
4. Citkovitz C Acupressure and acupuncture during birth. London: Singing Dragon; 2020.
5. Birch S, Felt RL Understanding acupuncture. Edinburgh: Churchill Livingstone; 1999.
6. Eckman P In the footsteps of the yellow emperor. San Francisco: Cypress Book (US) Company, Inc; 1996.
7. Flaws B Four LA blocks to therapy and TCM. Traditional Acupuncture Society 1989;6:5–7.
8. British Journal of Family Medicine; 2013. Available from: www.bjfm.co.uk/half-a-million-uk-cancer-survivors-faced-with-disability-and-poor-health
9. de Valois B, Peckham R Treating the person and not the disease: acupuncture in the management of cancer treatment-related lymphoedema. Eur. J. Orient. Med. 2011;6(6):37–49.
10. de Valois B Turning points: clearing blocks to treatment in women with early breast cancer. Eur. J. Orient. Med. 2008;5(6):10–15.
11. The National Cancer Survivorship Initiative: new and emerging evidence on the ongoing needs of cancer survivors. Br. J. Cancer 2011;105 (Suppl. 1):S1–S4.
12. de Valois B, Glynne-Jones R Acupuncture in the supportive care of colorectal cancer survivors: four case studies, Part 2. Eur. J. Orient. Med. 2018;9(1):10–22.
13. Hatton CL Acupuncture point compendium. Leamington: College of Traditional Acupuncture; 2004. Available from: www.dropbox.com/s/eso5a5mm2vpgod7/Acupuncture%20Point%20Compendium%202014.pdf?dl=0
14. Maciocia G The channels of acupuncture: clinical use of the secondary channels and eight extraordinary vessels. Edinburgh: Churchill Livingstone; 2006.
15. Maciocia G The foundations of Chinese medicine. London: Churchill Livingstone; 1989.
16. Deadman P, Al-Khafaji M, Baker K A manual of acupuncture. Hove: The Journal of Chinese Medicine; 2007.
17. de Valois B, Young T, Robinson N, et al. Using traditional acupuncture for breast cancer-related hot flashes and night sweats. J. Altern. Complement. Med. 2010;16(10):1047–1057.
18. Oleson T Auriculotherapy manual: Chinese and Western systems of ear acupuncture. 3rd ed. Edinburgh: Churchill Livingstone; 2003.
19. Landgren K Ear acupuncture: a practical guide. Edinburgh: Churchill Livingstone; 2008.
20. Bemis R Evidence for the NADA ear acupuncture protocol: summary of research. Laramie, WY: NADA; 2013. Available from: https://acudetox.com/wordpress/wp-content/uploads/2014/07/Research_Summary_2013-2.pdf

21. Brumbaugh AG Transformation and recovery: a guide for the design and development of acupuncture-based chemical dependency treatment programs. Santa Barbara: Stillpoint; 1994.

22. Peckham R The role and the impact of the NADA protocol (daily group acupuncture treatment used in addiction): explanatory case studies [MSc Thesis]. London: University of Westminster; 2005.

23. de Valois B, Young T, Robinson N, et al. NADA ear acupuncture for breast cancer treatment-related hot flashes and night sweats: an observational study. Med. Acupunct. 2012;24(4):256–268.

24. Harding C, Harris A, Chadwich D Auricular acupuncture: a novel treatment for vasomotor symptoms associated with luteinizing-hormone releasing agonist treatment for prostate cancer. Br. J. Urol. 2008;103:186090.

25. NADA National Acupuncture Detoxification Association. Laramie, WY; 2018–2019. Available from: https://acudetox.com

26. de Valois B Serenity, patience, wisdom, courage, acceptance: reflections on the NADA protocol. Eur. J. Orient. Med. 2006;5(3):44–49.

27. de Valois B, Degun T Using the NADA protocol to improve wellbeing of prostate cancer survivors: five case studies. Eur. J. Orient. Med. 2015;8(1):8–18.

28. National Acupuncture Detoxification Association (NADA), Medical Reserve Corps (MRC) Ear Acupoints for Trauma Recovery and Healing. Laramie, WY: National Acupuncture Detoxification Association; no date. Available from: https://acudetox.com/wordpress/wp-content/uploads/2017/04/MRC-NADA-Handout-Ear-Acupoints-for-Trauma-Recovery-Finalv2.pdf

29. Maciocia G The psyche in Chinese medicine. London: Churchill Livingstone; 2009.

30. de Valois B, Glynne-Jones R Acupuncture in the supportive care of colorectal cancer survivors: Four case studies, Part 1. Eur. J. Orient. Med. 2017;8(6):34–43.

31. Yim Y-K, Lee H, Hong K-E, et al. Electro-acupuncture at acupoint ST36 reduces inflammation and regulates immune activity in collagen-induced arthritic mice. Evid. Based Complement. Alternat. Med. 2007;4(1):51–57.

32. Johnston M, Sanchez E, Vujanovic NL, et al. Acupuncture may stimulate anticancer immunity via activation of natural killer cells. Evid. Based Complement. Alternat. Med. 2011;2011:481625.

33. Wong R, Sagar SM Acupuncture and moxibustion for cancer-related symptoms. In: Cho WCS, editor. Acupuncture and moxibustion as an evidence-base therapy for cancer. Dordrecht: Springer; 2012. pp. 83–120.

34. Wilcox L Moxibustion: the power of mugwort fire. Boulder, CO: Blue Poppy Press; 2008.

35. Abbate S An overview of the therapeutic application of moxibustion. J. Chinese Med. 2002;69:5–12.

36. Xiaorong C, Jing H, Shouxiang Y Illustrated Chinese moxibustion: techniques and methods. London: Singing Dragon; 2012.

37. Lesi G, Razzini G, Musti MA, et al. Acupuncture as an integrative approach for the treatment of hot flashes in women with breast cancer: a prospective multicenter randomized controlled trial (AcCliMaT). J. Clin. Oncol. 2016;34(15):1795–1802.

38. Park J-E, Lee MS, Jung S, et al. Moxibustion for treating menopausal hot flashes: a randomized clinical trial. Menopause 2009;16(4):660–665.

Chapter 6

Cancer-Related Fatigue

Introduction

The prevalence of cancer-related fatigue, and the potential for acupuncture to alleviate its impact on cancer survivors are expressed below:

> Fatigue is the most common side effect of cancer treatment. (National Cancer Institute)[1]

> Now getting up in the morning, I have energy all day, whereas before I was on the couch in front of the telly, I couldn't be bothered... And, you know, now I'm back and I'm doing, you know, my everyday life is normal. I feel like I've been given my life back. (Breast cancer survivor after a course of acupuncture treatment)

Everyone may feel fatigued at times; this is nature's way of telling us to rest. Cancer-related fatigue (CRF) is different. Unlike 'normal' fatigue, CRF is not relieved by rest. It is chronic, exhausting, and debilitating, depriving people of the energy to enjoy or even participate in daily activities.

People with CRF describe a range of symptoms. Exhaustion, heavy limbs, inability to concentrate, lack of motivation, abnormal sleep, and feeling low, irritable, and/or frustrated are characteristics of CRF.[2] Carrying out usual daily tasks is exhausting or impossible. CRF significantly impacts quality of life.

Survivors perceive CRF to be the most distressing symptom of cancer and its treatments, even more than pain or nausea and vomiting.[3] Most survivors experience CRF at some stage in the cancer trajectory. It is usually temporary, lasting a few months, but it may persist for many years after treatment ends.

As cancer treatment has become more successful, and the number of cancer survivors grows, healthcare professionals are likely to see people with prolonged states of CRF. It is difficult to treat; there are few effective interventions.

Acupuncture has attracted attention in the biomedical and research communities. While studies show mixed results, acupuncture is regarded as an option to treat a condition for which there are few solutions.[4,5]

People who have acupuncture often say they have more energy – sometimes as a 'side effect' of treatment for other symptoms. This is also true for some cancer survivors, even when treatment is not aimed specifically at CRF.

This chapter focuses on the potential of acupuncture to address CRF as experienced by people who have completed active primary cancer treatment and who are disease-free.

TERMINOLOGY

CRF is defined as:

> a distressing, persistent, subjective sense of physical, emotional and/or cognitive tired-ness or exhaustion, related to cancer or cancer treatment that is not proportional to recent activity and interferes with usual functioning.[3]

CRF is described as more severe and debilitating than fatigue experienced by healthy individuals. It is less likely to be relieved by rest.

Incidence and prevalence

CRF is one of the most common problems reported by people with cancer, affecting 65–90% of patients at some point in the cancer trajectory.[6,7] Fatigue at diagnosis is reported by 40%, and by up to 80–90% during chemotherapy and/or radiotherapy.[7]

CRF is associated with surgery, chemotherapy, hormone therapy, endocrine therapy, and radiotherapy. Survivors receiving trimodal treatment (surgery, chemotherapy, and radiotherapy) report higher levels of CRF than those receiving other treatment combinations.[8]

Survivors on hormonal therapies such as adjuvant endocrine therapy or androgen deprivation therapy (ADT) are also more likely to experience CRF. Studies report that 56% of breast cancer patients taking aromatase inhibitors experience moderate to severe CRF symptoms, while prostate cancer survivors with current or previous use of ADT are more likely to experience CRF than those who had never used ADT.[8]

Although CRF typically abates in the year following cancer treatment, it may persist for months or years, with 20–30% of cancer survivors experiencing symptoms five or more years post treatment.[9,10] In the short term, up to 60% of breast cancer survivors report moderate to severe tiredness one year after diagnosis, while 21–52% of cancer survivors report severe CRF three years from diagnosis.[8]

Longer term, in a UK survey 43% of people diagnosed with breast, colorectal, or prostate cancer or non-Hodgkin lymphoma up to five years previously reported always feeling tired.[11] Among testicular cancer and Hodgkin disease survivors, 16–24% reported fatigue 12 years or more after treatment, with some respondents experiencing it up to 30 years post treatment.[9] Long-term CRF is especially prevalent in survivors of adolescent and young adult cancers, with 25% still experiencing fatigue 5–30 years post diagnosis.[8]

Characteristics of CRF

CRF should not be confused with tiredness experienced by healthy individuals. Severe, distressing, and unlikely to be relieved by rest, it can be seriously debilitating. One survivor of a gynaecological cancer told me that for some time, it was all she could do in a day to muster the energy to move from lying on her bed to lying on the sofa in the same room.

This persistent tiredness may have wide-ranging consequences and be clustered with other debilitating symptoms. For example, pain, insomnia, depression, and fatigue have been identified as a symptom cluster in breast cancer survivors.[12] Affecting emotional, mental, and physical wellbeing, CRF can negatively impact survivors' ability to function in terms of their usual social activities and their ability to work.[13] As well as impacting quality of life, it is associated with shorter recurrence-free and overall survival.[14]

It affects people differently and may vary according to the stages of survivorship. Box 6.1 lists some common impacts of CRF.

Box 6.1: Some common effects of cancer-related fatigue[6]

- Difficulty doing simple things, such as brushing hair or getting dressed
- Feeling of having no energy or strength
- Difficulty concentrating and remembering things
- Difficulty thinking, speaking, or making decisions
- Feeling breathless after light activity
- Feeling dizzy or light-headed
- Difficulty sleeping (insomnia)
- Losing interest in sex
- Feeling low in mood and more emotional than usual

CRF has been under-acknowledged by healthcare providers and health agencies, causing serious financial difficulties for survivors whose struggle with fatigue continues even when they are considered 'cancer free'.[8,15] Such difficulties could be addressed if reimbursement for the management of CRF was made available, and if it ongoing impacts were covered by disability insurance.

Biomedical perspectives
Aetiology and risk factors
The aetiology of CRF is poorly understood. It is thought to have multiple causes and is accepted to be 'multifactorial', with contributions from physiological, clinical, and psychological factors.[8,9] Possible factors include:

- the cancer itself
- cancer treatments
- comorbid medical conditions (e.g. anaemia, hypothyroidism, sleep disorders)
- psychological factors (e.g. anxiety, depression, chronic stress)
- pain
- loss of functional status (the ability to perform daily activities).[9,13]

The cause(s) of CRF vary according to the individual, the phase of the disease, and the treatment(s) received. Causes of an individual's CRF may be multifactorial, or a single factor may trigger a cascade of events. For example, increased cytokine production (triggered by the tumour, or by cancer treatment, or both) may cause anaemia, which in turn may affect neuromuscular function, resulting in CRF.[9]

For survivors who are post treatment and disease-free, the causes of CRF are again unclear and thought to be multifactorial. Studies investigating molecular/physiological factors suggest that increases in serum levels of inflammatory markers (including C-re-active protein (CRP), lL-6, and IL-1 receptor antagonist (lL-1RA)) may be associated with increased fatigue.[10] A chronic inflammatory process involving the T-cell component may also cause persistent fatigue in survivors.

Risk factors associated with post-treatment survivors include:[10]

- Pre-treatment fatigue – individuals reporting high levels of fatigue before cancer treatment also report elevated fatigue after completing treatment.
- Anxiety and depression – pre-treatment anxiety and depression predict CRF before, during, and after cancer treatment.
- Physical activity – decreased levels of activity can lead to fatigue.
- Elevated BMI – also linked with fatigue and has been identified as a key predictor of fatigue in women with breast cancer.
- Coping methods and cancer-related stressors – psychological responses to cancer diagnosis and treatment can influence fatigue symptoms, particularly the tendency to catastrophise or engage in negative self-statements. Negative expectations and coping strategies early in the cancer trajectory appear to increase risk of post-treatment CRF.
- Comorbidities.
- Type of malignancy.
- Prior treatment patterns.
- Other late effects of treatment.

Sleep disturbance is also strongly associated with CRF. Pre-treatment levels of sleep disturbance have been shown to predict higher levels of CRF before, during, and after cancer treatment. However, while sleep disturbance may be a risk factor for CRF, the condition can persist even when survivors report adequate sleep.[10]

Similarly, depression is strongly correlated with CRF. In a complex relationship, fatigue may be a symptom of depression, and also trigger depressed mood because of its interference with normal daily activities.[10]

Assessment
Lack of knowledge about the aetiology and mechanisms underlying CRF hampers its treatment.[16] Furthermore, CRF is a subjective condition whose assessment relies on patient self-report. A range of questionnaires have been designed for assessment,[8] of which the ten-point Numeric Rating Scale for Fatigue (Box 6.2) is a recommended screening tool that can be used quickly and easily in clinic.[7]

Box 6.2: Numeric Rating Scale for Fatigue

Ask the question: 'How would you rate your fatigue on a scale of 0 to 10, with 0 being no fatigue and 10 being the worst possible fatigue?'

The assessment is:

- 0 = no fatigue
- 1–3 = mild fatigue
- 4–6 = moderate fatigue
- 7–10 = severe fatigue.

Expert guidelines recommend that survivors continue to be monitored long term, as CRF may develop or continue long after active treatment ends.[3,7]

Biomedical approaches to treatment

As a first step, contributing factors that are treatable should be addressed (Box 6.3). This may relieve the CRF partially or completely.

Box 6.3: Concurrent symptoms and treatable contributing factors[3]

Factors that may cause or contribute to CRF include:

- Hypothyroidism
- Anaemia
- Sleep disturbance
- Pain
- Emotional distress
- Medication adverse effects
- Malnutrition or nutritional imbalance
- Activity levels (low activity can lead to fatigue)
- Alcohol/substance abuse
- Comorbidities

Several treatment options exist for survivors who do not have these symptoms or treatable contributing factors, or if CRF persists after these have been addressed, although these may only yield moderate benefits.[8]

Pharmacological treatments for CRF

Many pharmacological products have been studied in relation to CRF, including psychostimulants, antidepressants, erythropoietin, steroids, and others. Apart from erythropoietin, which may be used for anaemia-related CRF in selected patients only due to safety considerations, these have shown little efficacy and are generally not recommended by expert panels on CRF.[7] For cancer survivors post treatment, the psychostimulant methylphenidate may be considered after other causes of fatigue have been ruled out.

Non-pharmacological treatments for CRF
Physical activity
Physical activity, sometimes called exercise (see Chapter 13, Reducing Risk of Recurrence and Subsequent Primary Cancers) is a Category 1 recommendation with the best evidence of all the non-pharmacological options to support its effectiveness for the management of CRF, both during and after cancer treatment.[1]

A Cochrane review recommended that aerobic exercise (especially walking or cycling) should be considered as a component of the multi-intervention strategy for managing CRF, particularly for survivors with solid tumours.[13] In addition to building strength, energy, and fitness, physical activity can facilitate the transition from patient to survivor, improve body image, and decrease anxiety and depression.[3]

Psychosocial/psychoeducation
Psychosocial interventions designed specifically for CRF, comprising education, self-care, and coping techniques, as well as activity management (balancing activities and rest) have shown some benefit for patients during active cancer treatment.[17]

Educational interventions may be helpful, even for survivors post treatment, especially as CRF may be a late- or long-term consequence. Many cancer survivors have beliefs about CRF that may prevent them seeking help, including perceptions that:

- fatigue is inevitable
- treating cancer is more important than addressing fatigue
- by reporting fatigue, the individual will be perceived as a complainer
- fatigue may be a sign of cancer recurrence.[1]

Thus, informing survivors that fatigue is a common consequence of cancer and its treatment can be beneficial.

Cognitive behavioural therapy (CBT) has been shown to be effective for reducing CRF, especially if provided at the end of active treatment. It is also useful for addressing insomnia, which is often a component of CRF.[8]

Mind–body therapies
Many mind–body practices have been studied, although evidence for effectiveness is equivocal. However, a randomised controlled trial (RCT) of yoga compared with standard survivorship care for CRF in breast cancer survivors reported significant benefit for yoga.[7] Meta-analyses of qigong and tai chi showed promising results for improving CRF, although evidence needs to be strengthened.[8]

The evidence for acupuncture, discussed in depth below, is generally regarded as low strength, and the European Society for Medical Oncology (ESMO) was unable to reach a consensus in its evaluation of acupuncture for CRF.[7] However, acupuncture is recommended in guidelines for supportive care of breast cancer patients to manage anxiety associated with ongoing fatigue and for treatment of CRF after cancer treatment ends.[18] Clinical practice guidelines for breast cancer suggest acupuncture may be helpful in managing post-treatment fatigue, although the studies reviewed suffered from design issues.[19]

Lifestyle

Managing CRF includes helping the survivor develop self-care strategies to manage energy and cope with fatigue in daily life. Healthcare professionals can support survivors to manage its chronic nature by helping them to:

- understand fatigue is a consequence of cancer and its treatment
- address aspects of daily living to manage fatigue.

Lifestyle changes should be supported, particularly physical activity, diet, and sleep behaviours. Box 6.4 lists examples of the many possible recommendations.

It is to be hoped that survivors have received educational interventions by the time they reach the end of primary cancer treatment, but this may not be the case.

Box 6.4: Some self-care strategies for managing CRF

- Plan ahead.
  Develop a realistic plan of what can be achieved in a day, including rest.
- Prioritise activities.
  Decide on which activities are important and which are not.
- Balance rest and activity.
  Plan rest breaks, including short naps of 30 minutes or less, into the day.
- Stay active.
  Regulate moderate exercise, especially walking, to ease fatigue.
- Get help.
  Ask family and friends to help.
- Eat well and drink sufficient fluids.
- Establish good sleep habits.
- Keep a regular schedule, and try to sleep seven to eight hours per night, or long enough to wake feeling refreshed. Keep the bedroom for sleeping and avoid staying in bed for too long.

East Asian medicine perspectives
Chinese medicine theories

Biomedicine differentiates several possible causes of CRF; so too does the theory of Chinese medicine (CM). Maciocia defines numerous syndrome patterns for tiredness and exhaustion, which may all be applicable to CRF (Table 6.1).[20]

We might deduce from the common effects of CRF (Box 6.1) that deficiency patterns are associated with CRF, especially those related to qi. However, the complexity of cancer and its treatments makes it unwise to associate any syndrome or set of syndromes as solely responsible for CRF. Furthermore, the syndrome(s) presented by any individual will be influenced by the specifics of their cancer (type and stage), the nature of their cancer treatments, their underlying constitution, comorbidities, and age.

When considering CRF we should expect to observe any of the syndromes listed in Table 6.1. This reflects the profound and various effects of cancer and its treatments on the vital substances. Within this range, any individual may present with one or more of the syndromes listed below. Diagnosis and treatment for these syndromes should proceed according to usual CM principles.

Table 6.1: Chinese medicine patterns for exhaustion (*Xu Lao*)

Deficiency patterns	Excess patterns
Lung qi deficiency	Liver qi stagnation
Lung yin deficiency	Liver yang rising
Heart qi deficiency	Liver fire blazing
Heart yin deficiency	Liver wind
Heart yang deficiency	Phlegm
Heart Blood deficiency	Dampness
Spleen qi deficiency	
Stomach and Spleen yin deficiency	
Spleen yang deficiency	
Spleen Blood deficiency	
Liver yin deficiency	
Liver Blood deficiency	
Kidney yin deficiency	
Kidney yang deficiency	
Combined deficiency patterns	**Mixed patterns (deficiency and excess)**
Lung qi and Spleen qi deficiency	Spleen qi deficiency with damp
Lung yin and Kidney yin deficiency	Spleen qi deficiency with phlegm
Spleen yang and Kidney yang deficiency	Spleen qi deficiency with Liver qi stagnation
Spleen Blood and Liver Blood deficiency	Liver Blood deficiency with Liver qi stagnation
	Liver Blood deficiency with Liver yang rising
	Liver Blood deficiency with Liver wind
	Kidney yin deficiency with Liver yang rising

Research perspectives
The evidence-base for using acupuncture for CRF

Evidence for using acupuncture to manage CRF is accumulating, as this is a condition that attracts much research interest globally. Research conducted in the West mainly comprises feasibility studies with small numbers of participants,[21-26] while the authors of two larger studies reach contradictory conclusions.[27,28]

Systematic reviews

Systematic reviews conclude that more research is required to determine whether acupuncture has any specific effect on CRF, citing methodological issues such as small number of participants and lack of robust research design.[29-31] Two systematic reviews acknowledge these limitations, and also propose that there is sufficient data to support the use of acupuncture as an effective treatment option for people with CRF.[31,32]

Research studies

Selected details of studies conducted in the West, focusing on cancer survivors who have completed active treatment and remain disease-free, are listed below:

- Table 6.2 summarises the acupuncture points used.
- Table 6.3 summarises study design and outcomes.

A study examining electro-acupuncture for breast cancer treatment-related arthralgia, reporting improvements in fatigue, psychological health, and pain, is discussed in Chapter 10, Chronic Cancer-Related Pain.[33]

Studies conducted in China are not discussed here as they focus on CRF during active treatment, or in advanced cancer, or use herbal interventions.[34] Studies using moxibustion are discussed separately below.

Commentary on acupuncture methods and point selection

Rationale: All studies cite TCM as the rationale.

Standardisation: Three studies incorporate individualisation.[21,23,28] Smith *et al.*[23] and Johnston *et al.*[21] carry out differential diagnosis, with only the latter providing a further breakdown of treatment approach according to symptoms associated with CRF.

Dose: The number of treatments is similar across studies, ranging from six to nine. Frequency of treatment varies considerably, ranging from three treatments per week for two weeks, to one treatment per week for eight weeks.

Needle techniques: Most aimed to elicit sensation (deqi). Smith *et al.*[23] specify tonification and reduction techniques; Molassiotis *et al.* specify using both tonification and even techniques in the 2007 study.[26] All studies retain needles for 20–30 minutes.

Points used: There is a remarkable consistency of core points, with ST-36 *Zusanli* used in all studies, and SP-6 *Sanyinjiao* by all but Vickers *et al.*[25] While none of the papers discusses the rationale for choosing the individual points, the protocols seem to be good broad-spectrum tonics to address the general symptoms of CRF and relate to the patterns of exhaustion (Table 6.1).

- ST-36 *Zusanli* is a major point to tonify qi and Blood, rectify the Stomach, Spleen, and Kidneys and the three jiao; stimulate qi and Blood. It supports the correct qi and is used to strengthen the mind and body in debilitated people and after chronic illness.[35,36]

- SP-6 *Sanyinjiao* tonifies the Spleen, Stomach, and Kidneys, harmonises the Liver, nourishes Blood and yin, and calms the spirit.[35,36]
- KID-3 *Taixi*, the principle point on the Kidney channel, addresses deficiencies of Kidney yin and yang.[35]

A variety of additional points supplement these 'energy-associated points', including:[21]

- REN-4 *Guanyuan* and REN-6 *Qihai*, which fortify original qi and tonify the Kidney, with the former benefitting the Essence and Spleen, while the latter regulates qi and strengthens yang.
- LI-4 *Hegu* and LI-11 *Quchi* may have been chosen for their role in strengthening Lung qi.

Safety considerations: Except for Johnston *et al.*[21] and Smith *et al.*,[23] all studies specify avoiding needling in a limb with or at risk of lymphoedema (see Chapter 9, Cancer Treatment-Related Lymphoedema).

Reporting of adverse events: Johnston *et al.*[21] assessed for adverse events after each treatment, specifying numerous possible adverse events from bruising to puncture of an internal organ, and report that no adverse events were recorded. However, the sample was small, with only 40 treatments delivered to five participants. Molassiotis *et al.*,[26] reporting on 90 acupuncture sessions delivered to 13 participants, recorded spot bleeding in two cases, with one participant each reporting bruising at one point, discomfort at one point (SP-6), and nausea at the end of treatment. Interestingly, bruising and pain in the points after pressure were recorded in the acupressure comparison group. Smith *et al.*[23] report that therapists assessed for adverse events, but do not report whether any occurred.

Additional information: In a further development of the 2012 study, Molassiotis *et al.* explored the value of maintenance therapy in a three-arm RCT comparing therapist-delivered acupuncture, self-acupuncture, and no further treatment.[37] After receiving six weekly therapist-delivered acupuncture treatments in the main study, participants were further randomised. Those in the acupuncture groups continued acupuncture for four weeks.

The self-needling group were taught to needle bilateral ST-36 *Zusanli* and SP-6 *Sanyinjiao*. Apart from a small number of cases of spot bleeding and minor pain and discomfort, no adverse events were reported. While the study showed no extra maintenance effect for managing CRF (there were no further improvements in CRF symptoms in either acupuncture group), the researchers concluded that self-needling was feasible, acceptable, safe, and useful for self-management.

Table 6.2: Studies using acupuncture in the management of CRF: Acupuncture points used

Author (Publication date)	Vickers et al. (2004)[25]	Molassiotis et al. (2007)[26]	Johnston et al. (2011)[21]		Deng et al. (2013)[27]	Smith et al. (2013)[33]	Molassiotis et al. (2012)[28]
Points used	Bilateral LI-11* ST-36 SP-8 SP-9 Unilateral REN-4 REN-6 *Participants at risk of lymphoedema not needled in the at risk/affected arm.	Bilateral LI-4* ST-36 SP-6 *Participants at risk of lymphoedema not needled in the at risk/affected arm.	Bilateral LI-4 ST-36 SP-6 KID-3 Plus points according to 4 syndrome patterns (in the adjacent column).	**A. Gastrointestinal** SP-4 P-6 **B. Emotional** LU-7 KID-4 LIV-3 DU-20 M-HN-3 Yintang **C. Sleep** HE-7 BL-62 KID-4 **D. Pain** SI-3 BL-62 TB-5 GB-20 GB-29 GB-30 GB-40 GB-43 Plus points specific to sites of pain.	Bilateral LI-11 ST-36 SP-6 HE-6* KID-3 Auricular point: antidepression Unilateral REN-4 REN-6 *Participants at risk of lymphoedema not needled in the at-risk/affected arm.	Bilateral ST-36 SP-6 KID-3 KID-27 REN-4 REN-6 Plus up to 3 secondary points, selected according to TCM differential diagnosis (unspecified).	Bilateral LI-4* ST-36 SP-6 *Not needled in participants who had undergone axillary dissection and in lymphoedematous limbs. Alternative points used to 'ensure an equal dose of treatment' were: SP-9 GB-34.

Table 6.3: Studies using acupuncture in the management of CRF: Summary of study design and outcomes

Author (Publication date)	Vickers et al. (2004)[25]	Molassiotis et al. (2007)[26]	Johnston et al. (2011)[21]	Deng et al. (2013)[27]	Smith et al. (2013)[33]	Molassiotis et al. (2012)[28]
Country	USA	UK	USA	USA	Australia	UK
Study design	Single arm observational	RCT	RCT	RCT	RCT	RCT
Tumour type	Various	Various	Breast	Various	Breast	Breast

cont.

Author (Publication date)	Vickers et al. (2004)[25]	Molassiotis et al. (2007)[26]	Johnston et al. (2011)[21]	Deng et al. (2013)[27]	Smith et al. (2013)[23]	Molassiotis et al. (2012)[28]
Cancer stage	≥ 3 weeks post chemo	≥ 1 month post chemo	Primary therapy completed	≥ 60 days post chemo	≥ 1 month post chemo	≥ 1 month post chemo (up to 5 years)
Participants	31	47	12	101	30	302
Comparison (Comparison/Acu)	None	Acupressure vs sham acupressure vs acupuncture 16/16/15	Patient education only vs acupuncture plus patient education 7/5	Sham acupuncture vs acupuncture 52/49	Sham acu vs waitlist control vs acupuncture 10/10/9	Usual care vs acupuncture plus usual care 75/227
Treatment frequency/ duration	Initially 2x/week for 4 weeks (8 total) Adjusted to 1x/week for 6 weeks (6 total)	3x/week for 2 weeks (6 total)	1x/week for 8 weeks (8 total)	1x/week for 6 weeks (6 total)	2x/week for 3 weeks, then 1/week for 3 weeks (9 total)	1x/week for 6 weeks (6 total)
Follow-up after end of tx (EOT)	None	2 weeks after EOT	None	6 months	None	None
Rationale	TCM	TCM	TCM	TCM plus expert opinion	TCM	Not stated
Protocol	Fixed	Fixed	Semi-individualised	Fixed	Semi-individualised	Semi-individualised
Adverse events	None attributable to acupuncture	Spot bleeding (2), bruise at point (1), nausea post tx (1), discomfort on ST-36 (1)	No adverse events associated with acupuncture	11 serious adverse events recorded; none deemed to be related to study interventions	Not addressed in the paper	Not addressed in the paper
Summary of results	Mean Brief Fatigue Inventory scores improved by 31% (sd 28). 12 participants improved by ≥ 40%, 3 improved by > 75%, 3 worsened. No evidence that frequency of treatment affected results; weekly treatment recommended.	Multidimensional Fatigue Inventory scores at EOT showed improvements of 36% for acu, 19% for acupuncture, 6% for sham acupressure. Improvement observed at follow-up, although to a lesser degree (22%, 15%, 7% respectively).	A 66% reduction in fatigue as measured on the Brief Fatigue Inventory. Low recruitment to the study was a problem – only 12 of the intended 80 participants were recruited.	Although both groups showed improvements in scores on all measures, there was no significant difference between the groups. No long-term reduction in fatigue scores was observed at 6-month follow-up.	Fatigue declined over time for all 3 groups, with significant improvements in the acu group after 2 weeks (p=.05), and in wellbeing at 6 weeks (p=.006).	Improvements in fatigue (mental, physical, overall), activity, motivation, psychological distress, quality of life after 6 weeks of acupuncture. This was the first large scale multi-centre RCT for acupuncture in the management of CRF.

The evidence-base for using moxibustion for CRF

Research into moxibustion is conducted rarely in the West. English language systematic reviews of studies published in the Chinese language provide insights into using moxibustion for CRF although the studies focus on cancer patients undergoing active treatment (usually chemotherapy) or with advanced cancers.[29,34,38] Authors of systematic reviews concede there is 'limited evidence indicating that moxibustion may be effective for improving fatigue in cancer patients'.[38] Many of the studies administer daily treatment to hospital in-patients; such intensive treatment may be difficult to administer to outpatients, particularly in the West.

One Korean RCT, published in English, focused on survivors of any tumour type who were at least 12 weeks post active treatment.[39] This three-arm study design compared moxibustion, sham moxibustion (using sham devices on non-acupuncture points), and usual care. Thirty-minute treatments were given twice weekly for eight weeks, for a total of 16 treatments.

The study recruited 96 participants, whose average time since cancer diagnosis was 51 months, and who with CRF for at least four weeks, measured as over four points on the Brief Fatigue Inventory.

While both the moxibustion and sham groups showed significant improvement in CRF during the treatment period, the moxibustion group:

- maintained improvement four weeks after the end of treatment, suggesting a prolonged treatment effect
- showed improvements in fatigue, dyspnea, appetite loss, and diarrhoea scores compared with the usual care group.

The researchers found that moxibustion could be applied for excess as well as deficiency conditions. Two instances of mild burns at the moxibustion site were reported; there were no serious adverse events.

Clinical perspectives

Developing a toolkit for CRF

Chinese medicine approaches to CRF

Possible syndromes implicated in CRF are presented in Table 6.1. Practitioners should choose treatment principles and points according to diagnosis of the individual.

Five Element approaches to CRF

Five Element techniques may be very helpful in managing CRF. Maxine's case study (later in this chapter) demonstrates the importance of clearing blocks to treatment for relieving fatigue.

Treating the element or constitutional factor can also alleviate CRF. Again, the specific Five Element treatment used at any given time depends on the patient characteristics and on individual diagnosis.

Moxibustion for CRF

I use moxibustion extensively when working with survivors with CRF. The points and procedures vary according to the Chinese medicine diagnosis, the patient's preference, and the environment I am working in – some hospital settings do not allow moxibustion, or clinics may only allow smokeless moxa.

I also use a wide range of applications of moxa, including moxa stick, warm needle, moxa box, Korean moxa device, and direct moxa. When using direct moxa, I avoid using blistering techniques.

Some approaches I use frequently to address CRF are listed in Table 6.4. This is not an exhaustive list, and many more points may be appropriate for moxa. Treatment approaches should be tailored to the diagnosis and the treatment principles selected for the individual patient. Moxibustion is discussed at length in Chapter 5, Toolkit, and Chapter 12, Supporting Resilience and the Immune System.

Table 6.4: Examples of points to moxa for the treatment of CRF

Points	Indication	Method
Ren-8 *Shenque*	Exhaustion; to warm and rescue yang	Moxa box, moxa cones on salt, moxa on ginger
ST-36 *Zusanli*	General tonic; to nourish Blood, tonify qi and yang, to tonify qi of the entire body, and support the upright qi	Stick, warm needle, or direct (7–20 cones). It is useful to teach patients to self-moxa this point
BL-43 *Gaohuangshu*	General tonic; to tonify and nourish the Lung, Heart, Kidney, Spleen, and Stomach; to nourish yin; to treat all types of deficiency taxation	Direct (7–50 cones, usually 15 bilaterally)
REN-4 *Guanyuan*	General tonic, especially for those in later life; nourish Blood; fortify original qi; tonify and nourish the Kidney; warm and strengthen the Spleen; benefit the Bladder; restore the yang	Stick, warm needle, or direct (7–20 cones)
Back shu points	As appropriate for the patient; to warm, tonify and nourish at a deep level	Stick, warm needle, or direct moxa using cones
Kidney chest points Usually: KID-24 *Lingxu*, or combined KID-25 *Shencang* and KID-27 *Shufu*	For fatigue with an emotional or spiritual component; to revive the spirit, stabilise the emotions, and calm	Usually direct (3–5 cones)

Classical texts recommend moxibustion on many of these points:[35]

- **BL-43 *Gaohuangshu*:** Sun Si-mao wrote that 'there is no [disorder] that it cannot treat' and 'once moxibustion is completed, it causes a person's yang to be healthy and full'.

- **REN-4 *Guanyuan*:** *The True Lineage of Medicine* states, 'When Kidney origin (yuan) is abundant, then life is long, when Kidney origin (yuan) is in decline, life is short', thus regular moxa on this point is recommended, particularly in later life. (Use of REN-4 for supporting cancer survivors is indicated also for its power to address Kidney deficiency caused by fear, as 'fear depletes the essence'.)
- **ST-36 *Zusanli*:** regular moxa on this point is a renowned practice, with great classical doctors such as Sun Si-mao, Wang Zhi-zhong, and Ma Dan-yang advocating its use for preserving and maintaining health. Its profound tonifying effects are mentioned in the *Great Compendium of Acupuncture*, which advocates moxibustion on ST-36 *Zusanli* and REN-6 *Qihai* in 'young people whose qi is feeble'. The *Spiritual Pivot* also recommends its use for the seven injuries, of which three may be particularly relevant to cancer survivors, including great anger which injures the Liver, worry and anxiety which injure the Heart, and excessive fear which injures the emotions.

I often teach patients to self-moxa ST-36 *Zusanli*. This gives them a self-management option that can be used as frequently as daily to improve energy levels (see Chapter 5, Toolkit).

Lifestyle advice

Acupuncturists can support the lifestyle advice given by biomedical healthcare professionals (Box 6.4) to develop self-care strategies to manage energy and cope with fatigue in daily life.

As well as helping the survivor to understand that fatigue is a consequence of cancer and its treatment, acupuncturists can facilitate the survivor in making lifestyle changes, particularly physical activity, diet, and sleep behaviours. Maintaining a balance of rest and activity is often challenging for patients to comprehend, and acupuncture can help survivors to develop good habits of rest (see Chapter 5, Toolkit, for a discussion of prescribing rest).

Additional notes about treating CRF

For many survivors, CRF may diminish or resolve without addressing it specifically. In my research studies, many participants specify 'tiredness' as a secondary complaint. Often, mild to moderate cases of CRF resolve as the individual is brought back 'into balance' through acupuncture and improved lifestyle practices.

Non-cancer patients often report their energy levels improve with acupuncture treatment. This also applies to cancer survivors with CRF, who may notice improvements in their energy as a 'side effect' of acupuncture treatment for other aspects of their health. This is not true for all cases, and CRF may remain intransigent and difficult to resolve, as illustrated in the vignette of Keith (below).

Finally, both the survivor and practitioner should be aware that CRF can fluctuate, varying throughout the day, and over time.[40] Developing an awareness of any individual's pattern will help to monitor, evaluate, and improve management and treatment.

VIGNETTE: KEITH AND A CASE OF PERSISTENT CRF

Keith, aged 58, was referred to the hospital outpatient acupuncture clinic by his oncologist. Keith had received chemoradiation the previous year for squamous cell carcinoma of the oesophagus. The oncologist noted that Keith had 'a difficult time but did get through' and that he was 'really troubled by debilitating fatigue' which hampered his ability to work.

At his intake interview, Keith reported that he felt 'great' apart from the fatigue. Confident of the success of his cancer treatment, he had no concerns about recurrence. In terms of the fatigue:

- he 'no longer had a reserve' and experienced 'sudden loss of energy'
- he was 'constantly tired' and did not feel refreshed even after 11 hours of good sleep
- his legs felt heavy and tired; lifting them took a lot of effort.

He had given himself a year to recover from cancer treatment and reported that he was feeling better than a year previously. However, his energy was 'still not good', which was 'frustrating'.

Keith was an active person; his work was a trade involving physical activity and he walked every day. He took care of his health, having a good diet and daily habits. He went to bed at 9–10pm, sleeping through until 6.30am. He was in a relationship and had a circle of friends. He was troubled by financial constraints due to his inability to work and had challenging relationships with his family and a neighbour.

- **Diagnoses: CM diagnosis:** included Spleen qi deficiency with Liver qi stagnation.
- **CF diagnosis:** I did not identify a CF but assessed that clearing blocks was indicated.

Keith had regular treatment, having 64 sessions over nearly three years. While he made gradual progress, fatigue remained a significant problem. This was disheartening for both of us, although the oncologist observed improvements when he reviewed Keith nearly two years into the acupuncture treatment.

Over the course of those treatments, I tried nearly 'everything in the book'. Keith also learned to self-moxa ST-36 *Zusanli* and was committed to carrying this out regularly. At times, he would seem to make progress; then something would happen, and Keith would slip back. Nevertheless, he valued the acupuncture, writing:

> I feel the acupuncture is doing something, but…it is more a maintenance than a noticeably 'wow' thing. I notice when I don't receive it, things come back quite quickly, so it must be 'doing' something positive.

Keith and I stayed in touch after the clinic closed. He remains cancer free seven years after his cancer diagnosis. He still experiences fatigue, saying:

> It's never really recovered, but I've learnt to live with it really. I accepted it was my personal

payment for the actual physical [cancer] treatment and I make the most of the energy I do have. Of course, I'm very happy to be alive.

Keith's is an example of persistent, intransigent CRF, which remained despite biomedical and acupuncture treatment.

Reflections on my clinical experience

It is my clinical observation that acupuncture can be beneficial in alleviating CRF, either in the short or long term. In some cases, it may eliminate this troublesome symptom. For most of the survivors I see, CRF is part of a bundle of symptoms, rather than the main or sole complaint. Therefore, I rarely have occasion to focus on fatigue as a single presenting symptom, and I find it often reduces or resolves as treatment for other complaints progresses.

This corresponds with what we observe and hear from our patients in general clinical practice, who often report improved energy. In the accumulating database of acupuncture research results at the Lynda Jackson Macmillan Centre, we are finding that outcome measures frequently record improvements in energy or vitality. It is always encouraging when research data supports what we observe routinely in clinic!

Many of the case studies in this book have CRF as a component of the survivor's presenting symptoms, as does the case study below. Maxine's case also illustrates how CRF responded to an unexpected and novel acupuncture approach, demonstrating how listening to patient preferences and feedback can engender surprising results.

Patient perspectives

CASE STUDY: MAXINE AND CRF

Introduction

Maxine was a breast cancer survivor with lymphoedema, who participated in a study of acupuncture to improve wellbeing for people with lymphoedema. She was a gentle, articulate woman, and I am very grateful for her consent to share her story and for her very informative written comments.

During the study's 13 acupuncture treatments, Maxine reported beneficial results in her lymphoedema, aches and pains, and chronic thrush (see Chapter 9, Cancer Treatment-Related Lymphoedema for details of the study and a vignette discussing Maxine's acupuncture experience). This case study focuses on CRF.

Background and main complaints

Maxine, aged 57, was diagnosed four years previously with carcinoma of the left breast with axillary node involvement, with 4 out of 14 nodes containing malignant cells. Treatment involved radical mastectomy, chemotherapy, radiotherapy, and adjuvant hormonal therapy with tamoxifen.

Case history details

At her initial consultation, Maxine spoke of feeling very tired. She 'used to have more energy' before the cancer diagnosis. A full-time teacher, she now was 'finished' by 5pm, having no energy to deal with anything else, and her husband managed the household. She went to bed at 8.30pm, was fast asleep by 9pm, and woke at 6am having slept through the night. Dreaming had ceased during cancer treatment.

Maxine had a good diet; her weight was within normal BMI range. Since cancer treatment, she no longer suffered monthly debilitating migraines.

Tongue: Red, with very red sides, and slightly swollen; thick white coating thickened at the root; sublingual veins were thin but distended.

Pulse: Left side: middle position choppy; extremely deep and weak on rear position. Right side: overall stronger, with some slipperiness on the middle position; deeper and weaker on the rear position.

Diagnoses

CM diagnosis: Spleen qi deficiency with damp, Kidney yin deficiency, Liver qi stagnation, Blood deficiency.

CF diagnosis: CF not apparent at this stage: clearing blocks is indicated.

Treatment approach

Maxine's priority for treatment was to address musculoskeletal symptoms associated with her breast cancer surgery and lymphoedema. Chronic tiredness was her second priority.

My planned treatment approach was to focus on Maxine's discomfort relating to breast cancer surgery and lymphoedema, by promoting transformation, transportation, and excretion of fluids (see Chapter 5, Toolkit). Ultimately, this is what Maxine's treatment comprised.

However, the first six weeks of treatment took quite a different turn, shaped by my clinical observation, Maxine's feedback, and her stated treatment preferences.

Initial treatments

On this research study, my standard approach was to clear energy blocks as a matter of course, starting with an Aggressive Energy Drain (AE Drain) for the first treatment, and clearing Internal Dragons (IDs) at the second. These were appropriate treatments given Maxine's cancer treatment history (see Chapter 5, Toolkit, for details of these treatments).

Table 6.5: Maxine's first two treatments

Note:

All needling to obtain deqi, no further stimulation, needles retained for at least 20 minutes unless otherwise specified.

Abbreviations: Tx treatment; **RS** right side

Tx	Treatment principles	Points	Notes
1	Clear block to treatment: Aggressive Energy (AE) Drain	BL-13 *Feishu* BL-14 *Jueyinshu* BL-15 *Xinshu* BL-18 *Ganshu* BL-20 *Pishu* BL-23 *Shenshu* Plus 3 check needles	Superficial unilateral needling (RS).
2	Internal Dragons	Extra point 0.25 cun below REN-15 *Jiuwei* ST-25 *Tianshu* ST-32 *Futu* ST-41 *Jiexi*	
	Ground treatment	SI-4 *Wangu* HE-7 *Shenmen*	RS only, no retention.

Tx 1: While no erythema appeared around the needles during the AE Drain, there was a marked pulse change at the end of treatment.

At her next appointment, Maxine reported that she had felt drowsy on the drive home. (Drowsiness after treatment proved to be a characteristic response to acupuncture, and Maxine stayed for a cup of tea and a rest after treatment for the remainder of her acupuncture sessions.) She slept well that night and had the first dream since her diagnosis nearly four years before. The following day, she 'had a little energy', and accompanied her husband shopping, something she was not usually able to do.

Tx 2: During this treatment, Maxine had a marked response to the IDs. The pulses became much stronger, with the left side strengthening and becoming more even across the three positions than previously.

More remarkable was the state of deep repose Maxine experienced immediately after insertion of the needles. Neither of us was certain whether she had fallen asleep or into a deep state of relaxation. Nevertheless, I observed changes in her expression and physical state, as well as a sense of changed energy within the treatment room.

When I next saw her, Maxine reported that on arriving home, she began to feel different:

- There were noticeable changes in the sensations in her lymphoedematous arm.
- She felt 'very, very energised', was less sleepy, had more energy at the end of the working day, and all of this had lasted the full week!

Table 6.6: Maxine's third treatment

Abbreviations: Tx treatment; **RS** right side; **LS** left side

Tx	Treatment principles	Points	Notes
3	Promote transformation, transportation, and excretion of fluids	Open *Ren Mai*: LU-7 *Lieque* (RS) KID-6 *Zhaohai* (LS) Plus REN-9 *Shuifen* REN-12 *Zhongwan*	See Chapter 5, Toolkit, for method.

Tx 3: During this treatment, I introduced the protocol for transforming, transporting, and excreting fluids, to focus on her arm and chest sensations.

Again, her chronically weak pulses on the left side strengthened, and she experienced vagueness and giddiness immediately after treatment. There were no other major changes, apart from being able to have a late night out with colleagues – she was 'wide awake until 11pm!'

Table 6.7: Maxine's treatments 4 and 5

Abbreviation: Tx treatment

Tx	Treatment principles	Points
4	Clear block to treatment: Internal Dragons Support spirit	All points as per Tx 2, Table 6.5
5	Promote transportation, transformation, and excretion of fluids	All points as per Tx 3, Table 6.6

Tx 4: At this appointment, we discussed the way forward. Maxine really liked the changes after the IDs treatment and asked to have this repeated. I agreed that repeating IDs would be relevant for her.

Again, I observed the state of profound repose during treatment. She did not experience the giddiness after treatment, and the following day noticed improvements in her arm and chest sensations. Her energy remained good, and the quality of her sleep improved – she was no longer tossing and turning in the night. She was also able to do some activity every evening after work.

Tx 5: Her response after this treatment was unremarkable, but there were no setbacks.

Tx 6: In view of the unremarkable response to the previous treatment, I administered IDs as per Tx 2 (Table 6.5), and Maxine appeared to progress again.

A week later she said she 'felt good' after this treatment. She had the energy to deal with work, which was very busy prior to Christmas season. At a Christmas concert, she was required to stand for four hours, and reported that after this, she 'was tired, but no more than anyone else'.

Progress through treatment

Tx 7–13: At treatment 7, I returned the focus to address the discomfort of the lymph-oedema and chest, as per treatment 3 (Table 6.6).

Maxine opted to have another six acupuncture treatments as part of the study, and at her eighth session, we reviewed her aims for treatment. Whereas 'tiredness' had been her second most troublesome symptom when she joined the study, this was no longer a problem needing attention. In the remaining sessions, treatment focused on transforming, transporting, and excreting fluids, as well addressing her gynaecological issues.

Short- and long-term feedback

At the end of 13 treatments, Maxine responded to the question 'what has treatment affected most in your life?' with this written feedback:

> My energy levels. Prior to the treatment, I would return from work at 5pm and by 8.30pm I had to go to bed, I was very tired. After the treatment started, the tiredness decreased and I could stay awake till 10 or 11pm and still wake up refreshed in the morning.

In a follow-up questionnaire, she wrote:

> One month on, I am still feeling good about my work, social life and so on because I still have enough energy. The day normally ends at 9.30pm (instead of the previous 5.30pm and bed at 8.30pm).

Two months later, Maxine confirmed that her acupuncture treatment had been very worthwhile, saying, 'I still have a lot of energy and general feeling of wellbeing.' Again, she commented that the aspect of her life that having acupuncture most affected was:

> ...the general feeling of wellbeing – I have more energy, am able to stay up longer at night and cope with more varied activities.

Summary

Maxine's story illustrates how acupuncture can improve and even resolve CRF. It also demonstrates the use of an unusual approach, that is, clearing blocks using Internal Dragons. This approach evolved through close observation of Maxine's responses to treatment, and by responding to her feedback about the effects of treatment.

Conclusion

Fatigue is a common side effect of cancer and its treatments, and one that we are likely to encounter frequently in clinical practice. A wide range of options exist for using acupuncture and moxibustion to manage CRF. These may be used to good effect to reduce or eliminate the distressing and disabling symptoms of fatigue experienced by cancer survivors.

CHAPTER SUMMARY

- CRF is a complex, multifactorial condition that is difficult to manage and treat. It requires multiple concurrent interventions as well as multidisciplinary care.
- Although common in the cancer trajectory, it may be overlooked by healthcare professionals focused on addressing other important cancer-related issues.[15]
- Survivors may be reluctant to bring it to the attention of their healthcare team.
- Acupuncture may be an option in the management and treatment of CRF.
- Acupuncture may resolve CRF as part of treatment for other presenting symptoms or it may be used to target CRF specifically.
- CRF may be persistent and intransigent, responding to neither biomedical nor acupuncture interventions.

References

1. PDQ° Supportive and Palliative Care Editorial Board PDQ Fatigue – Health professional version. Bethesda, MD: National Cancer Institute; Updated 17 November 2021. Available from: www.cancer.gov/about-cancer/treatment/side-effects/fatigue/fatigue-hp-pdq#section_5.74

2. American Cancer Society Managing fatigue or weakness. Atlanta, Georgia: American Cancer Society; 2020. Available from: www.cancer.org/treatment/treatments-and-side-effects/physical-side-effects/fatigue/managing-cancer-related-fatigue.html

3. Campos MPO, Hassan BJ, Riechelmann R, et al. Cancer-related fatigue: a practical review. Ann Oncol. 2011 Jun;22(6):1273–1279.

4. Molassiotis A Managing cancer-related fatigue with acupuncture: is it all good news for patients? Acupunct. Med. 2013;31(3):3–4.

5. Di Meglio A, Charles C, Martin E, et al. Uptake of recommendations for posttreatment cancer-related fatigue among breast cancer survivors. J. Natl. Compr. Canc. Netw. 2022:1–13.

6. Macmillan Cancer Support Tiredness (fatigue). London: Macmillan Cancer Support; 2014. Available from: www.macmillan.org.uk/cancer-information-and-support/impacts-of-cancer/tiredness

7. Fabi A, Bhargava R, Fatigoni S, et al. Cancer-related fatigue: ESMO clinical practice guidelines for diagnosis and treatment. Ann. Oncol. 2020;31(6):713–723.

8. Thong MSY, van Noorden CJF, Steindorf K, et al. Cancer-related fatigue: causes and current treatment options. Curr. Treat. Options Oncol. 2020;21(2):17.

9. Ng AB, Alt CA, Gore EM Fatigue. In: Feuerstein M, editor. Handbook of cancer survivorship. New York: Springer; 2007. pp. 133–150.

10. Bower JE Cancer-related fatigue – mechanisms, risk factors, and treatments. Nat Rev Clin Oncol 2014;11(10):597–609.

11. Macmillan Cancer Support Throwing light on the consequences of cancer and its treatment. Macmillan Cancer Support; 2013. Available from: www.macmillan.org.uk/Documents/AboutUs/Research/Researchandevaluationreports/Throwinglightontheconsequencesofcanceranditstreatment.pdf

12. Ruiz-Casado A, Álvarez-Bustos A, de Pedro CG, et al. Cancer-related fatigue in breast cancer survivors: a review. Clin. Breast. Cancer 2021;21(1):10–25.

13. Cramp F, Byron-Daniel J Exercise for the management of cancer-related fatigue. Cochrane Database Syst. Rev. 2012; 11:CD006145.

14. Bower JE Treating cancer-related fatigue: the search for interventions that target those most in need. J. Clin. Oncol. 2012;30(36):4449–4450.

15. Kober KM, Yom SS Doc, I feel tired...oh really, so how's your mucositis? Cancer 2021;127(18):3294–3297.

16. Bennett S, Purcell A, Meredith P, et al. Educational interventions for the management of cancer-related fatigue in adults. Cochrane Database Syst. Rev. 2009;4: CD008144.

17. Goedendorp M, Gielissen W, Verhagen C, et al. Psychosocial interventions for reducing fatigue during cancer treatment in adults (Review). Cochrane Database Syst. Rev. 2009;1:CD006953.

18. Greenlee H, Balneaves LG, Carlson LE, *et al.* Clinical practice guidelines on the use of integrative therapies as supportive care in patients treated for breast cancer. J. Natl. Cancer Inst. Monogr. 2014;2014(50):346–358.

19. Greenlee H, DuPont-Reyes MJ, Balneaves LG, *et al.* Clinical practice guidelines on the evidence-based use of integrative therapies during and after breast cancer treatment. CA Cancer J Clin. 2017 May 6;67(3):194–232.

20. Maciocia G The practice of Chinese Medicine. London: Churchill Livingstone; 1994.

21. Johnston M, Hays R, Subramanian S, *et al.* Patient education integrated with acupuncture for relief of cancer-related fatigue randomized controlled feasibility study. BMC Complement. Altern. Med. 2011;11(49).

22. Balk J, Day R, Rosenzweig M, *et al.* Pilot, randomized, modified, double-blind, placebo-controlled trial of acupuncture for cancer-related fatigue. J. Soc. Integr. Oncol. 2009;7(1):4–11.

23. Smith C, Carmady B, Thornton C, *et al.* The effect of acupuncture on post-cancer fatigue and well-being for women recovering from breast cancer: a pilot randomised controlled trial. Acupunct. Med. 2013;31:9–15.

24. Mao J, Styles T, Cheville A, *et al.* Acupuncture for non-palliative radiation therapy related fatigue: a feasibility study. J. Soc. Integr. Oncol. 2009;7(2):52–58.

25. Vickers A, Straus D, Fearon B, *et al.* Acupuncture for postchemotherapy fatigue: a phase II study. J. Clin. Oncol. 2004;22(9):1731–1735.

26. Molassiotis A, Sylt P, Diggins H The management of cancer-related fatigue after chemotherapy with acupuncture and acupressure: a randomised controlled trial. Complement. Ther. Med. 2007;15(4):228–237.

27. Deng G, Chan Y, Sjoberg D, *et al.* Acupuncture for the treatment of post-chemotherapy chronic fatigue: a randomised, binded, sham-controlled trial. Support. Care Cancer 2013;21:1735–1741.

28. Molassiotis A, Bardy J, Finnegan-John J, *et al.* Acupuncture for cancer-related fatigue in patients with breast cancer: a pragmatic randomized controlled trial. J. Clin. Oncol. 2012;30(36):4470–4476.

29. He XR, Wang Q, Li PP Acupuncture and moxibustion for cancer-related fatigue: a systematic review and meta-analysis. Asian Pac. J. Cancer Prev. 2013;14(5):3067–3074.

30. Posadzki P, Moon T-W, Choi T-Y, *et al.* Acupuncture for cancer-related fatigue: a systematic review of randomized trials. Support. Care Cancer 2013;21:2067–2073.

31. Zhang Y, Lin L, Li H, *et al.* Effects of acupuncture on cancer-related fatigue: a meta-analysis. Support. Care Cancer 2018;26(2):415–425.

32. Jang A, Brown C, Lamoury G, *et al.* The effects of acupuncture on cancer-related ratigue: updated systematic review and meta-analysis. Integr. Cancer Ther. 2020;19:1534735420949679.

33. Mao JJ, Xie SX, Farrar JT, *et al.* A randomised trial of electro-acupuncture for arthralgia related to aromatase inhibitor use. Eur. J. Cancer 2014;50(2):267–276.

34. Zhao Y, Wang S, Li J, *et al.* Effectiveness and safety of traditional Chinese medical therapy for cancer-related fatigue: a systematic review and meta-analysis of randomized controlled trials. J. Tradit. Chin. Med. 2020;40(5):738–748.

35. Deadman P, Al-Khafaji M, Baker K A manual of acupuncture. Hove: The Journal of Chinese Medicine; 2007.

36. Maciocia G The foundations of Chinese medicine: a comprehensive text for acupuncturists and herbalists. Edinburgh: Churchill Livingstone; 1989.

37. Molassiotis A, Bardy J, Finnegan-John J, *et al.* A randomized, controlled trial of acupuncture self-needling as maintenance therapy for cancer-related fatigue after therapist-delivered acupuncture. Ann. Oncol. 2013;24(6):1645–1652.

38. Lee S, Jerng UM, Liu Y, *et al.* The effectiveness and safety of moxibustion for treating cancer-related fatigue: a systematic review and meta-analyses. Support. Care Cancer 2014;22(5):1429–1440.

39. Han K, Kim M, Kim EJ, *et al.* Moxibustion for treating cancer-related fatigue: a multicenter, assessor-blinded, randomized controlled clinical trial. Cancer Med. 2021;10(14):4721–4733.

40. Jean-Pierre P, Figueroa-Moseley CD, Kohli S, *et al.* Assessment of cancer-related fatigue: implications for clinical diagnosis and treatment. Oncologist 2007;12(Suppl. 1):11–21.

Chapter 7

Dry Mouth

Introduction

The fact that dry mouth presents as part of a complex presentation, and there is potential for acupuncture to address this, is expressed below:

> As every clinician knows, patients rarely present with only one symptom. (Professor Christine Miaskowski)[1]

> The dryness is reduced a lot. ('Joe', head and neck cancer survivor)

Few treatments exist to cure dry mouth. A common condition, it has wide-ranging consequences with potentially serious implications for quality of life. Consequences not mentioned in the medical literature, but arising clinically, include the impact on personal relationships and intimacy, such as not being able to kiss a partner because of dry mouth (R Simcock, personal communication, 8 March 2021)

'Dry mouth' is dryness of the oral cavity. Affecting 10–33% of adults in the general population,[2] it is also associated with cancer and its treatments, and is a troublesome consequence specific to treatment for head and neck cancers.

It is likely that acupuncturists regularly encounter patients who experience dry mouth. Despite its frequent occurrence, patients usually do not reported it as a primary complaint.[3] This reticence should not undermine the potentially serious complications relating to this condition.

This chapter looks at dry mouth as it may affect survivors of cancers of any type as well as its specific relationship to head and neck cancers.

TERMINOLOGY

Dry mouth refers to two distinct conditions that may be interrelated and are often confused:

- Xerostomia, which is a subjective feeling of dryness in the mouth.
- Salivary gland hypofunction (SGH), which is a decrease in salivary production that can be *objectively measured*.

People may experience xerostomia even if there is no reduction in their salivary flow rate.

Conversely, people with SGH may or may not experience dry mouth. However, individuals with SGH having a greater than 50% reduction in salivary flow usually also experience xerostomia.[4]

Use of these terms in the medical literature is confusing. In this chapter, I refer to the condition of 'dry mouth' as an umbrella term, except when discussing references that specifically use the terms xerostomia or SGH.

Xerostomia

Xerostomia is a subjective feeling of dryness in the mouth. A common side effect of prescribed medicines, it is experienced widely by the general population. Its prevalence is reported to be increased in women (particularly menopausal) and individuals above 65 years of age.[5] It is also associated with specific diseases, such as Sjögren's syndrome, a condition where the immune system destroys tissues in the saliva-producing glands.

Pharmacotherapy (taking medication) and older age are characteristics associated with cancer survivorship, so it is reasonable to expect that xerostomia may be experienced by cancer survivors generally.

Radiotherapy-induced xerostomia (RIX)

RIX is a chronic, troublesome condition affecting 64–91% of head and neck cancer patients treated with radiotherapy.[6] Although called xerostomia, salivary gland hypofunction may also be associated with this condition.

Salivary gland hypofunction (SGH)

SGH occurs when production of saliva is significantly reduced. This can be measured objectively using tests that measure the output of saliva from the salivary glands (salivary flow).

The parotid, submandibular, and sublingual glands (Figure 7.1), responsible for 90% of saliva production, may be affected by numerous causes. Survivors most likely to be affected by SGH are those treated for head and neck cancers, where surgery, radiotherapy, and sometimes chemotherapy can cause temporary or permanent damage to the salivary glands.

Differentiating between xerostomia and SGH

Historically, medical literature made little or no distinction between xerostomia and SGH. Contemporary medical literature remains confusing in its use of these terms. Thus, xerostomia is often reported as SGH and vice versa. Furthermore, in some conditions or individuals, there is considerable overlap between the two. However, these conditions have specific characteristics:

- SGH is characterised by reduction in stimulated or unstimulated salivary flow which can alter the chemical composition of saliva. Both the rate of flow and chemical composition of saliva can be measured.
- Xerostomia can be assessed only by questioning patients. It cannot be assessed using measurements of salivary flow.[7]

Biomedical perspectives

Aetiology

There are many causes of dry mouth. Some are specific to diseases, including Sjögren's syndrome, diabetes mellitus, and HIV.[4] Box 7.1 lists causes and contributors most likely to affect cancer survivors. A survivor may experience several of these factors concurrently, and be affected by other causes of dry mouth not listed here.

Box 7.1: Common causes of dry mouth experienced by cancer survivors

Factors that may cause or contribute to xerostomia in cancer survivors (listed alphabetically) include:

- Anxiety or depression
- Cancer treatments, including radiotherapy and chemotherapy
- Dehydration
- Malnutrition or nutritional imbalance
- Medication side effects
- Mouth breathing
- Trauma to the salivary glands (including surgery)
- Tumours in the salivary glands

There are many more causes of dry mouth; this is a select list of those most likely to affect cancer survivors.

Table 7.1: Medications causing dry mouth[5]

Class of medication	Medication
Antidepressants	amitriptyline, imipramine, reboxetine, bupropion hydrochloride
Antihistaminic agents	clemastine
Antimigraine drugs	rizatriptan
Anxiolytics	benzodiazepine derivatives: diazepam, oxazepam, lorazepam
Appetite suppressants	sibutramine
Bronchodilators	B2-andrenomimetics, inhalatory glucocorticoids, inhalatory cholinolytics (ipratropium)
Cholinolytic agents	atropine, homatropine, scopolamine
Diuretics	chlorothiazide, hydrochlorothiazide
Hypotensive agents	angiotensin-converting enzyme inhibitors: enalapril, captopril, lisinopril, perindopril
Immunostimulants	interferon-alpha
Neuroleptics	derivatives of phenothiazine, butyrophenone, thioxanthene
Opioids	morphine, codeine, methadone, pethidine

Prescribed medication is a major cause of dry mouth in the general population, with medical literature reporting over 500 agents causing or increasing mouth dryness as a side effect. These medications are called xerogenic, that is, they cause dry mouth (Table 7.1).

Given the large numbers of xerogenic medications in widespread use, we might expect many of our patients (both cancer and non-cancer) to be experiencing dry mouth. In addition to the pharmaceuticals listed in Table 7.1, many chemotherapy agents may be implicated in dry mouth, as well as hormonal therapies such as Arimidex® (anastrozole).[8]

Furthermore, polypharmacy (taking two or more medications daily), may increase the likelihood of dry mouth. One study reported that two medications taken in combination (thyroxine and diuretics) showed a high incidence of xerostomia, while taken independently of each other showed no significant link, suggesting that interactions between certain drugs may increase the likelihood of dry mouth.[7]

Dry mouth is also common among older adults, with studies reporting 30% or more of the population aged 65 and over being affected.[4] This is not thought to be due to age-related deterioration of the salivary glands, as healthy older individuals do not demonstrate significant decreases in salivary gland flow. Rather, dry mouth among older adults may result from the increase in other systemic disorders that occur with age and/or the associated (often multiple) medications taken to manage these.[2,4,7]

This is pertinent to cancer survivorship, as many survivors are older, have multiple comorbidities, and may be using polypharmacy to manage these comorbidities and the consequences of cancer treatment. Many also experience anxiety or depression. Some may also have experienced trauma to the salivary glands, through surgery and radiotherapy, as discussed under 'Radiotherapy-induced xerostomia' below.

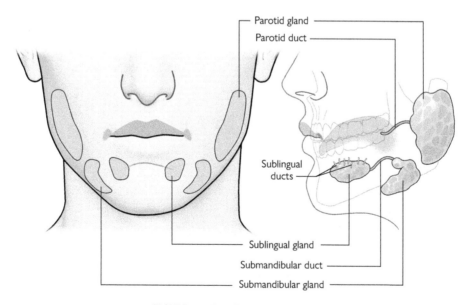

FIGURE 7.1: THE SALIVARY GLANDS

The importance of saliva

Potential consequences of dry mouth are wide-ranging and may have serious implications. Saliva, a key element in maintaining aspects of health (Table 7.2), is produced in healthy individuals at a rate of 0.5-1.5 litres per day. About 90% of saliva is produced by three major pairs of salivary glands – the parotid, submandibular, and sublingual, with the remaining 10% produced by other minor glands distributed in the mouth (Figure 7.1).

Table 7.2: Saliva's many functions in maintaining health[2,3,4]

Function of saliva	How saliva achieves this
Moisten oral mucosa and maintain oral health	• Antibacterial, antifungal, and antiviral agents in saliva balance oral flora, helping to prevent oral infections. • Minerals present in saliva help to maintain tooth enamel. • Saliva washes food residue from the teeth.
Facilitate digestive processes	• Saliva enhances taste and lubricates food making it easier to chew and swallow; it neutralises potentially damaging food, drink, and bacterial acids. • Enzymes in saliva initiate digestion of starches and fats.
Aid the immune system	• Numerous salivary components have protective antimicrobial effects against harmful microorganisms.
Facilitate speech	• Lubricates and moistens the inside of the mouth.
Retain removable prostheses (such as dentures)	• The layer of saliva between the gums and the denture helps keep oral health devices in place.

Consequences of dry mouth

Dry mouth can have a profound effect on daily living, impacting quality of life. People with severe xerostomia are reported to be two to five times more likely to experience negative impacts on health.[7] Box 7.2 lists some common effects of dry mouth. Head and neck cancer survivors may experience more troublesome effects, associated with the consequences of surgery (such as excision of the tongue) and radiotherapy.

Box 7.2: Some common effects of dry mouth[2,4,5,7]

Oral health

- Increased risk of dental caries
- Periodontal (gum) disease
- Oral infections such as candidiasis
- Salivary gland infections
- Halitosis
- Oral soreness and burning
- Difficulty or impossibility of wearing denture

Impaired daily activities

- Difficulty chewing and swallowing food

- Need for frequent consumption of fluids during meals
- Impaired taste
- Self-consciousness, embarrassment, and discomfort while eating
- Reduced nutritional uptake
- Difficulty speaking
- Impaired sleep

Quality of life

- Increased worry, tension
- Difficulty relaxing
- Depressive thoughts
- Less satisfaction with life
- Inability to function
- Feeling self-conscious
- Having to interrupt meals
- Inability to carry out usual activities
- Difficulty doing usual jobs

Treatments for dry mouth

Few treatments exist to cure dry mouth. Most available remedies aim to avoid or alleviate discomfort and pain and prevent complications. It may be necessary for healthcare providers to collaborate in offering individuals a range of approaches to manage dry mouth.[3] Some measures that may reduce or prevent mouth dryness are listed in Box 7.3.

Box 7.3: Measures to reduce or prevent dry mouth

- Avoid dehydration – increase fluid intake.
- Avoid irritants – including smoking, alcohol, and drinks containing caffeine.
- Breathe through the nose instead of the mouth.
- Manage anxiety and depression (counselling may be appropriate).
- Practise good oral hygiene – regular dental check-ups are essential, as is oral hygiene to prevent tooth decay, gum disease, and other infections.
- Review medication – whenever possible, xerogenic medications should be replaced with substitutes (e.g. serotonin reuptake inhibitors cause less mouth dryness than tricyclic antidepressants). Alterations to the timing or dosing schedules, such as avoiding taking medications at night when salivary flow is lowest, may reduce symptoms of dry mouth.[4]
- Using a humidifier, especially at night, may ease discomfort.

See also 'Salivary substitutes and stimulants' below.

The importance of oral hygiene

Oral health is a primary concern for people experiencing dry mouth. Patient education and support in establishing systematic, consistent oral hygiene is a priority for managing the condition and preventing complications.

This is especially important for people with SGH, as lowered saliva production results in a lowered pH, enabling bacteria to flourish in the mouth. This can lead to dental caries, periodontal disease, and erosion of dental enamel; acute oral mucositis and candidiasis are common conditions that may impact people treated for head and neck cancers.[3]

ESSENTIALS

Individuals with low salivary output can reduce the risk of oral complications by:[4]

- having frequent (every four to six months) dental examinations
- practising meticulous oral hygiene
- maintaining a low-sugar diet
- using a topical fluoride (toothpaste, mouthwash) regularly.

Individuals should work with their dentists to develop the specific healthcare regimen required; acupuncturists can reinforce the message of the importance of good dental care.

Salivary substitutes and stimulants

Measures offering temporary symptomatic relief include:

- Salivary substitutes, in the form of gels, liquids, sprays, pastilles or tablets.
- Taking sips of water or sugar-free fizzy drinks to help keep the mouth moist.
- Rinsing the mouth with fat (a teaspoon of vegetable oil or a small amount of softened butter or spread) may also be helpful, especially at night.[9]

Salivary stimulants may be non-pharmaceutical or pharmaceutical products. For those individuals who can produce some saliva, saliva production can be encouraged by sucking sugar-free sweets, chewing sugar-free gum, or trying food items such as pineapple chunks, ice cubes, yogurt, and buttermilk.

Prescription medications that influence salivary glands to increase saliva production (called secretagogues or sialagogues) include:

- pilocarpine
- cevimeline
- bethanechol.

These are effective if damage to the glands is partial or temporary; their relief lasts for only a few hours after intake, so they must be taken frequently. Two to three months of continuous pilocarpine may be needed before temporarily damaged salivary glands are restimulated. Medication side effects may include dizziness, sweating, flushing, urinary urgency, nausea, and vomiting.[3,9]

Other remedies

Other approaches include major interventions, such as surgical transfer of the submandibular gland in survivors with RIX and neuroelectrical stimulation. Pre-clinical and experimental trials are investigating interventions such as proton beam radiotherapy (PBRT), gene therapy, and stem cell transfer. Less dramatic interventions include hyperbaric oxygen treatment, hypnosis, massage of the salivary glands, mouth exercises, and acupuncture.[3,6,10,11]

Radiotherapy-induced xerostomia (RIX)

TERMINOLOGY

Head and neck cancer is a term that includes a variety of cancers arising in the head or neck region, including in the nasal cavity, sinuses, lips, mouth, salivary glands, throat, or larynx. It is the sixth most common cancer worldwide, with 890,000 new cases and 450,000 deaths in 2018.[12]

Dry mouth is significantly associated with treatment of head and neck cancer. As it is caused by radiation damage to the salivary glands (Box 7.4), it is called radiotherapy-induced xerostomia (RIX). However, the condition involves both xerostomia and SGH, as reduction in salivary flow is present.[10,13] Estimates suggest that about 9% of head and neck cancer patients report xerostomia prior to radiotherapy, while over 80% show signs of xerostomia and SGH following radiotherapy.[6,11]

RIX may arise in the first week of conventional radiotherapy, with salivary flow decreasing by up to 60%. This may then diminish to as low as 20% of normal flow in the subsequent five to seven weeks, with possible continued decline for some months after the end of radiotherapy.[14]

Partial or full recovery, possible for some survivors, may occur during the 12–18 months following cancer treatment. There are also some reports that salivary output can recover many years after radiotherapy. However, 41% of head and neck cancer survivors may still be affected five years after radiotherapy,[15] and RIX usually becomes an irreversible, life-long consequence of treatment, with wide-ranging effects on physical function and quality of life.[14]

To minimise the risk of xerostomia and SGH, guidelines for the treatment of head and neck cancers recommend the use of conformal radiotherapy techniques such as intensity modulated radiotherapy (IMRT), including tomography, or volumetric modulated arc therapy (VMAT).[10] Conformal radiotherapy shapes the radiation beams to closely fit the area of cancer.[16] This allows a more accurate delivery of radiation dose to the tumour, while better sparing the surrounding tissues, including the salivary glands. This reduces damage, and increases potential recovery, but is not always an option when treating head and neck cancers.

Box 7.4: An oncologist explains

Dr Richard Simcock, consultant clinical oncologist, explains how radiotherapy doses are adjusted to preserve the salivary glands in curative intent treatments for head and neck cancers.

In the treatment of head and neck cancer, the high dose of radiotherapy to cure a cancer often lies within a volume that is very close to, or encompasses, the nearby salivary glands. This dose of radiotherapy is damaging to the salivary glands, leading to changes to flow in the composition of saliva.

Damage to the salivary glands may be temporary or permanent, depending on a variety of factors, including the dose of radiotherapy. There are well-recognised thresholds to radiotherapy and modern radiotherapy techniques, such as intensity modulated radiotherapy, that are designed to respect (as much as possible) these thresholds.

In planning modern radiotherapy, the salivary glands (particularly the two large parotid glands) are considered an 'organ at risk' (OAR). As an example, a dose of radiotherapy required to treat most squamous cell cancers of the head and neck would be 65 Gray in 30 Fractions. We recognise that an average dose of greater than 26 Gray received by the salivary glands during this treatment would be enough to render them permanently non-functional.

While we focus our intention on preserving large parotid glands from radiotherapy, it is currently not common practice to be able to protect the smaller salivary glands (submandibular and sublingual), and some authors believe that salivary recovery comes from preservation of the multiple tiny salivary glands that are present throughout the oral cavity.

Assessment

SGH can be measured objectively using a variety of methods ranging from the use of saliva-collecting strips to highly technological imaging techniques.[4] As a subjective condition, xerostomia (the 'perception of dry mouth') is assessed by questioning the patient.[7]

The Xerostomia Index (XI) was developed to assess severity of dry mouth and to measure changes in the condition over time.[7,17,18] Its 11 statements provide an insight into the symptoms of dry mouth.

Acupuncturists can easily administer this questionnaire (Table 7.3) to measure changes in the condition. To use, have the patient score each item according to the value indicated in the respective column. The total possible score is 55. Higher scores indicate more troublesome symptoms. For follow-up, repeat the questionnaire.

A change in total score of six or more points is clinically significant, which means the patient can notice a difference.[18]

Table 7.3: The Xerostomia Inventory[7]

	Never	Hardly ever	Occasionally	Frequently	Very often
Item/score	I	2	3	4	5
My mouth feels dry					
I have difficulty in eating dry foods					
I get up at night to drink					
My mouth feels dry when eating a meal					
I sip liquids to aid in swallowing food					
I suck sweets or cough lollies to relieve dry mouth					
I have difficulties swallowing certain foods					
The skin of my face feels dry					
My eyes feel dry					
My lips feel dry					
The inside of my nose feels dry					
TOTAL SCORE /55					

Lifestyle advice

In addition to the measures listed in Box 7.3, survivors experiencing dry mouth should ensure they have a well-balanced diet. This is challenging for head and neck cancer survivors, who may experience difficulties with chewing and swallowing.

Additional resources

Cancer information websites offer information about managing dry mouth, particularly RIX. As dry mouth has serious implications for oral health, dental health professionals also provide information and tips for managing xerostomia and SGH.

Acupuncture in the medical literature

Medical literature generally takes a positive view of the role of acupuncture in the management of xerostomia, specifically RIX. Acupuncture is regarded as safe intervention, with minimal side effects, and is reported to be clinically effective for some patients.[5,10,19] There is advice to health professionals to 'explore the use of acupuncture for the management of their cancer patients with xerostomia'[3] and to manage RIX by using acupuncture 'to stimulate salivary gland secretion and to alleviate xerostomia'.[10]

Some commentators say the evidence from studies is poor and further research is needed.[2,13,20,21] One systematic review concludes that evidence is lacking for acupuncture's effect on objective salivary flow, but it improves the symptoms of cancer-induced xerostomia.[22]

East Asian medicine perspectives
General management of dry mouth
Dry mouth is a condition experienced by many patients other than those treated for head and neck cancer, so it is worth exploring some points that address the problem generally. Deadman *et al.* list numerous points indicated for dry mouth (Table 7.4),[23] which could be used as appropriate to the diagnosis of the individual patient.

Table 7.4: Points indicated for dry mouth as listed in Deadman *et al.*[23]

Point	Commentary
LU-5 *Chize*	Clears heat from the Lung in cases of deficiency heat where there may be tidal fever or taxation fever and dry mouth and tongue.
Ll-1 *Shangyang*	Clears heat.
Ll-2 *Erjian*	Expels wind, clears heat; especially for dry throat arising from accumulated heat in the Stomach and Large Intestine.
ST-19 *Burong*	No commentary supplied relating specifically to dry mouth.
BL-13 *Feishu*	Tonifies Lung qi and nourishes Lung yin.
BL-18 *Ganshu*	Spreads Liver qi.
BL-27 *Xiaochangshu*	For dry mouth that is hard to endure.
P-3 *Quze*	Clears heat which has reached the nutritive and Blood levels giving rise to agitation and restlessness, dry mouth, and haemorrhage from the Lung and Stomach.
TB-1 *Guanchong*	Clears upper jiao heat; particularly for when exterior pathogenic heat penetrates deeper to attack the Pericardium and the heat condenses the body fluids to form phlegm. Phlegm heat then obstructs the Pericardium and disturbs the spirit, giving rise to a range of symptoms including dry mouth with a bitter taste.
TB-4 *Yangchi*	For dry mouth with agitation, oppression.
LIV-14 *Qimen*	No commentary supplied relating specifically to dry mouth.
REN-23 *Lianquan*	Regulates the production of fluids in the mouth, either in the case of excess spittle or for dryness of the mouth and thirst. For this purpose, the needle is directed alternately towards the extraordinary points M-HN-20 *Jinjin* and *Yuye* located below the tongue.
REN-24 *Chengjian*	Can affect the production of fluids in the mouth and is indicated for excessive production of watery saliva, dry mouth.
DU-12 *Shenzhu*	Clears heat from the Lung and Heart.

Chinese medicine theories
In *Management of Cancer with Chinese Medicine,* Professor Li Peiwen provides detailed information from a CM perspective about radiotherapy-induced dry mouth and tongue in head and neck cancers.[24]

In CM theory, dry mouth belongs to the Fire Dryness type of Dryness patterns. The five *zang* organs store Essence, Blood and Body Fluids, and 'spittle' is generated from the transformation of qi and Blood. Li cites the *Su Wen: Xuan Ming Wu Qi Lun Pian* (Plain Questions: Xuan Ming's discussion on Five Qi), which says that '...the Spleen forms saliva and the Kidneys form spittle...'. The aetiology and pathology of dry mouth are summarised in Table 7.5.

Table 7.5: Aetiology and pathology of Fire Dryness implicated in dry mouth and tongue[24]

Note:

Capitalisation in this table is as per Li Peiwen's text.

Aetiology	Pathology
Dryness resulting from damage to the internal organs	• Failure of the Spleen and Stomach to send Body Fluids upwards causes saliva to diminish and the mouth to become dry. • Insufficiency of Kidney Yin depletes Body Fluids. • Yin is damaged by Deficiency of Liver-Blood and Lung-Dryness.
Dryness related to invasion of pathogenic factors	• Pathogenic Fire flames upward; this is the strongest factor in creating Dryness. • Invasion of pathogenic Warmth, Heat, and Dryness consumes Body Fluids and Blood, preventing adequate moistening of the orifices and passages.
Yin deficiency	• Kidney Yin may be consumed by constitutional Yin Deficiency, injury to the Essence, loss of Blood and Body Fluids. • Yin Deficiency generates internal Heat, which transforms into Fire. Deficiency Fire flaming upwards scorches Yin Liquids. • Prolonged Yin Deficiency affects Yang, causing deficiency of the Zang organs, Qi, and Blood.
Emotional disturbances	• Liver Depression and Qi Stagnation result from emotional disturbances. • Heat transforms into Fire, which scorches the Yin Liquids and prevents Body Fluids rising to the mouth.
Summary	Factors generating Dryness can be summarised as: • Deficiency of or damage to the Zang-Fu organs depriving the Body Fluids of their source • Spleen Deficiency causing failure of distribution of the Body Fluids throughout the body. • Heat and Fire scorching Yin, damaging Body Fluids and consuming the Blood. • Excessive loss of Blood and Body Fluids consuming Kidney Yin.

To reduce atrophy of the oral glands in patients undergoing radiotherapy to the neck and upper chest, Li supplies a list acupuncture points (Box 7.5) to use in general treatment to:

- clear Heat and relieve Toxicity
- nourish yin and moisten the Lungs.

> ### Box 7.5: Commonly used points to reduce oral atrophy of the glands caused by radiotherapy
>
> - LU-7 *Lieque*
> - LU-10 *Yuji*
> - Ll-4 *Hegu*
> - Kl-6 *Zhaohai*
> - P-4 *Ximen*
> - TB-17 *Yifeng*
> - GB-20 *Fengchi*
> - REN-23 *Lianquan*

Li does not provide rationale or commentary for these points. His general needling technique is to perform lifting and thrusting manipulation until qi is obtained and retain the needles for 20–30 minutes, manipulating at intervals during retention. He suggests treatment should be every day or every other day.

The items on the Xerostomia Inventory (Table 7.3) suggest yin deficiency is implicated in dry mouth, and this is confirmed by Li's pattern identification (Table 7.6), listing four yin deficiency patterns.

Table 7.6: Li's pattern identification for dry mouth

Yin deficiency patterns	Other patterns
- Lung Yin - Stomach and Spleen Yin - Liver Yin - Kidney Yin	- Liver Depression, Qi stagnation, and Blood stasis - Deficiency of Yin and Yang - Stomach and Spleen Qi Deficiency

Table 7.7 presents Li's pattern identification, with detailed treatment principles and recommended points. For further information on signs and symptoms I refer the reader to his excellent book.[24]

Table 7.7: Summary of Li's TCM patterns, treatment principles, and points for treating xerostomia

Note: The main principles and points for treating yin deficiency patterns are highlighted in **bold**. Additional points are added according to differentiation.

	Yin Deficiency predominately of the:				Liver Depression, Qi stagnation, Blood Stasis	Yin and Yang Xu*	Spleen/ Stomach Qi Xu*
	Kidney	Lung	Spleen/Stomach	Liver			
Enrich Yin, moisten dryness			**KID-6 LU-7**				
Generate body fluids, alleviate thirst (local points)			**TB-17 GB-20 REN-23**		GB-20 REN-23 DU-14	TB-17 DU-14	REN-23 DU-14
Promote upward movement of Body Fluids			**REN-17**				REN-17
Tonify Kidney Yin (clear heat)	KID-3 KID-7	KID-3		KID-3		KID-3 (HE-6)	
Tonify Kidney Qi	BL-23 GB-25						
Tonify Kidney Yang						BL-23 REN-4	
Tonify Lung Yin, regulate Lung Qi		BL-13 LU-1 LU-10					
Tonify Stomach/Spleen Qi, strengthen transformation and transportation			BL-20 BL-21 LIV-13 ST-36 REN-12		ST-36	BL-20 ST-36	BL-20 BL-21 LIV-13 ST-36
Regulate Liver, tonify Liver Yin				BL-18 LIV-3	LIV-3 LI-4		
Dredge Liver, relieve Depression					BL-18 LIV-14 GB-34 P-6		
Invigorate Blood, resolve Blood Stasis					SP-6 BL-17		
Tonify Liver, Spleen, Kidney	SP-6			SP-6			
Clear deficiency heat, treat dry mouth				P-4			
Resolve damp, turbidity							SP-9 ST-25

*Moxibustion is indicated, although Li is not specific about points.

Five Element approaches

With its focus on body, mind, and spirit, Five Element acupuncture is indicated for addressing anxiety associated with dry mouth, as well as for addressing the emotional aspects listed by Li.

In the research cited below, Blom *et al.*[25] point out that salivary flow may be affected by changes to the individual's overall health condition, including stress, depression, and the common cold. Strengthening the constitution, a fundamental principle of Five Element acupuncture, is beneficial here. Furthermore, Pfister *et al.*[26] found that xerostomia can be addressed within more generalised treatment using a minimal number of points, suggesting that this can be easily incorporated into Five Element treatments.

Moxibustion for dry mouth

Li advocates the use of moxibustion when the mixed pattern of deficient yin and yang is related to xerostomia, and when it is the result of Spleen and Stomach qi deficiency (Table 7.7). As he does not provide instructions, one assumes moxa is applied to body points, to avoid the possibility of burning the face.

Head and neck cancer patients may lack sensitivity to heat, due to tissue damage from surgical scarring and/or radiotherapy. Even tiger warmers should be used with caution, as illustrated in Joe's case study at the end of this chapter. Clinically, we have found that head and neck cancer patients fitted with a breathing stoma may be sensitive to moxa smoke, even from smokeless moxa.[27]

Research perspectives

The evidence base for using acupuncture to manage dry mouth

Using acupuncture to manage RIX has attracted much research effort, with several papers in the scientific literature. A range of acupuncture approaches have been researched, including electrical acupuncture and acupuncture-like transcutaneous electrical nerve stimulations (ALTENS).[28]

Of the studies published, I have selected five that demonstrate a variety of approaches and results (Table 7.8). These reveal important information about the nature and progress of acupuncture treatment of dry mouth.

Several studies investigate using acupuncture to prevent RIX during radiotherapy; I have not included these as this book focuses on survivorship post active treatment.

Table 7.8: Five studies using acupuncture in the management of RIX

Author (Publication date)	Blom et al.[25] (1996)	Cho et al.[29] (2008)	Garcia et al.[30] (2009)	Simcock et al.[35] (2013)	Pfister et al.[36] (2010)
Country	Sweden	South Korea	USA	UK	USA
Research design	RCT	RCT	Single arm pilot	RCT	RCT
Total participants	38	12	19	145	58
Time from RT	5 months–12.5 years	2–60 months	5–96 months	18–104 months	≥ 3 months since RT
Treatment frequency/ duration	2x/week for 6 weeks (12 treatments), repeated after a 2-week break (24 total)	2x/week for 6 weeks (12 total)	2x/week for 4 weeks (8 total)	1x/week for 8 weeks (8 total)	1x/week for 4 weeks (4 total) with additional 5th treatment post assessment
Points chosen	**AURICULAR** 2–4 from: *Kidney Mouth Parotid gland Shenmen Stomach Subcortex Sympathetic* **LOCAL/DISTAL** 5–8 chosen from: LI-4 LI-10 LI-11 LI-18 ST-3 ST-5 ST-6 ST-7 ST-36 SP-3 SP-6 SP-8 HE-7 SI-3 SI-17 KID-3 KID-5 KID-7 P-6 LIV-3 DU-20	**LOCAL/DISTAL** LI-4 ST-6 ST-36 SP-6	**AURICULAR** *Point Zero Salivary gland 2 Shenmen* **LOCAL/DISTAL** LU-7 LI-1 *(primed)* ST-36 REN-24	**AURICULAR** *Modified Point Zero Salivary gland 2 Shenmen* **LOCAL/DISTAL** LI-20 LI-2	**AURICULAR** *Shenmen* **LOCAL/DISTAL** LI-4 SP-6 DU-20 Extra point *Luozhen* Plus: LI-2 *Erjian* for patients with dry mouth And: Individualised points for pain treatment according to patient's pain and its locations.
Improvements	Improved salivary flow rates after 12 treatments, with improvement lasting for a year.	Real acu increased unstimulated salivary flow rates, and improved score for dry mouth on a xerostomia questionnaire.	Significant improvement at end of treatment and 1 month later, on Xerostomia Inventory (p=.0004, p=.0001), with improved physical wellbeing at follow-up. No significant changes in salivary flow rates.	Significant reductions in patient reports of severe dry mouth (p=.03), sticky saliva (p=.048), needing to sip fluids to swallow food (p=.011), and in waking at night to drink (p=.013). No significant changes in salivary flow rates.	Although, xerostomia was a secondary outcome in this study designed to measure pain and dysfunction, there were significant improvements on Xerostomia Inventory scores (p=.02).

Blom et al.: Early pioneers of acupuncture for RIX

In a randomised controlled trial (RCT) focusing on increase in salivary flow rates, 20 participants received true acupuncture and 18 received superficial acupuncture. They were followed up for one year after the end of acupuncture treatment (EOT).[25]

After 12 treatments, salivary flow rates increased by more than 20% in over half the true acupuncture group. The research team made important observations, finding that factors influencing the outcome included:

- the size of the radiated area
- the patient's history of surgery and radiotherapy
- the time interval between radiotherapy and the commencement of acupuncture
- the general health of the patient
- medications taken.

They observed that acupuncture was effective only when the function of the salivary glands was diminished, and not destroyed. However, they found that recovery was possible in patients who had had severe xerostomia for a long time (15 months to over seven years), although in such cases, it took longer to stabilise the condition.

Finally, they observed that sudden decreases in salivary flow following a pattern of improvement were related to changes in the patient's overall health condition, including factors such as depression, stress, common cold, changes in medication, metastases, hormonal cancer treatments, and surgery.

Garcia et al.: Can acupuncture reverse RIX?

This small pilot study aimed to investigate whether RIX could be reversed using acupuncture.[30] It reported improvements in the subjective symptoms of dry mouth as early as two weeks after starting acupuncture, and recorded benefits remaining for four weeks after EOT.

Showing no significant changes in objectively measured salivary flow rates, this study reported significant improvements in subjective reports of dry mouth symptoms: the overall Xerostomia Inventory score decrease by 6.3 points (p=.0004) EOT, thus showing a clinically significant change.

The study also reported some significant improvements in physical wellbeing and symptoms related to head and neck cancer.[30]

Simcock et al.: acupuncture for RIX in a group setting

This RCT compared a standardised acupuncture protocol using body and auricular points delivered in a group setting with patient education about oral care.[15] Acupuncture compared with oral care produced significant reductions in patient reports of severe dry mouth (p=.031), sticky saliva (p=.048), needing to sip fluids to swallow food (p=.011) and waking up at night to drink (p=.013). There were no significant changes in stimulated or unstimulated saliva flow over time.

The researchers found that subjective sensations of oral dryness were unrelated to salivary flow rates. This supports the view that xerostomia and SGH are independent of each other, and that symptoms of dry mouth may be improved even if salivary rates are not.

In a feasibility study preparatory to the RCT, the researchers reported the benefits of the group aspect of acupuncture treatment:[31]

- Having one acupuncturist treat many patients at one time reduced costs of treatment.
- Patients benefitted from being in a group of people with similar healthcare experiences, finding it both comforting and useful for sharing information and experiences.

Pfister *et al.*: acupuncture for pain and dysfunction

I have included this RCT as it most nearly resembles the clinical reality of treating head and neck cancer patients (see Joe's case study later in this chapter).[26] That is, they present with a complex symptom burden, of which dry mouth is merely a part, and their priorities for treatment may focus on symptoms such as pain and lack of function.

In this RCT, 28 head and neck cancer patients received four acupuncture treatments and were compared with 30 patients who received usual care. The primary outcome was reduction of pain and dysfunction; dry mouth was a secondary outcome.

Only one acupuncture point, Ll-2 *Erjian*, was chosen to specifically address xerostomia. Significant reduction in scores on the Xerostomia Inventory suggest that RIX can be treated alongside other troublesome symptoms, using a minimal number of points.

Commentary on the point selection for these studies

The outstanding characteristic is the range of points used, with very little consistency in point selection across the studies. The authors provide scant detail about the rationale for point selection. Few of the points accord with those recommended by Li and Deadman *et al.* (discussed previously) and all the studies supplement body points with auricular acupuncture. In addition, Simcock *et al.* and Blom *et al.* use facial points.

Ll-2 *Erjian* is the only body point repeated across studies, and in wider reading of research papers, this is a most popular point. As a ying-spring point, it clears heat, and as a water point on the Large Intestine Metal channel, it is used for the treatment of deficiency patterns of the Kidney.[23] Thus, Ll-2 *Erjian* fulfils two of Li's general treatment principles – clearing heat and nourishing yin.

Auricular *Shenmen* is used in four studies (all except Cho *et al.*). Oleson classifies this as a 'primary master point', one that is used in almost all treatment plans for alleviating a vast variety of health disorders.[32] Abbate calls it the 'foremost point in the treatment of virtually every disease'. Likening it to HE-7 *Shenmen* – the Earth point and sedation point of the Heart meridian – she suggests it adds 'dampness' to the body, which calms, grounds, and increases receptivity to treatment, and it should therefore be the first point treated in an ear acupuncture prescription.[33]

The evidence base for using moxibustion for xerostomia

There are no studies published in the English language about moxibustion for xerostomia.

Clinical perspectives
Tips from my clinical experience

- Although dry mouth considerably impacts quality of life, patients usually do not present this as a main complaint.[3] I find survivors may mention it in passing, or it is identified through specific questioning. Even for head and neck cancer survivors (nearly all of whom experience dry mouth), other consequences of treatment may take priority for treatment.
- Considerable improvements in dry mouth symptoms are possible, even when treated as part of managing more pressing symptoms, as demonstrated in Joe's case study (see below).
- I find using extraordinary meridians is a beneficial approach.
- I tend to avoid needling head and neck cancer patients in facial areas that are scarred from surgery or radiotherapy. If possible, I use contralateral face points; if this is not possible, I rely on distal points.
- Similarly, for head and neck cancer patients, I avoid using moxa on skin damaged by cancer treatments, even tiger warmers. (Many patients also report they have suffered burning from wheat bags heated in the microwave, so these too should be used with caution.)
- I teach patients with dry mouth to self-manage by applying acupressure to REN-24 Chengjiang (*Container of fluids*), which is indicated for dry mouth. Many patients report this is helpful for stimulating salivary flow, and it offers temporary relief.
- Tongue diagnosis may be difficult or impossible to conduct with some head and neck cancer patients, who may have trouble opening the mouth and/or protruding the tongue. In some survivors, part or all the tongue may be excised, and replaced by a 'flap' made from muscle taken from elsewhere in the body.

Patient perspectives

CASE STUDY: JOE AND USING THE EXTRAORDINARY MERIDIANS TO MANAGE RIX
Background

Joe participated in a study investigating using acupuncture to manage cancer treatment-related lymphoedema. Participants were offered a series of seven acupuncture treatments with the option to have a further six treatments (see Chapter 9, Cancer Treatment-Related Lymphoedema). Joe worked with me to write a previously published case study, of which this is an adapted version.[27]

As with many head and neck cancer survivors, Joe presented with complex physical and emotional symptoms, and my treatment plan attempted to address as many of these as possible. In this case study, I focus mainly on the changes in mouth dryness.

Cancer history

Joe, aged 61, was diagnosed with squamous cell carcinoma of the right mandible nine months before joining the study. Surgery, during which a bone graft from the right leg was used to reconstruct his jaw, was followed by radiotherapy. Three months from completing these treatments, Joe felt the lymphoedema that developed post surgery was well managed by the lymphoedema service and his own self-management.

His priorities for acupuncture treatment focused on other symptoms. Numbness affected his lower lip, chin, neck, and half of his tongue on the right side. Joe hoped acupuncture would make his face feel 'more vibrant'. Joe found eating difficult due to the loss of teeth removed during surgery, combined with his inability to open his mouth fully.

Mouth dryness (xerostomia) added to his discomfort. This was more troublesome at night than during the day and Joe woke every two hours to sip water and apply mouth-moistening gel.

Questioning the systems

Sleep: A light sleeper, managed six to seven hours of broken sleep; occasional disturbing dreams.

Appetite: 'Okay'; Joe, a vegetarian, maintained his weight at about 80 kilos during treatment by consuming 2500 calories a day. Food needed to be mashed or ground.

Thirst: Although not thirsty, drank a lot of fluid to counteract the 'sticky dryness' in his mouth.

Bowels: Occasionally sluggish since cancer treatment.

Other information: Joe worked abroad in business his entire career, bringing his family back to England on his retirement two years previously. Having led a 'simple life' with no history of smoking or other carcinogenic habits, he was bewildered by having cancer. He strove to maintain an attitude of acceptance of his diagnosis and treatment.

Physical examination: Tongue: Very red, peeled in patches, with thick white curds at the root, and a distended blue vein on the left underside. **Pulses:** Big middle pulse on left; slippery middle pulse on right.

Diagnosis: CF: Sadness of demeanour and a whitish hue around the eyes suggested Joe was a Metal CF.

Treatment approach

Although Joe reported having dry mouth, his treatment priorities were to:

- alleviate the numbness of his right lip, tongue, and neck
- improve opening his mouth.

His priority activity was to improve chewing and sensation when eating.

In the first seven treatments, my treatment plan was primarily to relieve as much physical distress as possible.

Extraordinary meridians are particularly beneficial when working with head and neck cancer survivors, as they have a wide range of influence on the body (see Chapter 5, Toolkit). I often use the Yang Linking Vessel for its influence over the lateral side of the head and neck, and for its indications for problems of the mouth, tongue, teeth, gums, and neck.[34] It also addresses problems along the leg, often affected by removal of bone for implantation in the jaw.

As Joe was participating in a lymphoedema study, I also used the Directing Vessel and Triple Burner to promote transformation and transportation of fluids to deal with the swelling (see Chapter 9, Cancer Treatment-Related Lymphoedema, and Chapter 5, Toolkit).

To deal with the numbness, restricted movement, and mouth dryness, I used points on the Stomach channel; facial points were needled contralateral to the affected side. Treatments and progress through his first seven treatments are detailed in Table 7.9. As per the research protocol, I cleared blocks to treatment (Aggressive Energy and Internal Dragons) in the first two treatments (see Chapter 5, Toolkit).

I avoided needling the affected side of his face (right side). In general, I tend to avoid needling the affected area in head and neck cancer patients, even when they do not have lymphoedema. I prefer to avoid needling areas that have been severely traumatised by surgery and radiotherapy and I use the principle of treating the opposite side to address issues. (During this study, I also avoided using body points on the affected side of the upper body in head and neck cancer survivors. I think this may have been over-cautious, and now would use body points below the neck on the affected side.)

Treatment and progress – the first seven treatments

Table 7.9: Joe's treatments 1–7

Notes:

For details of treatments see Chapter 5, Toolkit.

For the functions of the individual points, refer to Deadman *et al. A Manual of Acupuncture*.[23]

Abbreviations: Tx treatment; **RS** right side; **LS** left side

Tx	Tx principles	Points: no needles in RS of face and neck	Notes
I	Clear block to treatment: Aggressive Energy (AE) Drain	BL-13 *Feishu* (LS) BL-14 *Jueyinshu* (LS) BL-15 *Xinshu* (LS) BL-18 *Ganshu* (LS) BL-20 *Pishu* (LS) BL-23 *Shenshu* (LS) Plus 3 check needles	Needled unilaterally on unaffected side.
2	Clear block to treatment: Internal Dragons (IDs)	Master point 0.25 cun below REN-15 *Jiuwei* ST-25 *Tianshu* ST-32 *Futu* ST-41 *Jiexi*	
	Support spirit (using yuan source points of Fire)	SI-4 *Wangu* (LS) HE-7 *Shenmen* (LS)	

3	Promote transportation, transformation and excretion of fluids	Open *Ren Mai*: LU-7 *Lieque* (LS) and KID-6 *Zhaohai* (RS) Plus REN-9 *Shuifen* REN-12 *Zhongwan* TB-5 *Waiguan* (LS)	
	Address xerostomia, facial swelling and stiffness	REN-24 *Chengjiang* ST-4 *Dicang* (LS) ST-5 *Daying* (LS) ST-6 *Jiache* (LS)	
	Tonify qi	ST-36 *Zusanli* (LS)	
4	Promote transportation, transformation, and excretion of fluids	As per Tx 3	
	Address xerostomia, facial swelling and stiffness	As per Tx 3 Plus: LI-6 *Pianli* (LS)	
5	Influence lateral aspect of head and neck	Open Yang Linking Vessel: TB-5 *Waiguan* (LS) GB-41 *Zulinqi* (RS)	
	Influence facial sensation and oedema	ST-4 *Dicang* (LS) ST-5 *Daying* (LS) ST-6 *Jiache* (LS) ST-43 *Xiangu* (LS) ST-44 *Neiting* (RS)	
	Promote transportation, transformation, and excretion of fluids	REN-9 *Shuifen* REN-12 *Zhongwan* REN-24 *Chengjiang*	
6	Support spirit	KID-25 *Shencang* KID-27 *Shufu*	Direct moxa, 3 cones, left side only, no needling.
	Influence lateral aspect of head and neck Influence facial sensation and oedema Promote transportation, transformation, and excretion of fluids	As per Tx 5	
7	Clear block to treatment: Internal Dragons (IDs) (to address dreams)	As per Tx 2	
	Calm shen	REN-17 *Shanzhong*	Direct moxa, 3 cones, no needling.
	Improve facial sensation	ST-7 *Xiaguan* (LS)	
	Regulate flow of saliva	REN-24 *Chengjiang*	

Progress through treatment

Tx 1: After this treatment, Joe felt a sensation of warmth in the affected areas of his head and neck, which lasted for about an hour afterwards; otherwise, he noticed no major changes.

Tx 2: Joe experienced 'moistness' in his mouth after this treatment, but dryness increased as the week progressed.

Tx 3: Again, dryness improved, especially at night, enabling him to sleep longer than his usual two hours (sometimes for three to four hours).

Tx 4–7: After Tx 4, he only needed to use mouth gels twice during the night for the dryness. At Tx 6, he reported a 'big improvement'; he was usually getting up once a night. At Tx 7, he was still reporting improvements, and could sleep regularly for three to four hours at a stretch.

Improvements in facial sensations

Acupuncture improved the sensations in Joe's face, and over this period, the numbness diminished. After Tx 2, Joe experienced sensations in his tongue. During subsequent sessions, he reported feelings of movement like those experienced when he carried out his simple lymphatic drainage exercises to move lymph; that is, he felt sensations of movement in his face, tongue, and neck. During treatments, his mouth felt moister.

These treatments were during an usually cold winter in the south of England, and Joe's face was extremely sensitive to cold. I taught him to use a tiger warmer, hoping moxa would alleviate discomfort and stimulate healing. Joe tried the tiger warmer at home but did not feel comfortable using it. He feared burning himself because of his inability to register sensation in his face, so we discontinued this. However, he applied a hot water bottle, which he found comforting.

Treatment and progress: treatments 8–13

Joe continued having acupuncture for another six treatments, resetting his priorities to:

- improving movement of the neck
- reducing numbness in the tongue and cheek.

His priority was to improve his concentration, especially when reading.

Summary of treatments, progress, and changing priorities

At Joe's 11th treatment, he reported he was still experiencing 'tremendous improvement' in the dry mouth. He applied oral gel before going to bed, and mouth dryness only woke him once or twice during the night.

As the sensations in his mouth improved, Joe's attention turned to the pain in his left leg, caused by the removal of bone to rebuild his jaw. I addressed this, utilising the Yang Linking Vessel in conjunction with local points along the Gall Bladder channel.

He also began to reveal his emotions. Initially self-contained, Joe began to open up, and at the end of Tx 7, he was beginning to shift 'from symptom to self' (see Chapter 4, Offering Complex Patients a Simple Piece of Heaven). He talked about avoiding depression by keeping active and involved in business projects. He strove for acceptance of his condition; however, Joe was anxious and felt cut adrift when follow-up appointments with his surgeon were reduced to once every three months.

Around this time, Joe began to talk about nightmares, and I cleared blocks to treatment, administering Internal Dragons and External Dragons (see Chapter 5, Toolkit). I also focused on supporting Metal, using points on the Lung and Large Intestine channels. His sleep improved, he felt more positive, and he continued to improve physically and emotionally.

After Tx 12, which coincided with the advent of spring after a cold winter, he felt full of energy and optimism, and able to embark on a programme of home improvements. It was a cruel blow, then, to return home after a shopping trip to buy DIY items, to find his home had been burgled. This caused a resurgence of symptoms, and in his last treatment, I focused on treating shock and calming the shen.

Long-term feedback

In feedback at end of treatment (EOT), Joe wrote that being in the study had been beneficial. At the top of his list of beneficial changes, he wrote '[acupuncture] helped in reducing the dryness in my mouth'.

Joe experienced gradual, continuous improvements in his overall health. Originally sceptical about acupuncture, he came to value its supportive aspects most. At EOT, he wrote 'it is important to recognise the motivational support this treatment gave' and he valued the 'good care and support' offered.

For Joe, continuous professional support was important; it provided reassurance that 'I am not alone', and the acupuncture sessions were a place where he could discuss aspects of his illness that he could not raise with his family. Twelve weeks after EOT, he wrote that acupuncture brought 'comfort and knowledge on how to control your own health'.

Summary

Joe's case exemplifies the complex issues experienced by head and neck cancer patients. It demonstrates what I often observe in clinical practice: although mouth dryness is a troubling symptom, it is overwhelmed by numerous other symptoms experienced concurrently by these survivors. Few report it as a primary symptom; as in Joe's case, it is mentioned but not seen as a major focus for treatment.

Fortunately, it can be addressed as part of treatment for the complex symptoms associated with surgery and radiotherapy. Joe's dry mouth was not resolved in 13 treatments; however, it was reduced sufficiently to allow him to noticeably improve his sleep. Perhaps with a longer course of treatment, it might have resolved.

CHAPTER SUMMARY

Dry mouth is a complex condition, comprising xerostomia or SGH, or both. Research and clinical experience suggest that acupuncture can temporarily alleviate the symptoms. Long-term treatment may have more lasting benefits, and this needs to be explored clinically and in research.

In summary:

- Dry mouth is a troublesome symptom with potentially serious consequences on overall health that may affect many patients, whether cancer or non-cancer patients, as well as being a specific consequence of treatment for head and neck cancer.
- Dry mouth may be xerostomia, a subjective feeling of mouth dryness, or salivary gland hypofunction, which is reduced salivary flow that can be objectively measured.
- Patients may suffer the effects of dry mouth, but not report it as a primary symptom.
- Maintaining good oral health is a primary consideration.
- Acupuncture may be beneficial in improving the condition, especially the subjective feelings of xerostomia.
- Dry mouth may be addressed specifically, as the main treatment principle, or within the context of the wider issues affecting the patient.

References

1. Miaskowski C, Dodd M, Lee K Symptom clusters: the new frontier in symptom management research. J. Natl. Cancer Inst. 2004;32:17–21.
2. Furness S, Bryan G, McMillan R, *et al.* Interventions for the management of dry mouth: non-pharmacological interventions. Cochrane Database Syst. Rev. 2013;9: CD009603.
3. Borgnakke W, Taylor G, Anderson P, *et al.* Dry mouth (xerostomia): diagnosis, causes, complications and treatment. Michigan: Delta Dental Plans Association; 2011.
4. Napeñas JJ, Brennan MT, Fox PC Diagnosis and treatment of xerostomia (dry mouth). Odontology 2009;97(2):76–83.
5. Tanasiewicz M, Hildebrandt T, Obersztyn I Xerostomia of various etiologies: a review of the literature. Adv. Clin. Exp. Med. 2016;25(1):199–206.
6. Jasmer KJ, Gilman KE, Muñoz Forti K, *et al.* Radiation-induced salivary gland dysfunction: mechanisms, therapeutics and future directions. J. Clin. Med. 2020;9(12).
7. Hopcraft M, Tan C Xerostomia: an update for clinicians. Aust. Dent. J. 2010;55(3):238–244.
8. Breastcancer.org Dry mouth. Ardmore, PA: Breastcancer.org; 2019. Available from: www.breastcancer.org/treatment/side_effects/dry_mouth
9. Macmillan Cancer Support Mouth care during radiotherapy – coping with a dry mouth (xerostomia). London: Macmillan Cancer Support; 2012. Available from: www.macmillan.org.uk/Cancerinformation/Livingwithandaftercancer/Symptomssideeffects/Mouthcare/Radiotherapy.aspx
10. Jensen SB, Pedersen AML, Vissink A, *et al.* A systematic review of salivary gland hypofunction and xerostomia induced by cancer therapies: prevalence, severity and impact on quality of life. Support. Care Cancer 2010;18(8):1039–1060.
11. Porter SR, Fedele S, Habbab KM Xerostomia in head and neck malignancy. Oral Oncol. 2010;46(6):460–463.
12. Johnson DE, Burtness B, Leemans CR, *et al.* Head and neck squamous cell carcinoma. Nat. Rev. Dis. Primers 2020;6(1):92.

13. Mercadante V, Al Hamad A, Lodi G, *et al*. Interventions for the management of radiotherapy-induced xerostomia and hyposalivation: A systematic review and meta-analysis. Oral Oncol. 2017;66:64–74.

14. Dirix P, Nuyts S, Van den Bogaert W Radiation-induced xerostomia in patients with head and neck cancer. Cancer 2006;107(11):2525–2534.

15. Simcock R, Fallowfield L, Monson K, *et al*. ARIX: A randomised trial of acupuncture v oral care sessions in patients with chronic xerostomia following treatment of head and neck cancer. Ann. Oncol. 2013;24(3):776–783 %R 10.1093/annonc/mds515.

16. Cancer Research UK Intensity modulated radiotherapy techniques. London: Cancer Research UK; 2020. Available from: www.cancerresearchuk.org/about-cancer/cancer-in-general/treatment/radiotherapy/external/types/intensity-modulated-radiotherapy-imrt

17. Thomson WM, Chalmers JM, Spencer AJ, *et al*. The Xerostomia Inventory: a multi-item approach to measuring dry mouth. Community Dent. Health 1999;16(1):12–17.

18. Thomson WM Measuring change in dry-mouth symptoms over time using the Xerostomia Inventory. Gerodontology 2007;24(1):30–35.

19. Visvanathan V, Nix B Managing the patient presenting with xerostomia: a review. Int. J. Clin. Pract. 2010;64(3):404–407.

20. O'Sullivan EM, Higginson IJ Clinical effectiveness and safety of acupuncture in the treatment of irradiation-induced xerostomia in patients with head and neck cancer: a systematic review. Acupunct. Med. 2010;28(4):191–199.

21. PDQ® Integrative A, and Complementary Therapies Editorial Board, PDQ Acupuncture. Bethesda, MD: National Cancer Institute; 2021. Available from: www.cancer.gov/about-cancer/treatment/cam/hp/acupuncture-pdq

22. Ni X, Tian T, Chen D, *et al*. Acupuncture for radiation-induced xerostomia in cancer patients: a systematic review and meta-analysis. Integr. Cancer Ther. 2020;19:1534735420980825.

23. Deadman P, Al-Khafaji M, Baker K A manual of acupuncture. Hove: The Journal of Chinese Medicine; 2007.

24. Li P Management of cancer with Chinese medicine. St Albans: Donica; 2003.

25. Blom M, Dawidson I, Fernberg J-O, *et al*. Acupuncture treatment of patients with radiation-induced xerostomia. Oral Onc. E. J. Cancer 1996;32(3):182–190.

26. Pfister DG, Cassileth BR, Deng GE, *et al*. Acupuncture for pain and dysfunction after neck dissection: results of a randomized controlled trial. J. Clin. Oncol. 2010;28(15):2565–2570.

27. de Valois B, Peckham R Treating the person and not the disease: acupuncture in the management of cancer treatment-related lymphoedema. Eur. J. Orient. Med. 2011;6(6):37–49.

28. Cho W, editor Acupuncture and moxibustion as an evidence-based therapy for cancer. Dordrecht: Springer; 2012.

29. Cho JH, Chung WK, Kang W, *et al*. Manual acupuncture improved quality of life in cancer patients with radiation-induced xerostomia. J. Altern. Complement. Med. 2008;14(5):523–526.

30. Garcia M, Chiang J, Cohen L, *et al*. Acupuncture for radiation-induced xerostomia in patients with cancer: a pilot study. Head Neck 2009;31(10):1360–1368.

31. Simcock R, Fallowfield L, Jenkins V Group acupuncture to relieve radiation induced xerostomia: a feasibility study. Acupunct. Med. 2009;27(3):109–113.

32. Oleson T Auriculotherapy manual: Chinese and Western systems of ear acupuncture. 2nd ed. Los Angeles: Health Care Alternatives; 1998.

33. Abbate S Advanced techniques in oriental medicine. Stuttgart: Thieme; 2006.

34. Maciocia G The channels of acupuncture: clinical use of the secondary channels and eight extraordinary vessels. Edinburgh: Churchill Livingstone; 2006.

Chapter 8

Cancer Treatment-Related Hot Flushes and Night Sweats (HFNS)

Introduction

The general biomedical attitude to menopausal hot flushes and the impact of these incidents on cancer survivors are encapsulated in these quotations:

> Perhaps because no one has ever died from a hot flush, this most characteristic and distressing symptom of the menopause has not received the attention that it might otherwise have done. (Sturdee *et al.*)[1]

> I went from 26 (flushes) in 24 hours day and night and I was almost awake the whole night soaking wet…to about three or four (flushes) in 24 hours. (Participant in a study of acupuncture for breast cancer related hot flushes)[2]

Hot flushes and night sweats (HFNS) are not directly life-threatening. However, they may be disruptive of daily life and are often accompanied by troublesome symptoms. These may affect many aspects of a sufferer's life, from sleeping to the ability to work. They impact quality of life and the ability to cope.

A common symptom of natural menopause, HFNS are also a consequence of treatments for many cancers, especially breast, gynaecological, and prostate cancers. The discomfort of HFNS may cause cancer survivors to take holidays from, or discontinue, adjuvant hormonal treatments. This has potential to reduce long-term survival.

HFNS are a powerful driver for people to seek interventions offering relief, and acupuncture can help. It is a useful intervention, especially for cancer survivors who do not wish to take additional medications to manage the consequences of their cancer treatments.

Studies show acupuncture to be as effective as commonly used pharmaceuticals for managing HFNS, while having no serious side effects. As well as reducing HFNS, acupuncture may simultaneously improve other concurrent symptoms and overall quality of life.

This chapter focuses on hot flushes and night sweats that are the consequences of cancer treatment and will be referred to as HFNS.

TERMINOLOGY

Hot flushes (UK English) or flashes (American English) are defined as: 'recurrent transient periods of flushing, sweating and the sensation of heat, often accompanied by palpations and feeling of anxiety, and sometimes followed by chills'.[3]

They are also referred to as *vasomotor*, *climacteric*, or *menopausal* symptoms. Night sweats, or *nocturnal flushes*, are hot flushes that occur during the night. These are often encompassed in the terms for hot flushes.

Terms for treating cancer with hormones include *hormone therapy*, *hormonal therapy*, and *endocrine therapy*. For women, these may also be referred to as *oestrogen therapy*. For prostate cancer, hormone therapy is also referred to as *androgen deprivation*, *androgen ablation*, *androgen suppression*, and *chemical castration*.

Incidence and prevalence of HFNS
General notes

- Hormone replacement therapy (HRT) (or menopausal hormone therapy (MHT)) is contraindicated for women diagnosed with hormonally mediated cancers (including high-risk endometrial and most breast).[4,5] Most women stop taking HRT on diagnosis of these cancers, and may experience an upsurge in HFNS (called 'rebound effect').
- Chemotherapy can suppress the ovaries and cause a sudden onset menopause, often with aggressive HFNS. In younger women, menses may return; for older women, this may be permanent.
- Both men and women undergoing hormonal therapy may experience debilitating HFNS.

Breast cancer

- Associated with adjuvant endocrine therapies, over 80% of women taking tamoxifen report troublesome HFNS,[6] which are also associated with aromatase inhibitors (AIs) (e.g. anastrozole (Arimidex®), exemestane (Aromasin®), and letrozole (Femara®)).[7]
- The minimum duration of adjuvant endocrine therapy is currently five years, with some women recommended a further five years of treatment.[5] Many women experience HFNS for the duration, and HFNS may continue after endocrine therapy ceases.[8]
- For pre-menopausal women with breast cancer, the symptoms resulting from ovarian suppression induced by chemotherapy or gonadotrophin-releasing hormone agonists (GnRHa) (e.g. goserelin) are reported to be more severe than those of tamoxifen.[9]
- Adjuvant endocrine therapies (chiefly tamoxifen) are also used in the treatment of male breast cancer, with potential for HFNS.

Prostate cancer

Fifty to eighty per cent of prostate cancer patients experience andropause ('male menopause') with associated HFNS. These are a consequence of treatments including surgical castration (orchiectomy), luteinising hormone (LH) blockers, anti-androgens, gonadotrophin-releasing hormone (GnRH), or oestrogen.

Some men find HFNS the most troublesome consequence of prostate cancer treatment. HFNS may continue for the duration of treatment (which may range from up to three years to lifelong) and are associated with high levels of cancer-related distress. Some men choose to discontinue androgen deprivation therapy (ADT) because of persistent, troublesome HFNS.[10,11]

Gynaecological cancers

HFNS are reported by women treated for any of the five gynaecological cancers – womb, ovarian, cervical, vulval, and vaginal. HFNS may be severe due to earlier age of onset of the menopause, abruptness of onset (as a consequence of surgery, radiotherapy, and/or chemotherapy), and/or the use of anti-oestrogen medications as adjunctive hormonal therapy.[12]

Other cancers

HFNS may be a consequence of treatment for other cancers, especially when surgery, radiotherapy, and/or chemotherapy affect ovarian function or inhibit testosterone production, triggering menopausal symptoms.

Side effects of pharmaceuticals

HFNS are a side effect of some pharmaceuticals, for example opioids, tricyclic antidepressants, and steroids.[13]

Characteristics of HFNS

Some people experience HFNS merely as a mild irritation. For many female cancer survivors, they are troublesome and may be more severe, frequent, and persistent than those of natural menopause.[14,15] Cancer treatment-related HFNS may occur regardless of natural menopause status:

- Young women may experience menopausal symptoms prematurely because of cancer treatment.
- Women whose cancer diagnosis coincides with menopause may have exacerbated symptoms, especially if they have discontinued HRT.
- Post-menopausal women may experience an unwelcome return of symptoms.

HFNS may be distressing for male cancer survivors as well.

Variability of HFNS

HFNS cannot easily be measured objectively. They are largely subjective, and vary from person to person and within the individual:

- **Duration** – lasting on average three to four minutes, their perceived duration may be from a few seconds to as much as an hour.[1]
- **Frequency** – HFNS may be as infrequent as a few per week or as frequent as many per hour throughout day and night.[1]
- **Severity** – HFNS range from being mild (facial warmth lasting less than five minutes) to severe (intense heat, likened to 'a raging furnace'), with associated profuse sweating, increased heartbeat, and feeling faint. At their most severe, they may be experienced as severe heat ('boiling eruption') and drenching perspiration, requiring changing of clothing and bed linen.[16]
- **Triggers** – they may occur spontaneously or be triggered by known stimuli, including embarrassment, stress, alcohol, caffeine, warm drinks, and changes in ambient temperature.[1]

Physical sensations

Accompanying physical sensations include chills before and/or after the flush, dizziness, feelings of suffocation, flushing or redness, nausea, palpitations, sweating, and tingling sensations in the hands.

Emotional impact

Emotional symptoms include annoyance, anxiety, feelings of panic, frustration, irritation, and even suicidal feelings. Night sweats may disturb sleep patterns, causing fatigue and irritability.[8,17,18]

Effect on quality of life

HFNS may be distressing, disabling, and socially embarrassing. Their serious impact on quality of life is often underrated. Menopausal symptoms layered on other cancer treatment-related issues contribute to poor body image, self-esteem, and self-confidence.[15] Women experiencing cancer treatment-related HFNS have worse quality of life than those who do not, while prostate cancer survivors with HFNS register higher levels of distress than those without.[19,20]

Longevity of HFNS

Cancer survivors are often advised that HFNS will reduce or become less severe in the first few months to a year after hormonal therapy commences.[9,21] However, a study reported that of 84% of breast cancer survivors taking tamoxifen who experienced HFNS, 60% described them as severe, with severity remaining high until the fourth year of treatment.[6] Studies report that HFNS remain problematic for women who are five years post cancer diagnosis, persisting even after endocrine therapy ends.[8,22]

Potential adverse consequences of HFNS

Cancer survivors are often advised that little can be done, and they must put up with HFNS. The distress they cause may lead people to take 'holidays' from medication or to abandon taking it all together. This has potential consequences for long-term survival, as these therapies are prescribed to reduce risk of cancer recurrence.[23]

Biomedical perspectives
The pathophysiology of HFNS

The mechanisms for HFNS in women are not known. One theory suggests that HFNS are caused by a disturbance in the temperature-regulating mechanism, in which hormones are implicated.

The precise role of oestrogen, previously seen as a major cause, has yet to be established, particularly as HFNS may cease spontaneously after natural menopause when oestrogen levels continue to decline. However, the rate at which oestrogen declines appears to be a contributing factor; HFNS are often more severe for premenopausal women experiencing the acute withdrawal associated with bilateral oophorectomy (surgical removal of the ovaries) than for women undergoing natural menopause, as hormone levels drop suddenly rather than gradually.

Cultural factors, environment, and stress are also implicated, adding to the complexity of the phenomenon.[17,24,25]

Similarly, the mechanisms for male HFNS are not clear. As with women, a contributory factor may be the rate of withdrawal of significant hormones, such as sudden deprivation or significant reductions in androgen levels associated with prostate cancer treatments.[11]

Biomedical approaches to treatment
Pharmacological treatments for breast cancer treatment-related HFNS

HRT, also known as MHT, is considered the most effective treatment for HFNS during natural menopause. Its use by women with breast cancer is controversial, with concerns that it increases the risk of disease progression or recurrence, and of venous thromboembolic disease.[26] Therefore, it is not recommended for women with:

- hormone receptor positive breast cancer
- oestrogen-dependent gynaecological cancers
- a history of venous thromboembolic disease.[26]

While HRT may be prescribed for women with other cancers (e.g. ovarian and some cervical cancers),[27] women with breast cancer are usually advised to stop taking HRT, and many stop voluntarily on receiving a breast cancer diagnosis.[28,29]

Consequently, women and their medical professionals are keen to seek alternative means of managing HFNS.[28,30] Recommended pharmacological preparations that may be prescribed include:[9,26,31]

- **Selective serotonin reuptake inhibitors (SSRIs):** for example, citalopram, escitalopram, paroxetine, fluoxetine. Some SSRIs may inhibit the anti-cancer properties of tamoxifen, and it is recommended that paroxetine and fluoxetine be used with caution or avoided in women treated with tamoxifen.[32]
- **Serotonin noradrenaline reuptake inhibitors (SNRIs):** for example, venlafaxine, desvenlafaxine. Venlafaxine is reported to reduce hot flushes in breast cancer patients by 10–40%, although it is associated with side effects of dry mouth, nausea, and constipation.

- **Antihypertensives:** for example, clonidine. Often of limited effectiveness, women may not tolerate side effects which include dizziness, hypotension, headache, constipation, and dry mouth.
- **Anticonvulsants:** for example, gabapentin, pregabalin. Frequently experienced side effects include somnolence, dizziness, and fatigue as well as psychological side effects such as anxiety and depression.

Pharmacological treatments for prostate cancer treatment-related HFNS

Medications prescribed for women have been explored (e.g. clonidine, gabapentin, estradiol, SSRIs, SNRIs); however, these may not be active in androgen-deprived men.

National Institute for Health and Care Excellence (NICE) guidance for the treatment of prostate cancer treatment-related HFNS recommends:[33]

- medroxyprogesterone as first-line therapy
- cyproterone acetate as second-line therapy, if medroxyprogesterone is not effective or well tolerated.

In the US, recommended medications include:[34]

- **antidepressants:** for example, venlafaxine (Effexor®) and sertraline (Zoloft®)
- **nonhormonal treatments:** for example, gabapentin (Gralise®, Neurontin®)
- **progesterone:** for example, megestrol acetate (Ovaban®, Pallace®).

Non-pharmacological remedies

There are low levels of evidence for the safety and efficacy of over-the counter preparations, of which Vitamin E, alfalfa, and evening primrose oil are frequently considered.[9,26,35,36]

Black cohosh, red clover, and soy are used frequently for natural menopause remedies, with some evidence they are useful for HFNS. However, the active ingredients may include substances that mimic the action of oestrogen, called phytoestrogens. It is not known whether these are safe for people with breast cancer as there are concerns that phytoestrogens may increase the likelihood of cancer recurrence.[37,38]

St John's wort should be used cautiously, as there are risks of interaction with tamoxifen, docetaxel, and anti-coagulants.[9]

Behavioural interventions

Therapies recommended include:

- Cognitive behavioural therapy (CBT): there is a growing body of evidence that CBT is effective for reducing the impact and frequency of HFNS for women and men with cancer.[39]
- Yoga: weekly sessions have been shown to reduce HFNS frequency and severity in the short term.
- Hypnosis, breathing exercises, mindfulness, and relaxation.[36,40]

Exercise has not been observed to be beneficial in studies of healthy women experiencing HFNS, although anecdotally some women report it is helpful.[14] Acupuncture is discussed later in this chapter.

Lifestyle advice

HFNS may be improved by lifestyle changes, of which the recommendations in Box 8.1 are an example.

Box 8.1: Lifestyle recommendations for managing HFNS[41]

- Keep rooms cool – use a fan if necessary.
- Wear layers of light clothing so clothes can be removed if the individual feels hot.
- Have layers of bedclothes to remove (and replace) as needed.
- Wear natural fibres (silk, cotton, linen) instead of synthetic fabrics.
- Have a lukewarm shower or bath instead of a hot one.
- Put a towel over the mattress if there is night sweating.
- Use cooling pads to keep cool, including a chilled pillow (Chillow®).
- Learn to stay calm under pressure, as heightened emotions can trigger HFNS.

Identifying and avoiding triggers, such as caffeine, alcohol, spicy foods, and hot drinks in general, may also be helpful.

Higher body mass index (BMI) has been related to higher risk for vasomotor symptoms for women.[26]

East Asian medicine perspectives
Chinese medicine theories

In Chinese medicine (CM), menopausal syndrome has been associated with ageing and therefore the decline of Kidney essence, which controls the important transitional stages in life, including birth, puberty, menopause, and death.[42] Symptoms associated with the menopause are attributed to 'decline of Kidney-Essence in its Yin or Yang aspect'. While Kidney deficiency may be combined with excess patterns such as 'Dampness, stagnation of Qi, stasis of Blood, Empty Heat, or Liver-Yang rising', Kidney deficiency is seen as the basic pathology of menopause.[43]

In Western CM literature in the early 21st century, hot flushes have been widely attributed to Kidney yin deficiency, although some sources noted that 'many [women] will have other associated symptoms that must be addressed'.[44] In a study of TCM diagnoses of post-menopausal women, researchers observed that 'practitioners of TCM who diagnose post-menopausal women with vasomotor symptoms are likely to make a diagnosis that includes Kidney yin deficiency'.[44]

In recent years, this interpretation began to change. Maciocia maintains it is a 'common misconception that menopausal symptoms are always due to Kidney-Yin deficiency because they are characterised by hot flushes'. Kidney yang deficiency may also be implicated, and in the early years of menopause, Kidney deficiency 'nearly always includes a deficiency of both Ying and Yang' (thus explaining the contradictory hot and cold symptoms experienced by some women).[45] Phlegm can also aggravate menopausal symptoms, especially hot flushes, and Maciocia identifies 13 different syndromes associated with 'feeling of heat in the face [which] includes menopausal hot flushes'.

Box 8.2: Maciocia's 13 syndromes for menopausal HFNS[45]

- Liver yang rising
- Liver fire
- Heart fire
- Heart yin deficiency with empty heat
- Kidney yin deficiency with empty heat
- Lung heat
- Lung yin deficiency with empty heat
- Stomach heat
- Stomach yin deficiency with empty heat
- Damp heat in the Spleen
- Spleen heat
- Spleen yin deficiency with empty heat
- Yin fire

VIGNETTE: AN ACUPUNCTURE RESEARCHER'S LEARNINGS ABOUT CM THEORY FOR HFNS

The rationale of Kidney yin deficiency guided the design of my first research project into using acupuncture to manage HFNS. Once in clinic I found that many women did not exhibit signs of Kidney yin deficiency. Rather than the peeled or thin tongue coat and thin rapid pulses characteristic of Kidney yin deficiency, I encountered a range of other presentations.[44] Many women had the pale, swollen tongues of yang deficiency and damp; others had red tongues with yellow coats of full heat, as illustrated by Figure 8.1. Pulse qualities were also many and varied. A colour version of Figure 8.1 is available to view and download from the Singing Dragon Library.

Although I continued with the protocol designed for this study, in my private clinic I began to expand my repertoire of treatments.[46] I discovered there were many, varied ways to approach the management of HFNS, as discussed below. The discrepancies between CM theory and my clinical observations suggested there was more to menopausal hot flushes than Kidney yin deficiency.

Norwegian researchers came to a similar conclusion in research into acupuncture for HFNS associated with natural menopause.[47] Analysing diagnoses made by ten TCM acupuncturists, they found that half of the 131 research participants were diagnosed with Kidney yin deficiency as their primary syndrome. In discussing possible diagnoses for HFNS, the researchers concluded:

> the current interpretation of menopausal symptoms as mainly a result of Kidney deficiency is only one of several possible understandings, and the correct TCM diagnoses for menopausal vasomotor symptoms remains unclear.[47]

In extensive work on the menopause, Professor Volker Scheid argues that rather than evolving from centuries of traditional doctrine and experience, treatment strategies for menopausal syndrome emerged in the 1960s as part of China's modernisation of CM. This process involved translating the biomedical view of menopause as a hormonal deficiency into the CM syndrome of Kidney deficiency, a translation Scheid says is problematic and may impact adversely on clinical practice.[48,49]

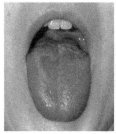 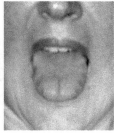 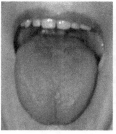 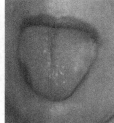

(A) Stomach yin xu with damp accumulating in lower jiao.

(B) Stomach and Spleen qi xu with damp accumulation.

(C) Liver Blood xu, general qi xu with Blood stasis lower jiao, Heart yin xu.

(D) Stomach dry with Spleen qi xu, heat in upper jiao.

FIGURE 8.1: KIDNEY YIN DEFICIENCY?

Research perspectives
The evidence base for using acupuncture to manage HFNS
In the 21st century, researchers have shown great interest in HFNS, with many studies investigating acupuncture's effects on vasomotor symptoms related to both natural menopause and cancer treatments. Research into the latter focuses mainly on breast cancer, with less attention paid to prostate cancer. I have not identified studies investigating gynaecological cancers.

Systematic reviews of using acupuncture to manage HFNS
A 'review of reviews' covering systematic reviews published up to 2016 concluded that evidence from RCTs supports the use of acupuncture for reducing vasomotor symptoms (menopausal and cancer treatment-related) and reducing their impact on women's activities and health-related quality of life.[50] Another review of 17 studies reported the majority of women had a reduction in HFNS of more than 50%, with beneficial effects continuing for up to six months.[51]

In contrast, the *British Medical Journal (BMJ)* cited a 2013 systematic review, which concluded that although acupuncture was more effective than no treatment, improvements in vasomotor symptoms could be due to placebo effect.[52] Nonetheless, the *BMJ* noted that acupuncture was free from adverse side effects.[40]

Focusing specifically on cancer treatment-related HFNS, Frisk *et al.*'s[53] analysis of prostate and breast cancer studies found reductions in HFNS of 43.2% after 5–12 weeks of treatment. This review also investigated long-term effects and reported the reduction from baseline was sustained at 45.6% in 153 of 172 patients who were followed up after the end of therapy (mean 5.8 months, range three to nine months).

Chinese researchers conducting systematic reviews and meta-analyses focus on breast cancer treatment-related HFNS. Their conclusions about the effects of acupuncture on HFNS frequency and severity are varied, with one review team reporting no benefit[54,55] and others reporting benefit during but not beyond the end of treatment.[56-58] However, most of these reviews report alleviation of 'menopause-related symptoms' for up to three months after the end of acupuncture treatment. These symptoms include palpitations, vertigo, headache, sleep disturbance, vaginal dryness, arthralgia, fatigue, nervousness, and depression. These reviews concur with many other systematic reviewers, concluding that while acupuncture appears promising, more rigorous research is needed.

One systematic review focuses on HFNS related to prostate cancer. Published in 2009, it does not include subsequent studies (Table 8.3); however, as those are uncontrolled trials with small numbers, the reviewers' recommendations that future studies should be RCTs with sufficiently large samples and appropriate research design and methodology remain valid.[59]

Other reviews and clinical practice
Acupuncture is frequently mentioned in medical reviews discussing management of HFNS. In these, discussion usually focuses on the mixed results of studies and the need for further, more conclusive research.[9,26,31,35,41,60]

Clinically, acupuncture appears to be gaining popularity. A UK study found that acupuncture was the complementary therapy most frequently recommended to breast cancer survivors, with over 50% of healthcare professionals surveyed recommending it to their patients and over 50% of those patients finding it helpful.[61]

Research investigating acupuncture for breast cancer treatment-related HFNS
Most published studies have been conducted in Europe and the USA. Lack of research from China may be due to cultural perceptions of menopause; there is much debate in the medical and sociological literature about whether HFNS are a troublesome symptom for Asian women during natural menopause.[62,63] Breast cancer treatment-related HFNS have been investigated in Korea.[64]

While frequency and severity of HFNS are usually a primary outcome, many studies also investigate menopause-related symptoms as secondary outcomes, including sleep disturbance,[65,66] depression,[67] and health-related quality of life.[66,68-70] Long-term effects of acupuncture treatment on HFNS are also of interest.[67,70]

Randomised controlled trials comparing acupuncture with pharmacological products

Key RCTs comparing acupuncture with pharmacological products prescribed for breast cancer treatment-related HFNS include:

- **HRT:** as part of the HABITS (Hormonal Replacement Therapy After Breast Cancer – Is it Safe?) study, a randomised clinical trial conducted in Scandinavia in the 1990s that studied the relationship between HRT and breast cancer recurrence, Frisk et al.[68] compared 12 weeks of electro-acupuncture with 24 months of sequential or continuous combined oestrogen/progestogen therapy. The study showed that although electro-acupuncture decreased HFNS less than HRT, improvements in health-related quality of life and sleep improved to the same extent in both groups. (The HABITS study was closed in 2003 due to significantly increased breast cancer recurrence in the HRT group, leading to recommendations that HRT should be avoided by women with a history of breast cancer.)
- **Venlafaxine:** Walker et al.[70] found acupuncture as effective as venlafaxine in reducing HFNS at the end of treatment. In addition, women randomised to venlafaxine experienced a significant increase in HFNS two weeks after treatment ended (rebound effect), while the acupuncture group continued to maintain low levels of HFNS four weeks after treatment ended. Additional benefits observed in the acupuncture group included increased sex drive, higher energy levels, and improved clarity of thought and sense of wellbeing.
- **Gabapentin:** Mao et al.[71] found electro-acupuncture as effective as gabapentin at the end of active treatment. At a 16-week follow-up, the two groups reported improvements in HFNS of 55% and 21% respectively.

Safety and adverse effects

In these studies, participants randomised to acupuncture reported either no adverse events (Walker et al.) or mild bruising experienced by some participants (Mao et al.), while those randomised to pharmaceuticals reported side effects including gastrointestinal disturbances and fatigue.[70,71]

ESSENTIALS

These studies are promising indicators for acupuncture for individuals who:

- do not wish to use pharmaceuticals to manage HFNS
- find those products ineffective
- cannot tolerate their side effects.

As well as offering an alternative to these products, acupuncture may have several benefits. It appears to:

- be equal to or more effective than pharmacological products

- be safe, with only minor transient adverse effects
- confer longer-term benefit after treatment ends.

Acupuncture may also improve many menopause-related symptoms, with longer-term benefit after treatment ends.

Acupuncture points used in research for breast cancer treatment-related HFNS

Table 8.1 presents the acupuncture points used in RCTs published since 2009 that have included details about the point selection within the publication. Study design and results are also summarised.

Commentary

There is little commonality of points used and considerable variance in channels selected for treatment. Two studies, Walker et al.[70] and Lesi et al.[69] use semi-individualised protocols based on TCM theory: the latter is presented below (Table 8.2).

Concerns about needling arms with or at risk of lymphoedema (see Chapter 9, Cancer Treatment-Related Lymphoedema) are discussed by Hervik[72] and Lesi et al.,[69] who explicitly avoid the arm ipsilateral to the affected breast. Liljegren et al.[73] also needle points in the arm unilaterally, but do not discuss the rationale for this.

Using a semi-individualised treatment protocol for breast cancer treatment-related HFNS

Lesi et al.[69] describe their Italian multi-centre (six sites) RCT in a publication providing unusually comprehensive details about diagnosis and individualised treatment. (Mao et al.'s gabapentin RCT also used individualisation according to diagnosis; however, the six-page manual is difficult to locate and to summarise.)[71] Distinctive characteristics of this study design (summarised in Table 8.1) and its publication include:

- It is one of the few papers to detail individualised treatment according to diagnosis, following CM principles (citing the 'six menopausal syndromes according to Maciocia's recommendations').
- The authors report the number of participants with each CM diagnosis, as identified at the first treatment. In view of the previous discussion about Kidney yin deficiency, it is interesting that Kidney yin emptiness is the fourth most common syndrome, with only 16% of women diagnosed with it.
- The authors present data on the number of women receiving moxibustion, although no details about the method are provided.
- Enhanced self-care (ESC) only was used as a control, enabling researchers to focus on effectiveness (rather than efficacy) of acupuncture, an approach that best reflects the likely clinical response in practice.

Table 8.1: Acupuncture points used in selected RCTs investigation acupuncture for breast cancer treatment-related HFNS published since 2009

Author (Publication date)	Hervik & Mjåland (2009)[72]	Walker et al. (2010)[70]	Liljegren et al. (2012)[73]	Bokmand & Flyger (2013)[65]	Lesi et al. (2016)[59]	Bao et al. (2014)[66]
Country	Norway	USA	Sweden	Denmark	Italy	USA
Study design	RCT	RCT	RCT	RCT	RCT	RCT
Participants	59	50	84	94	190	45
Comparison (Comparison/Acu)	Sham acu (29/30)	Venlafaxine (25/25)	Non-insertive stimulation at non-acupuncture points 'CTRL' (42/42)	Sham acu and no treatment (29/34/31)	Enhanced self-care (ESC) (105/85)	Sham acu (24/23)
Treatment frequency/duration	2x/week for 5 weeks then 1x/week for 5 weeks (15 total)	2x/week for 4 weeks then 1x/week for 8 weeks (16 total)	2x/week for 5 weeks (10 total)	1x/week for 5 weeks (5 total)	1x/week over 12 weeks (10 total)	1x/week for 8 weeks (8 total)
Follow-up	12 weeks (2 years)	3, 6, 9, 12 months	Week 18 (13 weeks after EOT)	6 and 12 weeks	3 and 6 months	4 weeks
Rationale	TCM	TCM	Acu textbooks, previous reports, expert opinion	Acu textbook	TCM	Textbook and clinical experience
Protocol	Fixed	Semi-individualised	Fixed	Fixed	Semi-individualised	Fixed

Points used	Unilateral on opposite side to affected breast: LU-7 SP-6 KID-13 PER-7 GB-20 LIV-3 LIV-8 REN-4	All: SP-6 BL-23 KID-3 As per diagnosis: LU-9 ST-36 HE-7 PER-7 GB-20 REN-6 DU-14 DU-20	Unilateral: LI-4 ST-36 HE-6 LIV-3 Bilateral: SP-6 KID-7	Bilateral: SP-6 HE-6 KID-3 LIV-3	All: Bilateral LI-11 SP-6 REN-4 Plus points selected as per diagnosis – maximum 11 points in total. Moxa used as per TCM diagnosis. (See below for a detailed discussion.)	Bilateral: LI-4 ST-36 HE-6 BL-65 KID-3 GB-34 Unilateral: REN-4 REN-6 REN-12
Adverse events	Not reported	Zero in acu group; 18 in venlafaxine group.	Slight bleeding (1); bruising (1) in CTRL group.	Fatigue, pruritis, or nausea in 15% of all participants; mild temporary side effects in acu group.	Mild events in 12 acu participants including muscle ache, headache, and one menstrual bleed.	No adverse events in either group.
Summary of results	At EOT, HF reduced by 50%, NS by 60% in acu group, further 30% reduction in HFNS at 12 weeks.	50% decrease in HFNS frequency in both groups EOT. Acu group reported better post-tx maintenance of reduction and no adverse effects.	HFNS reduced in both groups; no difference between groups.	Acu significantly reduced HFNS and sleep disturbance; effects last at least 12 weeks after treatment ends.	Acu plus ESC reduced HFNS significantly more than ESC only (p<.001); effects maintained at 3- and 6-month follow-ups (p=.0028 and .01 respectively). Acu also associated with higher quality of life (p<.05).	HFNS reduced in both groups, no difference between groups.

Table 8.2: TCM syndromes and points used by Lesi *et al.*

Notes:

TCM syndromes recorded before session.

Needles in all points manipulated to evoke needle sensation (deqi), no further manipulation.

Total of 11 acupoints per session (bilateral or unilateral not stated).

Needles retained for 20 minutes.

Moxibustion provided as per CM diagnosis (type of moxibustion not stated).

Participants with lymphoedema not needled in the affected arm.

Minimal conversation between acupuncturists and participants.

TCM syndrome	Acupuncture points	Participants (n=85)	
		Number	**%**
All participants	Ll-11, SP-6, REN-4	85	100
	Supplementary points (in some cases)		
Kidney and Liver yin and yang deficiency and yang escape from Liver	LU-7, Ll-4, ST-37, KID-6, PC-7, LIV-2, LIV-3, DU- 20	31	36.40
Kidney yin and yang deficiency	LU-7, ST-36, HE-6, BL-2, BL-52, KID-3, KID-6, KID-7, REN-6, DU-20	15	17.65
Phlegm or qi stasis	LU-7, ST-28, ST-40, SP-9, SP-10, PC-6, TB-6, KID-6, REN-6, REN-10, REN-17	14	16.47
Kidney yin emptiness	LU-7, HE-6, KID-3, KID-6, KID-7, KID-10	14	16.40
Kidney and Heart disharmony	LU-7, ST-37, HE-6, HE-8, KID-2, KID-3, KID-6, KID-7, KID-13, PC-6, REN-14, REN-15, DU-24	9	10.59
Blood stasis	LU-7, SP-4, SP-10, BL-17, KID-14, PC-6, LIV-3, REN-4, REN-6	0	–
Not indicated		2	2.3
Use of moxibustion		29	34.2

Summary of key findings:

- At end of treatment (EOT), the acupuncture group showed a greater reduction in hot flushes (-20.8) than the ESC (-4.6) ($p<.001$). There was also a statistically significant difference between the two groups at three- and six-month follow-ups, in favour of acupuncture.
- Similar improvements were observed for menopause-related symptoms and quality of life.
- The ESC group recorded more frequent physical activity than the acupuncture group. The authors note the ESC group was significantly more compliant in following self-care recommendations and suggest that 'acupuncture alone was highly effective' in reducing HFNS.
- No serious adverse events were reported; mild adverse events were registered by 12 participants receiving acupuncture, including muscle pain, headache, and one menstrual bleed.

- The authors concluded that 'acupuncture is an effective and safe intervention for severe menopausal symptoms in women with breast cancer'.[69]

This study is unusual in its attempts to measure acupuncture as it would be practised (a pragmatic trial), rather than using a fixed protocol. It suggests that acupuncture is effective in reducing HFNS and improving quality of life with minimal mild adverse effects and no severe adverse effects. Offering acupuncture in combination with enhanced self-care is a useful integrative approach for managing consequences of breast cancer treatment.

Research investigating acupuncture for prostate cancer treatment-related HFNS

Research into prostate cancer-related HFNS is sparse. There have been very few RCTs, few studies published recently, and very small numbers of participants. Most research has been conducted in the USA. Table 8.3 summarises results of studies published since 2000 that include details about the point selection in the publication.

Commentary

These are all small exploratory, uncontrolled studies with fixed protocols. Although all report promising results, there has been no follow-up in this area with further RCTs. The exception is Frisk et al.'s[74] RCT comparing traditional body acupuncture and electro-acupuncture (discussed below).

Across the studies, there is no similarity in point selection. They use numerous points in each treatment, and there is a preference for electro-acupuncture, despite Frisk's early findings that there was no significant difference between electro-acupuncture and 'traditional' acupuncture (discussed below).

Comparing 'traditional' acupuncture with electro-acupuncture

Frisk et al.'s[74] Swedish multi-centre (three sites) RCT is the only published RCT on acupuncture for prostate cancer-related HFNS. The aim was to compare outcomes for electro-acupuncture (EA) with traditional acupuncture (TA) on:

- frequency of HFNS
- related distress.

Table 8.3: Acupuncture points used in published studies investigating acupuncture for prostate cancer treatment-related HFNS since 2000

Author (Publication date)	Harding et al. (2008)[75]	Frisk et al. (2009)[74]	Beer et al. (2010)[76]	Ashamalla et al. (2011)[77]	Capodice et al. (2011)[78]
Country	UK	Sweden	USA	USA	USA
Study design	Uncontrolled trial	RCT	Uncontrolled trial	Uncontrolled trial	Uncontrolled trial
Cancer stage	Advanced	Surgical or GnRH analogue castration at least 3 months previously	Not undergoing chemotherapy	Locally advanced, no metastatic disease	Advanced
Acupuncture	Auriculotherapy	Traditional acu (TA) vs electro-acupuncture (EA)	Body acu plus electrostimulation	Body acu plus electrostimulation	Body and auricular acupuncture
Participants	60	31 (16 TA, 15 EA)	25	17	17
Treatment frequency/duration	1x/week for 10 weeks (10 total)	2x/week for 2 weeks, then 1x/week for 10 weeks (14 total)	2x/week for 4 weeks, then 1x/week for 6 weeks (14 total)	2x/week for 4 weeks (8 total)	1x/week for 14 weeks (14 total)
Follow-up	None	6, 9, 12 months	None	8 months	28 weeks
Rationale	NADA protocol	Not stated	Prior published study plus TCM textbook	Not stated	Standard texts, informal practitioner query, and previous studies
Points chosen	NADA: Autonomic Shenmen Kidney Liver Lung	Unilateral: SP-6 SP-9 HE-7 PER-6 LIV-3 DU-20 Bilateral: BL-15 BL-23 (2Hz estim)* BL-32 (2Hz estim)* *For EA group only	Unilateral: SP-6 HE-7 PER-6 LIV-2 Bilateral: BL-15 BL-23 (2Hz estim) BL-32 (2Hz estim) GB-34	Bilateral: LI-11 ST-36 (2Hz estim) SP-6 (2Hz estim) HE-7 BL-15 (2Hz estim) BL-23 (2Hz estim) KID-3 PER-6 GB-34 Extra point Taiyang	Auricular: Shenmen Brain Kidney Liver Upper Lung Body: LU-7 SP-6 HE-7 BL-15 BL-23 BL-32 KID-6 LIV-3
Adverse events	Transient increase in HFNS which subsided in a few seconds (2 patients).	Distress (1), fatigue (1), haematoma (1).	Fatigue (6), mood changes (6), sweating (6), somnolence (5), dizziness (4), insomnia (4), dry mouth (4), and other mild events.	'No adverse events were encountered'	'No serious side effects… no reports of bleeding, bruising at any needle site, dizziness or vasovagal response(s)…'
Brief summary of results	95% of participants reported decreased severity of symptoms including frequency of daytime (p<.05) and night-time (p<.05) incidents. Wellbeing showed clinical improvement of 2.1 points on a 6-point scale (p<.05).	Both EA and TA lowered number of HFNS and related distress; hot flush scores decreased by 78% and 73% respectively.	After 4 weeks, 9 (41%) patients had > 50% HFNS reduction; all participants achieved this reduction at some point during the treatment. Quality of life and sleep also improved.	Mean HFNS decreases: 68.4% (p=.0001) at 2 weeks, 89.2% (p=.0078) at 6 weeks, and 80.3% (p=.002) at 8 months.	A trend toward improvement after 7 weeks and significant improvement at 14 weeks. HFNS frequency still lower at 28 weeks than at baseline.

The researchers expected the EA group to show more pronounced results due to the electrical stimulation. Details of study design and points are summarised in Table 8.3.
Key findings:

- At EOT (12 weeks), hot flushes per 24 hours decreased significantly in both groups, with hot flush scores reduced by 78% for the EA group and 73% for the TA group.
- Distress from flushes was significantly reduced in both groups at almost all measurement points.
- The effects continued to nine months after EOT.
- Adverse events reported were mild and included treatment-related distress (n=1), fatigue on the treatment day (n=1), and a centimetre-sized hematoma at the insertion site (n=1).
- The study included objective measures of calcitonin gene-related peptide (CGRP), a potent vasodilator and stimulant of cholinergic sweating. Changes in s-testosterone were also measured. No significant changes were observed in either measure for both groups.

Comparing the outcomes of EA and TA is an important feature of this study, and the results do support the hypothesis that EA is superior to TA. The researchers suggest this finding indicates that it is not the type of acupuncture that is important for the results, but rather the acupuncture as such.

Research into using moxibustion for cancer treatment-related HFNS

There are no studies published in the English language investigating moxibustion for managing cancer treatment-related HFNS, although Lesi et al.[69] incorporated its use according to TCM diagnosis.

This lack of studies may not be surprising given the predominant theory that Kidney yin deficiency underlies menopausal HFNS, thus contraindicating moxa (see discussion above). However, a Korean study published in 2009 reported promising outcomes after giving 14 moxibustion treatments to women experiencing HFNS related to natural menopause.[79]

Research case study: two observational studies of acupuncture to manage tamoxifen-related HFNS

My first research projects investigated using acupuncture to manage HFNS experienced by breast cancer survivors taking tamoxifen; my approach and findings are summarised below.

Study 1: Using a semi-individualised 'traditional' approach

I developed this approach for research into using body acupuncture to manage tamoxifen-related HFNS.[46] It is based on a core protocol (Table 8.4), supplemented with 'points for the patient' to provide semi-individualised treatment. This was administered weekly after the initial treatment, which was an Aggressive Energy (AE) Drain (see Chapter 5, Toolkit).

Developed in 2001, after seeking advice from eminent colleagues and textbooks, the core protocol assumes Kidney yin deficiency as the root of hot flushes, the prevailing view at the time. It incorporates strategies for managing night sweats and for clearing heat and damp, which were observed to be associated with tamoxifen.[46] Points for the patient were selected with regard for their stated treatment priorities; sometimes I reduced the number of points for women sensitive to needling.

In a study recruiting 50 women, this approach reduced HFNS frequency by an average of 49.8% (p<.0001) at EOT (eight treatments). Improvements in menopause-related symptoms, measured by the Women's Health Questionnaire (WHQ), included sleep, memory and concentration, anxiety, depressed mood, and other symptoms. Women found their HFNS to be less troublesome at EOT and 18-week follow-up.[46] Outcomes were measured mid-treatment (before the fourth treatment) and at EOT (before the eighth treatment), and at four and 18 weeks after EOT.

Table 8.4: A protocol for treating HFNS

Notes:

Insert all needles using even technique and obtain deqi.

All points are needled unilaterally; because of concerns about needling the arm at risk or affected by lymphoedema, arm points are needled contralateral to affected breast.

Treatment principle	Points	Method
Nourish Kidney yin	Open *Ren Mai*: LU-7 *Lieque* KID-6 *Zhaohai* SP-6 *Sanyinjiao* REN-4 *Guanyuan*	Open the *Ren Mai* (Directing Vessel): Insert needle into LU-7 first (on the side not affected by breast cancer) then KID-6 on the opposite side. Retain for at least 20 minutes. After LU-7 and KID-6, needle the remaining points. Do not manipulate the needles. After 20 minutes, remove all needles. KID-6 is penultimate needle removed, and LU-7 the last.
Stop night sweats	HE-6 *Yinxi* KID-7 *Fuliu*	
Clear heat	LI-11 *Quchi*	
Resolve damp	LU-7 *Lieque* LI-11 *Quchi* SP-6 *Sanyinjiao*	

Study 2: Using a fixed protocol – NADA ear acupuncture

Following Study 1, our team investigated a standardised approach, choosing the NADA (National Acupuncture Detoxification Association) protocol (see Chapter 5, Toolkit).[80]

Anecdotal evidence suggested this five-point ear acupuncture protocol, developed for use in detox centres, helped with the HFNS associated with addiction withdrawal.

In our study recruiting 50 women, NADA reduced HFNS frequency by an average of 36% (p<.0001) after eight treatments, delivered weekly. Improvements in menopausal-related symptoms, measured by the WHQ, included sleep, memory and concentration, anxiety, depressed mood, and other symptoms, and participants found their HFNS to be less of a problem.[80]

Comparing the studies

The NADA study did not attain the same levels of overall reduction in HFNS frequency as the semi-individualised approach. The difference at the primary endpoint (EOT) was significant (p=.038).[80] The NADA group also demonstrated a more gradual response, with a 23.6% reduction in HFNS after four treatments compared with the body acupuncture reduction of 40.8% (p=.008).

An interesting difference was observed during follow-up. The body acupuncture group demonstrated a gradual increase in HFNS as time from EOT increased, while the NADA group continued to decrease slightly at both follow-up points. However, the difference between the two groups at four- and 18-week follow-ups is not significant (p=.606 and 0.699 respectively).

Both groups showed good reduction and maintenance of menopause-related symptoms and HFNS as a problem.

Both studies suggest a good level of effectiveness for managing HFNS and associated symptoms. Clinically, NADA's slightly lower performance might be outweighed by its cost-effectiveness to deliver in a group setting, which is a consideration for organisations such as the UK's National Health Service (NHS) or charities, where resources are limited. As always, further research in the form of well-designed RCTs is needed.

Coda
Based on this research, the Lynda Jackson Macmillan Centre implemented a service offering NADA treatment for breast cancer treatment-related HFNS. In 2022, we analysed 15 years of service data, comprising over 2285 treatments given to 300 women. NADA performed similarly in the 'real world' to the research, and there were only two adverse events reported, neither of which was serious.[81,*]

Clinical perspectives

ESSENTIALS

Recommendations for approaching the treatment of HFNS
In view of my clinical experience and the discussion about Kidney yin deficiency (see earlier in this chapter), I proffer this advice:

- Treat what you see, which may not always accord with what textbooks suggest.
- Look at the symptom(s) in the context of the individual person and in the context of that person's experience of cancer diagnosis and treatment.
- Explore what works for the individual.

Developing a toolkit for cancer treatment-related HFNS
In this section, I revisit some approaches introduced in Chapter 5, Toolkit, in the context of HFNS. First, an important note:

---

*   The open access publication is available at https://link.springer.com/article/10.1007/s00520-022-06898-7

In the absence of clear evidence as to the benefit or harm of applying acupuncture to an affected limb, current practice would advise caution and avoid needling limbs with or at risk of lymphoedema. Refer to Chapter 9, Cancer Treatment-Related Lymphoedema, for a detailed discussion.

Protocol for treating hot flushes and night sweats

I often use the protocol designed for my research, presented in Table 8.4 and Chapter 5, Toolkit, finding it useful for individuals presenting with Kidney yin deficiency. It is also useful as a basis for those presenting with other syndromes, in which case I tailor it to their presentation. For example, I supplement it with moxa on relevant points for presentations of Kidney yin and yang deficiency.

NADA ear acupuncture

I use the NADA protocol flexibly in clinic, both in group settings and when treating patients individually. For the latter, I may use it on its own, or in combination with body acupuncture. For breast cancer survivors with bilateral risk of lymphoedema, I often combine NADA with points on the lower body.

Ear seeds or magnets can be applied to the ear points in addition to or instead of needles. I offer this to patients to facilitate symptom control between treatments. For individuals concerned about the appearance of ears seeds, I apply seeds to *Reverse Shenmen* (as detailed in Chapter 5, Toolkit).

Moxibustion

I find moxa very useful, especially for anxious patients, to calm the shen and support the spirit, and for those patients who actively enjoy moxa. (I do not use moxa on patients who clearly dislike it.) I also use it when working according to Five Element principles.

I apply it even when there is Kidney yin deficiency and empty heat (often contraindicated for moxa), although in these cases I use minimal moxa, such as three to five small cones on Kidney chest points and REN-17, and carefully observe the responses.

When working with patients with HFNS, I draw on the following techniques described in detail in Chapter 5, Toolkit:

- Treating the spirit, especially Kidney chest points (I moxa unilaterally and contralaterally to the affected side for breast cancer patients) and REN-17.
- 'Toasted Pericardium Sandwich' – moxa cones on BL-43 *Gaohuangshu* (usually 15 cones, bilateral) and REN-17 *Shanzhong* (three to five cones).

For patients with Blood deficiency, I also consider using moxa (seven cones each point bilaterally) on:

- Four Flowers – BL-17 *Geshu* and BL-19 *Danshu*
- Magnificent Six – BL-17 *Geshu*, BL-18 *Ganshu*, BL-20 *Pishu*.

Five Element acupuncture

Five Element approaches may be used very successfully in treating HFNS, as the case study of Alauda (below) demonstrates. The focus on strengthening the constitution is in harmony with supporting the body's qi so it can better withstand the impact of the adjuvant hormonal treatments. Supporting body, mind, and spirit also assists with this. Furthermore, Five Element techniques and the strong emphasis on the therapeutic relationship can be powerful interventions for addressing stress and anxiety that contribute to HFNS as a problem.

Clearing blocks to treatments can also be important when treating patients with HFNS, including:

- **Aggressive Energy (AE Drain):** many patients report alleviation of HFNS following an Aggressive Energy Drain (see Chapter 5, Toolkit). I discovered this through clinical practice, when patients specifically requested 'the treatment on the back' because it reduced their flushing incidents (this also applies to HFNS associated with natural menopause). I frequently use this in response to patient request; patients who have experienced improvements in HFNS after an AE Drain often suggest it as a treatment when they feel they need it.
- **Seven Dragons:** I use Internal (IDs) or External Dragons (EDs) especially when a patient hasn't made progress after three to four treatments. I also consider these approaches if a patient regresses for no apparent reason, after assessing possible reasons by using the checklist of factors affecting progress or relapse (Table 8.5).

  Seven Dragons are also indicated when HFNS accompany obsessive thoughts or disturbing dreams, as illustrated by Lily's vignette in Chapter 5, Toolkit. As in Lily's case, I use IDs and EDs flexibly and interchangeably, in instances where it may not be possible to needle an area of the body. For example, Lily's recent surgery made it difficult to needle the torso points for ID, so I used EDs instead.

Shen disturbance

Cancer survivors experiencing HFNS often present signs of shen disturbance. In these cases, I may focus solely on this disharmony or incorporate it as part of my treatment strategy. I select points from the:

- Pericardium and Heart channels
- associated back shu (BL-14 *Jueyinshu*, BL-15 *Xinshu*)
- associated front mu (REN-17 *Shanzhong*, REN-14 *Juque*) points
- outer Bladder line (BL-43 *Gaohuanshgu*, BL-44 *Shentang*).

For patients presenting with dream-disturbed sleep, Pericardium points may be especially useful (particularly REN-15 *Jiuwei* in combination with moxa on REN-17 *Shanzhong*). When dreams are distressing or develop into nightmares, I consider clearing IDs or use moxa on BL43 *Gaohuanshgu* and Ren17 *Shanzhong* (see 'Toasted Pericardium Sandwich' in Chapter 5, Toolkit).

Adapted Four Gates (Three Gates)

I frequently use Four Gates (LIV-3 *Taichong* and LI-4 *Hegu*) as a first treatment (adapted to Three Gates, see below). Clinically, I have observed that this can strongly affect HFNS (for both cancer treatment and natural menopause).

For patients who experience this, Four, or Three, Gates may remain the main treatment approach I use. Simple and elegant, its wide-ranging effects are often appropriate for addressing complex symptom patterns (as discussed in Chapter 4, Offering Complex Patients a Simple Piece of Heaven). Especially valuable when treating HFNS are its potential to:

- calm the mind
- alleviate anxiety
- promote sleep in insomnia.[42,82]

ESSENTIALS

Four Gates can be adapted as appropriate for cancer survivors with or at risk of lymphoedema, by excluding the point on the affected limb, thus making it 'Three Gates'. (Obviously, this is not suitable for patients who have, or are at risk of, bilateral lymphoedema, for whom other approaches may be found.)

Additional tools for your toolkit

See the discussions below for:

- prescription for rest
- HFNS Diary.

Lifestyle advice

Managing qi

In addition to conventional lifestyle advice (Box 8.1) patients should also take care to avoid over-extending their qi through activities such as overwork or play.

The importance of rest

Rest is of particular importance to these patients, and I usually 'prescribe' a daily rest (see Chapter 5, Toolkit). Patients who embrace this as a regular practice report that they experience an improvement in their energy levels as well as a reduction in HFNS. Sleep problems also may improve with this practice.

Managing stress

Research identifies a strong relationship between stress and HFNS in natural menopause, and methods that help to reduce stress can positively impact flushing incidents.[24,25,83,84] The stresses of modern life combined with those associated with cancer survivorship, such as fear of recurrence, may affect the frequency and severity of HFNS (as illustrated in the case studies of Alauda (below) and of Rose and Claire in Chapter 11, Survivorship: Navigating the Milestones).

In clinic, I aim to induce a state of deep relaxation during treatment and seek to calm the shen. Acupuncturists can work with patients to identify strategies to minimise and manage stress. A powerful factor in managing HFNS is when a person makes the connection between stress and their HFNS themselves, and then devises their own technique(s) for managing this. I regard this as one of the most effective self-management strategies an individual can harness.

Making progress and managing expectations

The distress caused by frequent, persistent HFNS means that patients desire immediate improvement in their condition. Often, they expect the effects of acupuncture to be instantaneous and complete. Practitioners will also wish to have quick, long-lasting effects from minimal interventions.

Treatment frequency and duration

Despite the research, there is little information about optimum dose of acupuncture for HFNS. As seen in Table 8.1, dose and duration ranges from:

- as few as five treatments delivered on a weekly basis – five treatments over five weeks[65]
- to 16 treatments delivered twice weekly for four weeks, then weekly for eight weeks – 16 treatments over 12 weeks.[70]

In a Korean study, dosage was three treatments a week for four weeks, that is, 12 treatments over four weeks.[64] In my research studies, treatments were weekly for eight sessions.[46,80]

While there is little consensus, these provide some guidelines. Practical factors for people attending for treatment are also a consideration, and include time for the treatment itself, time to travel to treatment, and cost of treatment, as well as cultural expectations of frequency of treatment (e.g. daily treatment appears customary in China, while in Western countries regular treatment is likely to be weekly).

In my private practice, I prefer weekly treatment, with reviews at four and eight weeks, spacing out treatments as the condition improves.

Managing expectations

Managing expectations is vital when treating HFNS. I explain to patients that acupuncture does not work like a tap that immediately turns off HFNS; instead, improvements may be gradual and cumulative. Responses vary according to the individual and I have observed:

- Instant changes, resulting in reduced frequency and/or severity.
- Gradual change, with cumulative improvement in frequency and/or severity.
- Reduced frequency and increased severity (or vice versa).

- Daytime flushes decrease and night sweats increase, or vice versa.
- No apparent change for some weeks, then a sudden dramatic improvement.
- Symptoms worsen severely for 24 hours, then improve dramatically.

There may be other permutations. Both practitioner and patient may need to exercise patience. I have met practitioners who discharge patients after three treatments, identifying them as non-responders or patients who cannot be helped. My advice is:

- Expect to see noticeable change after three to four treatments and set the patient's expectations to see a gradual improvement.
- Check for changes in other aspects of the patient's health. Is sleep improving? Is energy improving? Are there changes in any other symptoms?
- Check the patient's expectations. Patients may disregard gradual changes, considering anything less than complete and total cessation of HFNS as 'no change'.

Box 8.3 illustrates the variety of responses, taken from my Study 1, in which participants were invited to give feedback on their experiences after their third treatment.

Box 8.3: Breast cancer survivors' experiences after three body acupuncture treatments

I am sorry to say that I have not experienced any significant changes since starting acupuncture. The hot flushes are as yet unchanged. However, I think that I am sleeping better at night and am probably more relaxed during the day. (Participant 35)

Following the second treatment, the hot flushes continued in number, averaging approximately six over the day, but increased intensity significantly. However, since my third treatment last Wednesday, I have suffered no hot flushes at all since Thursday – Friday, Saturday, Sunday so far have been flush free! (Participant 40)

Still have hot flushes, still have problems sleeping. (Participant 45)

Amount of hot flushes reduced by approx. 50%. Intensity has also reduced. I have much more energy. (Participant 04)

I am convinced this treatment is slowly starting to work! Before...hot flushes during the day were quite unbearable and I was experiencing six to eight during the day. The night flushes too were just awful. Around three to five per night. Totally wet through and had to get up to change clothes. Since my treatment started the hot flushes have reduced in the length of each flush and also there is a reduction in how many hot flushes/night sweats I am experiencing. (Participant 13)

Patterns of change

In observing participants' experience of change in my research, three factors appeared to be a related: HFNS, sleep, and energy.

It seems obvious that if night sweats diminish, sleep will improve, with consequent improvement in energy. However, in many cases, participants reported improved energy before noticing changes in HFNS or sleep. For others, sleep improved before anything else changed.

Figure 8.2 illustrates these permutations. The entry point for change can be any-where in the cycle. Awareness of this can help practitioners and patients identify that change is happening. Even if HFNS are not showing immediate or noticeable change, improvements in sleep or energy are good predictors for improvement in HFNS. It is as if the body has its own priorities, using the changes effected by acupuncture to carry out fundamental repairs before dealing with HFNS.

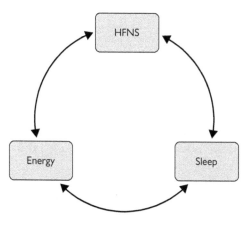

FIGURE 8.2: POSSIBLE PERMUTATIONS OF CHANGE

If there is no change, or if the patient regresses

If there really is no change on any level after three to four treatments, I check for blocks to treatment, and address any that may be blocking progress (see Chapter 5, Toolkit: 'Five Element blocks to treatment').

This assumes treatment is taking place sufficiently frequently. Also, check other factors that can affect progress (Table 8.5).

Other factors that affect progress

Many factors can affect progress or cause patients who have been improving to relapse. Use this checklist to identify possible contributors to this, and to help patients self-monitor.

Table 8.5: Checklist of factors affecting HFNS progress or relapse

If the answer to any of these questions is 'yes', discuss their potential impact on HFNS with the patient.	
• Is there a change in any existing non-cancer-related health conditions? Has a new health problem arisen?	
• Has the patient had an acute illness (colds, flu, or other)?	
• Had the patient undergone other medical events (surgery, other invasive investigations)?	
• Have there been changes in medication (either cancer or non-cancer-related, and including changes in brand of hormonal therapy)?	
• Have there been new or unusual life events that are stressful?	
• Has the patient increased activity levels (work, exercise, social)?	
• Is a cancer follow-up appointment imminent?	
• Is an anniversary of cancer diagnosis or treatment imminent?	
• Is acupuncture treatment too infrequent?	
• Is there a possibility of cancer recurrence (check Red Flags)?	

RED FLAG

Heavy drenching night sweats can be a sign of cancer and recurrence.

I have also observed (often in hindsight) that when cancer recurs or progresses, daytime and/or nocturnal HFNS can become intractable and do not respond to treatment.

It may be difficult to assess this. However, if the factors listed in Table 8.5 have been ruled out, it may be necessary to consider recurrence, especially if the patient presents with any other symptoms indicating cancer recurrence (see Chapter 13, Reducing Risk of Recurrence and Subsequent Primary Cancers). Refer the patient to their oncology health professional or physician. This may be a difficult topic and requires sensitivity.

VIGNETTE: YVES AND THE IMPACT OF STRESS ABOUT MEDICAL INTERVENTIONS ON HFNS

This vignette illustrates how stress about medical interventions can cause HFNS to dramatically flare.

Yves, aged 68, was experiencing HFNS as a consequence of anti-androgen therapy for prostate cancer. He had heard about NADA for HFNS and sought this treatment.

Yves was a charming and successful man, whose quiet assurance suggested he was accustomed to being in control. Now retired, he enjoyed family life and attended to his health. Walking a good five miles a day was his chosen physical activity, and his wife, a good cook, ensured that his diet was healthy and delicious. He appeared to have taken the cancer diagnosis in his stride.

His HFNS responded well to weekly NADA treatment. However, on attending for his sixth treatment, he reported they had flared up during the previous week and were worse than they had ever been.

There was no apparent reason, until Yves recounted his hospital visit earlier that week for brachytherapy (implants of radioactive seeds in the prostate). He recounted the alarm of the nurse when she took his blood pressure, how she summoned the consultant, and how the consultant dismissed the nurse's concerns. This was not pathological high blood pressure, he said, but rather a strong reaction of fear to the impending process. The intervention was administered successfully, and Yves's blood pressure returned to normal. However, his HFNS flared.

When I suggested this may have been a reaction to the intense experience at the hospital, Yves was not keen to admit to being anxious about the procedure. Nonetheless, on resuming NADA treatment, his HFNS immediately reduced.

Yves's case illustrates how medical interventions may exacerbate HFNS. It also shows how people may feel compelled to put on a brave face, not admitting to feeling frightened by medical procedures.

Empowerment and self-management

Acupuncture can reduce HFNS and make them more manageable. Generally, HFNS are unlikely to disappear completely in the short term. Acupuncturists can play a vital role in empowering patients and helping them to manage this (additional) chronic condition.

Keeping an HFNS diary

Keeping a diary of HFNS, such as that shown in the Appendices (online), can be beneficial to both practitioner and patient. I aim to have new patients keep this for one to two weeks before starting treatment.

Recording each HFNS incident and using a simple system to rate severity can give valuable information. Used prior to starting treatment, the diary provides a baseline measurement of HFNS. Comparing this with later diaries is a useful measure of progress and shows changes in flushing patterns.

Many patients appreciate the insight a diary gives them. By recording HFNS they may:

- gain insight into **how many incidents** they are experiencing ('I didn't realise I was having so many' is a frequent comment)
- see **patterns** in flushing
- identify **triggers**
- confirm **progress** over time.

Identifying triggers empowers survivors. For example, many find that alcohol triggers HFNS. Identifying this relationship gives the person choice; they may eliminate alcohol completely or they may choose to have that glass of wine and accept the consequence of HFNS. Whatever their decision, it becomes an active choice, putting the patient in control of managing their HFNS.

A person's attitude to diary keeping can also provide information about that person, as well as treatment progress. While some are diligent, others find diary keeping challenging (for some, it is not a suitable strategy and should be abandoned). Some find diaries useful learning tools and utilise the insights to facilitate self-management. A vital sign of progress is when a committed diary keeper finds it no longer worthwhile keeping the diary, as the HFNS are sufficiently under control for them to abandon close monitoring.

Patient perspectives

CASE STUDY: ALAUDA AND LONG-TERM MANAGEMENT OF HFNS

Introduction

Alauda's case tells the story of managing HFNS long term (she has chosen to continue having acupuncture for 13 years) and demonstrates many of the techniques discussed in this chapter. Alauda was actively involved in writing and reviewing this case study, contributing many comments.

Background and main complaints

Alauda, aged 46, had surgery and radiotherapy for invasive ductal carcinoma in the left breast diagnosed ten months before starting acupuncture in 2009. Tamoxifen commenced two weeks after surgery. She experienced no HFNS until convalescing from a subsequent total hysterectomy and bilateral oophorectomy for a large fibroid. Since then, she experienced up to 20 HFNS in 24 hours, many of which were severe night sweats that disrupted her sleep.

Poor concentration was also a concern. A senior medical professional, Alauda was also an internationally competitive sportswoman in a high-risk sport, so good concentration was vital to both her professional and leisure activities. She described herself as 'emotionally labile'; she had lost confidence, was feeling unmotivated, and was also subject to feeling low. Prior to the cancer diagnosis, her health was good.

Questioning the systems

Sleep: A 'night person', Alauda was reluctant to go to bed before midnight, after which she read. Wakened by night sweats at 3am.

Appetite: Eating habits irregular: 'not good' about eating breakfast, had tea and a biscuit on arriving at work; lunch irregular, either taken late or skipped; dinner, her only 'decent meal', was eaten late in the evening.

Drink: Did not drink much fluid during the day; drank water at night to cool off after night sweats.

Bowels: Experienced constipation, passing small dry stools with some difficulty.

Urination: Had returned to normal after the hysterectomy.

Sweating and temperature: Sensitive to cold, with chills following flushing incidents.

Other information: Alauda was single, with a demanding career and a deep commitment to her sport and to her ageing parents. On commencing acupuncture, she was working part time as part of phased return to work following the hysterectomy. She resumed full-time work a month later.

Physical examination: Tongue: Red and dry, with a thick white coat at the rear. **Pulses:** Deep and weak on both sides, with some wiriness on the Liver pulse.

Diagnoses
CM diagnosis: Symptoms, tongue, and pulse picture suggested Kidney yin deficiency.

CF diagnosis: CF not apparent at this stage. I prioritised clearing any blocks to treatment before addressing HFNS.

Treatment approach
Alauda's treatment priorities were to reduce HFNS and improve concentration. She also needed emotional support.

Lifestyle advice
I was concerned about Alauda's daily habits, especially eating, and sleeping. At her first treatment, I discussed the importance of:

- regular meals, particularly having a good breakfast
- a daily afternoon rest
- going to bed earlier.

HFNS diary
Alauda took to keeping a diary with great enthusiasm. It was her decision to keep an ongoing daily record on an Excel spreadsheet. She scored the flushes (1 for mild, 2 for moderate, and 3 for severe) and the weekly totals are referenced below.

Initial treatments
Table 8.6 details Alauda's initial six treatments; methods can be found in Chapter 5, Toolkit.

Table 8.6: Alauda's initial treatments

Notes:

No needles or moxa on the left limb or left torso quadrant.

All needling to obtain deqi, no further stimulation, needles retained for at least 20 minutes unless otherwise specified.

Abbreviations: Tx treatment; **RS** right side; **LS** left side

Tx	Treatment principles	Points	Notes
1	Clear block to treatment: Aggressive Energy (AE) Drain	BL-13 *Feishu* BL-14 *Jueyinshu* BL-15 *Xinshu* BL-18 *Ganshu* BL-20 *Pishu* BL-23 *Shenshu* Plus 3 check needles	Superficial needling RS only.
2	Internal Dragons	Extra point 0.25 cun below REN-15 *Jiuwei* ST-25 *Tianshu* ST-32 *Futu* ST-41 *Jiexi*	
	Ground treatment	SI-4 *Wangu* (RS) HE-7 *Shenmen* (RS)	
3–6	Treat spirit	KID-24 *Lingxu* OR: KID-25 *Shencang* AND KI-27 *Shufu*	Direct moxa (3 cones, no needling) RS only.
	Address HFNS (using protocol in Table 8.4)		
	Nourish Kidney yin	Open *Ren Mai*: LU-7 *Lieque* (RS) and KID-6 *Zhaohai* (LS) REN-4 *Guanyuan* SP-6 *Sanyinjiao* (RS)	
	Treat night sweats	HE-6 *Yinxi* (RS) KID-7 *Fului* (LS)	

Progress through treatment

Tx 1: Alauda reported feeling calmer after treatment 1 and thought daytime HFNS were reducing.

Tx 2–7: During treatment 2, she 'saw colours' (especially purple) on closing her eyes. Observing this was associated with deep relaxation, and we talked about the importance of getting 'purple time'.

Alauda started making lifestyle changes and ate breakfast before leaving for work. She reported feeling changes in herself: she felt brighter, in control, more capable and confident about work, and was getting less 'worked up' about things. She took time off work to recover from a cold, something she would not normally have done.

HFNS incidents were reducing and by treatment 7:

- frequency reduced from 17–20 per day to ten
- total weekly HFNS score was down from 195 at the first treatment to 90. (HFNS scores were calculated by adding up the ratings (1 for mild, 2 for moderate, 3 for severe) for all HFNS.)

She noticed that her HFNS were more frequent when she was 'mentally in turmoil' and when she was physically compromised by the cold.

Addressing the emotions

I was becoming familiar with Alauda's emotional states. Using our joint observation of the strong impact these had on her HFNS, I began to support her emotions.

I introduced strategies to calm shen and harmonise qi, supplementing the core protocol for treating HFNS (Table 8.4). These included the 'Toasted Pericardium Sandwich', Three Gates, and using moxa on the Kidney chest points to support the spirit (all as mentioned above and in Chapter 5, Toolkit). I administered these according to her presentation at her weekly treatments.

I also incorporated extra point M-HN-3 *Yintang* to calm the shen and address the intermittent sinus problems Alauda experienced when overtired.

Progress!

At treatment 9, Alauda triumphantly produced her diary, announcing her HFNS had reduced by 50% after eight treatments!

She aimed to have 'purple time' each day and was working on improving eating habits. Return to full-time work and sporting activities was tiring, getting sufficient rest was a struggle, and she was short-tempered at work. I introduced vaccaria ear seeds on the back of the ear (*Reverse Shenmen*, as described in Chapter 5, Toolkit) to give her emotional control. Alauda found this very helpful, pressing them whenever she felt irritable. An allergic reaction to the adhesive on the seeds was overcome by experimenting with different types until we found a brand she could tolerate.

The advantages of keeping a diary

A careful diary keeper, Alauda began noticing the impact of her lifestyle and emotions on her HFNS. She called this 'getting payback' – HFNS increased if she overexerted herself. She began to make changes to curb activities and get more rest. She was beginning to take control.

An emotional setback – the power of an anniversary

A spike in HFNS occurred around treatment 17, accompanied by feelings of 'melancholy' and 'apathy'. 'I can't be bothered' was her attitude; she was lacking motivation, over-sleeping, and arriving late for work.

This occurred a few weeks before the first anniversary of her diagnosis; it peaked the week before she was due for a check-up and mammogram. We discussed the potential impact of anniversaries of cancer diagnosis and treatments, and how fear of cancer recurrence could cause symptoms to flare (see Chapter 11, Survivorship: Navigating the

Milestones). An 'all clear' from the oncologist saw the HFNS reduce, but the melancholy remained.

Adjusting the strategy – treating the constitutional factor (CF)

As the melancholy persisted, I chose to switch to a Five Element approach.

CF diagnosis: Alauda's voice took on a deep groan, especially when tired or stressed. Groaning is the sound associated with the water element and I began to address this. I still frequently used the HFNS protocol, finishing the treatment with points for CF, as detailed in Table 8.7.

Table 8.7: Examples of Alauda's later treatments, focusing on treating the CF

Notes:

No needles or moxa on the left limb or left torso quadrant.

All needling to obtain deqi, no further stimulation, needles retained for at least 20 minutes. When treating the CF, needles not retained.

Abbreviations: Tx treatment; **RS** right side; **LS** left side; **NR** not retained

Tx	Treatment principles	Points	Notes
22	Strengthen will (motivation)	BL-13 *Feishu* BL-52 *Zhishi*	Bilateral, moxa (3 cones each point) followed by needling.
	Tonify qi and yang (for physical and mental exhaustion and depression)	REN-6 *Qihai*	Moxa on needle.
23	Treat spirit	KID-22 *Bulang* (RS)	Direct moxa (3 cones, no needling).
	Treat HFNS	See Tx 3–6, Table 8.6	
	Treat CF (Fire points of water)	BL-60 *Kunlun* KID-2 *Rangu*	Bilateral, NR.
24	Treat HFNS	See Tx 3–6, Table 8.6	
	Treat CF (Horary points of water)	BL-66 *Zutonggu* KID-10 *Yingu*	Bilateral, NR.
25	Treat HFNS	See Tx 3–6, Table 8.6	
	Treat sinusitis	M-HN-3 *Yintang* LI-20 *Yinxiang*	Bilateral.
	Treat CF (yuan source and earth point of water)	KID-3 *Taixi*	Bilateral, NR.
26	As per Tx 25 plus	BL-40 *Weizhong* (earth point of water)	Bilateral, NR.
27	Treat HFNS	See Tx 3–6, Table 8.6	
	Treat CF (yuan source points)	BL-64 *Jinggu* KID-3 *Taixi*	Bilateral, NR.

Progress through treatments 22–27

Alauda responded well; the melancholy began to lift. She felt positive, handled irritations at work, and performed well in her sport. HFNS scores were in the low 40s, well down from the initial score of 195. She used her diary to monitor and self-manage, always noting that physical and emotional overexertion caused HFNS to increase.

Long-term feedback

By the second anniversary of her cancer diagnosis, Alauda's weekly HFNS scores were in the 20s, and she was reasonably comfortable with her HFNS. She chose to continue having acupuncture, using it to manage the life's stresses: professional life became increasingly challenging, her parents' health was a growing concern, and she was focused on deeper issues of life as she approached her 50th birthday.

Anniversaries of cancer diagnosis and treatment

Transient increases in HFNS occurred when Alauda had scheduled follow-ups with her surgeon and oncologist, diminishing when she received the 'all clear'. Anniversaries of her cancer diagnosis and treatment triggered extreme anxieties, even as she approached the fourth anniversary of the end of cancer treatment. Alauda was able to identify and understand these triggers, and acupuncture focused on supporting her through these periods.

Lifestyle and self-needling

We continued to address improving her lifestyle – Alauda still struggles to get to bed early enough to ensure she has adequate rest. At treatment 63, I taught Alauda to self-needle KID-3 *Taixi*. This aimed to help her manage her energy, especially when competing abroad. I judged this was a safe strategy because of her medical training combined with her sensitivity to point sensation.

Summary

Alauda's case illustrates the interaction between lifestyle, emotions, and HFNS. Her diligent diary keeping also shows how acupuncture combined with improvements in lifestyle can reduce HFNS. The diary remains a valuable tool, enabling her to understand the relationship between her behaviours and HFNS.

Coda

Reviewing this case study during the Covid-19 (2020) pandemic, Alauda wrote:

> I continued to have semi-regular acupuncture sessions which were particularly helpful in managing work and life events, such as bereavement. I continue my hot flush diary to this day, finding it a useful aid memoir for physical and emotional feedback. I have become more aware of my physical signs of stress and/or fatigue, such as dry lips. I still carry out self-needling when faced with potentially challenging work or sporting events.
>
> Overall, as a medical professional I appreciate the holistic approach of acupuncture which has resulted in an improved lifestyle (although I still struggle to achieve

enough rest!). I have become more aware of my mental and physical signs of stress and fatigue, to recognise when intervention is required.

Unusually, Alauda continues to keep her HFNS diary, even though hormonal treatment ended three years ago. When asked to comment on this, she replied:

It has become a basic diary of my physiological response to what life throws me. I suppose when I start having more flushes or more intense flushing, it helps me to rationalise them, so they don't take over! Makes me reset!

CHAPTER SUMMARY

- Acupuncture can be used to successfully manage cancer treatment-related HFNS.
- Acupuncture has been shown to be as effective as pharmacological interventions for HFNS, with fewer side effects.
- HFNS respond to a variety of approaches. The art of successful treatment is to identify what works for each patient, considering the patient's overall physical and emotional state.
- Change may be gradual.
- It may not always be possible to eliminate HFNS, but they are likely to reduce and become less of a bother to the patient.
- Patients can be educated to self-manage to improve control.
- Lifestyle is an important factor in short- and long-term management.

References

1. Sturdee DW, Hunter MS, Maki PM, et al. The menopausal hot flush: a review. Climacteric 2017;20(4):296–305.
2. Walker G, de Valois B, Davies R, et al. Ear acupuncture for hot flushes – the perceptions of women with breast cancer. Complement. Ther. Clin. Pract. 2007;13(4):250–257.
3. Voda AM Climacteric hot flash. Maturitas 1981;3(1):73–90.
4. Rossouw JE, Anderson GL, Prentice RL, et al. Writing Group for the Women's Health Initiative Investigators. Risks and benefits of estrogen plus progestin in healthy postmenopausal women: principal results From the Women's Health Initiative randomized controlled trial. JAMA. 2002 Jul 17;288(3):321–333.
5. National Institute for Health and Care Excellence (NICE) Early and locally advanced breast cancer: diagnosis and management NICE guideline [NG101]. London: NICE; 2018.
6. Moon Z, Hunter MS, Moss-Morris R, et al. Factors related to the experience of menopausal symptoms in women prescribed tamoxifen. J. Psychosom. Obstet. Gynaecol. 2017;38(3):226–235.
7. Kligman L, Younus J Management of hot flashes in women with breast cancer. Curr. Oncol. 2010;17(1):81–86.
8. Fenlon DR, Corner J, Haviland JS Menopausal hot flushes after breast cancer. Eur. J. Cancer Care (Engl). 2009;18(2):140–148.
9. Marsden J British Menopause Society Consensus Statement: the risks and benefits of HRT before and after a breast cancer diagnosis. Post. Reprod. Health 2019;25(1):33–37.
10. Frisk J Managing hot flushes in men after prostate cancer: A systematic review. Maturitas 2010;65(1):15–22.
11. Hunter M, Stefanopoulou E Vasomotor symptoms in prostate cancer survivors undergoing androgen deprivation therapy. Climacteric 2016;19(1):91–97.

12. Capriglione S, Plotti S, Montera R, *et al.* Role of paroxetine in the management of hot flashes in gynecological cancer survivors: Results of the first randomized single-center controlled trial. Gynecol. Oncol. 2016;143(3):584–588.

13. PDQ° Supportive and Palliative Care Editorial Board PDQ Hot Flashes and Night Sweats. Bethesda, MD: National Cancer Institute; 2021. Available from: www.cancer.gov/about-cancer/treatment/side-effects/hot-flashes-hp-pdq

14. Tran S, Hickey M, Saunders C, *et al.* Nonpharmacological therapies for the management of menopausal vasomotor symptoms in breast cancer survivors. Support. Care Cancer 2021;29(3):1183–1193.

15. Fenlon DR, Rogers AE The experience of hot flushes after breast cancer. Cancer Nurs. 2007;30(4):E19–26.

16. Finck G, Barton DL, Loprinzi CL, *et al.* Definitions of hot flashes in breast cancer survivors. J. Pain Symptom Manage. 1998;16(5):327–333.

17. Miller HG, Li RM Measuring hot flashes: Summary of a National Institutes of Health Workshop. Mayo Clin. Proc. 2004;79:668–670.

18. National Institutes of Health State-of-the-Science Panel National Institutes of Health State-of-the-Science Conference statement: management of menopause-related symptoms. Ann. Intern. Med. 2005;142(12, pt 1):1003–1013.

19. Carpenter JS, Johnson DH, Wagner LJ, *et al.* Hot flushes and related outcomes in breast cancer survivors and matched comparison women. Oncol. Nurs. Forum 2002;29(3):16–25.

20. Ulloa EW, Salup R, Patterson SG, *et al.* Relationship between hot flashes and distress in men receiving androgen deprivation therapy for prostate cancer. Psychooncology 2008;18(6):598–605

21. Love RR, Feyzi JM Reductions in vasomotor symptoms from tamoxifen over time. J. Natl. Cancer Inst. 1993;85(8):673–674.

22. Davis SR, Panjari M, Robinson PJ, *et al.* Menopausal symptoms in breast cancer survivors nearly 6 years after diagnosis. Menopause 2014;21(10):1075–1081.

23. Atkins L, Fallowfield L Intentional and non-intentional non-adherence to medication among breast cancer. Eur. J. Cancer 2006;42:2271–2276.

24. Hunter M, Liao KL A psychological analysis of menopausal hot flushes. Br. J. Clin. Psychol. 1995;34:589–599.

25. Swartzman LC, Edelberg R, Kemmann E Impact of stress on objectively recorded menopausal hot flushes and on flush report bias. Health Psychol. 1990;9(5):529–545.

26. Szabo RA, Marino JL, Hickey M Managing menopausal symptoms after cancer. Climacteric 2019;22(6):572–578.

27. Biglia N, Bounous V, Sgro L, *et al.* Treatment of climacteric symptoms in survivors of gynaecological cancer. Maturitas 2015;82(3):296–298.

28. Hickey M, Davis SR, Sturdee DW Treatment of menopausal symptoms: what shall we do now? Lancet 2005;366:409–421.

29. Biglia N, Cozzarella M, Cacciari F, *et al.* Menopause after breast cancer: a survey on breast cancer survivors. Maturitas 2003;45(1):29–38.

30. Hickey M, Saunders CM, Stuckey BGA Non-hormonal treatments for menopausal symptoms. Maturitas 2007;57:85–89.

31. Johns C, Seav SM, Dominick SA, *et al.* Informing hot flash treatment decisions for breast cancer survivors: a systematic review of randomized trials comparing active interventions. Breast Cancer Res. Treat. 2016;156(3):415–426.

32. National Institute for Health and Care Excellence (NICE) Scenario: Tamoxifen – prescribing information. NICE; 2019. Available from: https://cks.nice.org.uk/topics/tamoxifen-managing-adverse-effects/management/tamoxifen-prescribing-information

33. National Institute for Health and Care Excellence Guideline NG131: Prostate cancer: diagnosis and management. 2019. Available from: www.nice.org.uk/guidance/ng131

34. American Society of Clinical Oncology Hormone deprivation symptoms in men. 2019. Available from: www.cancer.net/coping-with-cancer/physical-emotional-and-social-effects-cancer/managing-physical-side-effects/hormone-deprivation-symptoms-men

35. Johnson A, Roberts L, Elkins G Complementary and alternative medicine for menopause. J. Evid. Based Integr. Med. 2019;24:2515690X19829380.

36. Hutton B, Hersi M, Cheng W, *et al.* Comparing interventions for management of hot flashes in patients with breast and prostate cancer: a systematic review with meta-analyses. Oncol. Nurs. Forum 2020;47(4):E86–E106.

37. Macmillan Cancer Support Complementary therapies for managing menopausal symptoms. London: Macmillan Cancer Support; 2018. Available from: www.macmillan.org.uk/cancer-information-and-support/impacts-of-cancer/menopausal-symptoms-and-cancer-treatment

38. American Cancer Society Menopausal hormone therapy after breast cancer. Atlanta: American Cancer Society; 2019. Available from: www.cancer.org/cancer/breast-cancer/living-as-a-breast-cancer-survivor/menopausal-hormone-therapy-after-breast-cancer.html

39. van Driel CM, Stuursma A, Schroevers MJ, et al. Mindfulness, cognitive behavioural and behaviour-based therapy for natural and treatment-induced menopausal symptoms: a systematic review and meta-analysis. BJOG 2019;126(3):330–339.

40. Hickey M, Szabo RA, Hunter MS Non-hormonal treatments for menopausal symptoms. BMJ 2017;359:j5101.

41. Santen RJ, Stuenkel CA, Davis SR, et al. Managing menopausal symptoms and associated clinical issues in breast cancer survivors. J. Clin. Endocrinol. Metab. 2017;102(10):3647–3661.

42. Maciocia G The foundations of Chinese medicine: a comprehensive text for acupuncturists and herbalists. Edinburgh: Churchill Livingstone; 1989.

43. Maciocia G Menopausal syndrome. In: Obstetrics and gynecology in Chinese medicine. Edinburgh: Churchill Livingstone; 1998. pp. 741–762.

44. Zell B, Hirata J, Alon M, et al. Diagnosis of symptomatic postmenopausal women by traditional Chinese medicine practitioners. Menopause 2000;7(2):129–134.

45. Maciocia G Diagnosis in Chinese medicine: a comprehensive guide. Edinburgh: Churchill Livingstone; 2004.

46. de Valois B, Young T, Robinson N, et al. Using traditional acupuncture for breast cancer-related hot flashes and night sweats. J. Altern. Complement. Med. 2010;16(10):1047–1057.

47. Borud E, Alraek T, White A, et al. The acupuncture treatment for postmenopausal hot flushes (acuflash) study: traditional Chinese medicine diagnoses and acupuncture points used, and their relation to the treatment response. Acupunct. Med. 2009;27:101–108.

48. Scheid V Not very traditional, nor exactly Chinese, so what kind of medicine is it? TCM's discourse on menopause and its implications for practice, teaching, and research. J. Chinese Med. 2006;82:5–18.

49. Scheid V Traditional Chinese medicine: What are we investigating? The case of menopause. Complement. Ther. Med. 2007;15:54–68.

50. Befus D, Coeytaux RR, Goldstein KM, et al. Management of menopause symptoms with acupuncture: an umbrella systematic review and meta-analysis. J. Altern. Complement. Med. 2018;24(4 %R 10.1089/acm.2016.0408):314–323.

51. Alfhaily F, Ewies AA Acupuncture in managing menopausal symptoms: hope or mirage? Climacteric 2007;10:371–380.

52. Dodin S, Blanchet C, Marc I, et al. Acupuncture for menopausal hot flushes. Cochrane Database Syst. Rev. 2013;2013(7):CD007410.

53. Frisk JW, Hammar ML, Ingvar M, et al. How long do the effects of acupuncture on hot flashes persist in cancer patients? Support. Care Cancer 2014;22(5):1409–1415.

54. Chien TJ, Hsu CH, Liu CY, et al. Effect of acupuncture on hot flush and menopause symptoms in breast cancer – a systematic review and meta-analysis. PLoS One 2017;12(8):e0180918.

55. Chien TJ, Liu CY, Fang CJ, et al. The maintenance effect of acupuncture on breast cancer-related menopause symptoms: a systematic review. Climacteric 2020;23(2):130–139.

56. Chen YP, Liu T, Peng YY, et al. Acupuncture for hot flashes in women with breast cancer: A systematic review. J. Cancer Res. Ther. 2016;12(2):535–542.

57. Chiu HY, Shyu YK, Chang PC, et al. Effects of acupuncture on menopause-related symptoms in breast cancer survivors: a meta-analysis of randomized controlled trials. Cancer Nurs. 2016;39(3):228–237.

58. Wang XP, Zhang DJ, Wei XD, et al. Acupuncture for the relief of hot flashes in breast cancer patients: a systematic review and meta-analysis of randomized controlled trials and observational studies. J. Cancer Res. Ther. 2018;14(Suppl.):S600–S608.

59. Lee MS, Kim K-H, Shin BC, et al. Acupuncture for treating hot flushes in men with prostate cancer: a systematic review. Support. Care Cancer 2009;17:763–770.

60. Leon-Ferre RA, Majithia N, Loprinzi CL Management of hot flashes in women with breast cancer receiving ovarian function suppression. Cancer Treat. Rev. 2017;52:82–90.

61. Fenlon D, Morgan A, Khambaita P, et al. Management of hot flushes in UK breast cancer patients: clinician and patient perspectives. J. Psychosom. Obstet. Gynaecol. 2017;38(4):276–283.

62. Islam RM, Bell RJ, Rizvi F, et al. Vasomotor symptoms in women in Asia appear comparable with women in Western countries: a systematic review. Menopause 2017;24(11):1313–1322.

63. Yang D, Haines CJ, Pan P, et al. Menopausal symptoms in mid-life women in southern China. Climacteric 2008;11(4):329–336.

64. Jeong YJ, Park YS, Kwon HJ, et al. Acupuncture for the treatment of hot flashes in patients with breast cancer receiving antiestrogen therapy: a pilot study in Korean women. J. Altern. Complement. Med. 2013;19(8):690–696.

65. Bokmand S, Flyger H Acupuncture relieves menopausal discomfort in breast cancer patients: a prospective, double blinded, randomized study. Breast 2013;22(3):320–323.
66. Bao T, Cai L, Snyder C, *et al.* Patient-reported outcomes in women with breast cancer enrolled in a dual-center, double-blind, randomized controlled trial assessing the effect of acupuncture in reducing aromatase inhibitor-induced musculoskeletal symptoms. Cancer 2014;120(3):381–389.
67. Frisk J, Carlhäll S, Källström A-C, *et al.* Long-term follow-up of acupuncture and hormone therapy on hot flushes in women with breast cancer: a prospective, randomized, controlled multicentre trial. Climacteric 2008;11:166–174.
68. Frisk J, Kallstrom AC, Wall N, *et al.* Acupuncture improves health-related quality of life (HRQoL) and sleep in women with breast cancer and hot flushes. Support. Care Cancer 2012;20(4):715–724.
69. Lesi G, Razzini G, Musti MA, *et al.* Acupuncture as an integrative approach for the treatment of hot flashes in women with breast cancer: a prospective multicenter randomized controlled trial (AcCliMaT). J. Clin. Oncol. 2016;34(15):1795–1802.
70. Walker EM, Rodriguez AI, Kohn B, *et al.* Acupuncture versus venlafaxine for the management of vasomotor symptoms in patients with hormone receptor-positive breast cancer: a randomized controlled trial. J. Clin. Oncol. 2010;28(4):634–640.
71. Mao JJ, Bowman MA, Xie SX, *et al.* Electroacupuncture versus gabapentin for hot flashes among breast cancer survivors: a randomized placebo-controlled trial. J. Clin. Oncol. 2015;33(31):3615–3620.
72. Hervik J, Mjåland P Acupuncture for the treatment of hot flashes in breast cancer patients, a randomized, controlled trial. Breast Cancer Res. Treat. 2009;116(2):311–316.
73. Liljegren A, Gunnarsson P, Landgren BM, *et al.* Reducing vasomotor symptoms with acupuncture in breast cancer patients treated with adjuvant tamoxifen: a randomized controlled trial. Breast Cancer Res. Treat. 2012;135(3):791–798.
74. Frisk J, Spetz A, Hjertberg H, *et al.* Two modes of acupuncture as a treatment for hot flushes in men with prostate cancer – a prospective multicenter study with long-term follow-up. Eur. Urol. 2009;55(1):156–163.
75. Harding C, Harris A, Chadwich D Auricular acupuncture: a novel treatment for vasomotor symptoms associated with luteinizing-hormone releasing agonist treatment for prostate cancer. Br. J. Urol. 2008;103:186090.
76. Beer TM, Benavides M, Emmons SL, *et al.* Acupuncture for hot flashes in patients with prostate cancer. Urology 2010;76(5):1182–1188.
77. Ashamalla H, Jiang M, Guirguis A, *et al.* Acupuncture for the alleviation of hot flashes in men treated with androgen ablation therapy. Int. J. Radiat. Oncol. Biol. Phys. 2011;79(5):1358–1363.
78. Capodice J, Cheetham P, Benson M, *et al.* Acupuncture for the treatment of hot flashes in men with advanced prostate cancer. Int. J. Clin. Med. 2011;2(1):51–55.
79. Park J-E, Lee MS, Jung S, *et al.* Moxibustion for treating menopausal hot flashes: a randomized clinical trial. Menopause 2009;16(4):660–665.
80. de Valois B, Young T, Robinson N, *et al.* NADA ear acupuncture for breast cancer treatment-related hot flashes and night sweats: an observational study. Med. Acupunct. 2012;24(4):256–268.
81. de Valois B, Young T, Thorpe P, *et al.* Acupuncture in the real world: evaluating a 15-year NADA auricular acupuncture service for breast cancer survivors experiencing hot flushes and night sweats as a consequence of adjuvant hormonal therapies. Support. Care Cancer 2022;30(6):5063–5074.
82. Maciocia G The psyche in Chinese medicine. London: Churchill Livingstone; 2009.
83. Carmody JF, Crawford S, Salmoirago-Blotcher E, *et al.* Mindfulness training for coping with hot flushes. Menopause 2011;18(6):611–620.
84. Fenlon DR, Corner J, Haviland JS A randomized controlled trial of relaxation training to reduce hot flashes in women with primary breast cancer. J. Pain Symptom Manage. 2008;35(4):397–405.

Chapter 9

Cancer Treatment-Related Lymphoedema

Introduction

The enormity of the impact of cancer treatment-related lymphoedema is expressed in these quotations:

> One of the most troublesome and feared consequences of breast cancer treatment. (Professor Patricia Ganz)[1]

> You have to go through all this rubbish with the...cancer, and then to add insult to injury... you get lymphoedema, as a side thing, you know, it's awful. But you've got it for life, you know. (Cancer survivor with lymphoedema)

As expressed by Ganz, lymphoedema is one of the most significant and feared issues of survivorship for breast cancer survivors and is a chronic condition associated with many cancers. Generally regarded as incurable, lymphoedema requires lifelong care along with psychosocial support.[2]

Characterised by swelling of an area of the body, lymphoedema can be disfiguring, disabling, and distressing, and impact the quality of life of cancer survivors. It may affect daily functioning, psychological health, and quality of life, and has associated social and economic consequences.[3] Lifelong self-management of this chronic condition requires considerable motivation on the part of patients.

This chapter discusses lymphoedema, and how acupuncture can play an important role in its management by helping to reduce the symptom burden, improve quality of life, and increase patients' motivation for self-care. It also describes how acupuncturists can play a role in early identification and referral to specialist treatment.

TERMINOLOGY

Lymphoedema is a chronic inflammatory condition that results from failure of the lymphatic system. Consequences are swelling, skin and tissue changes, and predisposition to infection.

'Chronic oedema', a term that is often used interchangeably with the term 'lymphoedema', is swelling that lasts for more than three months. Its presence indicates that the lymphatic system is failing and the condition should be treated as lymphoedema.[4]

Many people confuse the word 'lymphoedema' with 'lymphoma'. These are completely different conditions: lymphoma is a cancer that starts in the lymph glands or organs of the lymph system.

Understanding lymphoedema
Primary and secondary lymphoedema
Lymphoedema is categorised as:

- **Primary** (or congenital) lymphoedema, which occurs because of an abnormality of the lymphatic system present from birth (although it may not become evident until later in life).
- **Secondary** lymphoedema, which results from damage to an otherwise normally functioning lymphatic system, and may be due to surgery, trauma, radiotherapy, infection, or inflammation.

Causes of secondary lymphoedema
Globally, the most common cause of secondary lymphoedema is filariasis, a parasitic infection carried by mosquitos, affecting people mainly in non-industrialised countries.[5] Cancer-related lymphoedema is the most common form in industrialised countries. It may be:

- caused by a tumour invading the lymphatic system
- a consequence of cancer treatments, including surgery, radiotherapy, and some chemotherapy agents. Surgery to remove the tumour cuts the lymphatic vessels, as does removal of lymph nodes. Removal of lymph nodes is the cancer treatment that is most damaging to the lymphatic system, followed by radiotherapy and chemotherapy.

There are many other causes of secondary lymphoedema, such as:

- recurrent cellulitis
- venous disease, including cardiac failure, varicose veins, and deep vein thrombosis
- inflammatory conditions
- non-cancer-related surgeries that include areas rich in lymph nodes, including orthopaedic surgery
- conditions affecting mobility and/or motor function, such as stroke, multiple sclerosis, and frailty ('dependency lymphoedema')
- medications, including calcium antagonists (amlodipine), corticosteroids, non-steroidal anti-inflammatory drugs (NSAIDS), hormones, anticonvulsants (pregabalin), and medications for Parkinson's disease
- poor skin integrity and poor hygiene, which increase risk of fungal infections and dry, cracked skin, leading to potential cellulitis

- lifestyle, especially obesity and inactivity.[6]

This chapter focuses on secondary lymphoedema resulting from cancer treatment. The practitioner should be aware of these other potential causes of lymphoedema, which may affect both cancer survivors and non-cancer patients attending for treatment.

Cancer treatment-related lymphoedema

In the remainder of this chapter, 'lymphoedema' refers to cancer treatment-related lymphoedema unless otherwise specified. Lymphoedema can occur with any cancer and is most associated with the following cancers:

- breast
- gynaecological, including uterine, cervical, vulvar, endometrial
- genitourinary, including penile, bladder, prostate
- head and neck cancers
- melanomas
- Stewart-Treves syndrome/angiosarcoma
- Kaposi's sarcoma.[7]

Generally, lymphoedema affects one (unilateral) (Figure 9.1A) or both (bilateral) arms or legs (Figure 9.1B), and this is known as **peripheral** lymphoedema. Lymphoedema affects other areas of the body, such as the head and neck (Figure 9.1C), breast, trunk, and genitalia, with the location(s) of the swelling related to the type of cancer.

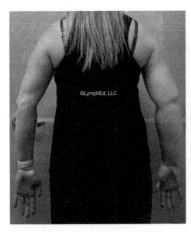 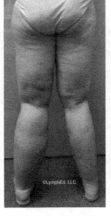 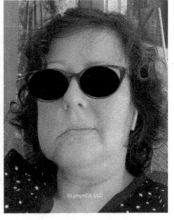

| FIGURE 9.1A: BREAST CANCER-RELATED LYMPHOEDEMA COMPARING UNAFFECTED (LEFT) WITH AFFECTED (RIGHT) ARM | FIGURE 9.1B: LOWER LIMB LYMPHOEDEMA COMPARING LEFT LEG AT STAGE IIB WITH RIGHT LEG CONTROLLED AT STAGE I | FIGURE 9.1C: CANCER TREATMENT-RELATED LYMPHOEDEMA OF THE HEAD AND NECK |

Biomedical perspectives
The pathophysiology of lymphoedema[5]

Lymphoedema is a low-output failure of the lymphvascular system, meaning that lymph transport is reduced.

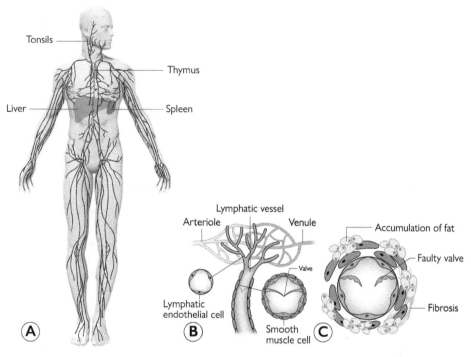

FIGURE 9.2: THE LYMPHATIC SYSTEM

A: The lymphatic system comprises vessels, nodes and lymphatic organs. B: shows the normally functioning lymphatic vessels; note the closed vessel which prevents retrograde flow of the lymph and the smooth muscle cell. C: shows the vessel in advanced disease; note the dysfunctional valve, subcutaneous tissue fibrosis and fat accumulation.

Disruption to the lymphatic system (whether congenital or through external factors) causes lymphatic transport to fall below the capacity needed to handle the microvascular filtrate (including plasma protein and other cells) that normally moves from the bloodstream into the interstitial spaces. Accumulation of materials (excess water, plasma proteins, blood cells, and other cell products) in the extracellular spaces causes swelling.

Chronic lymph stasis can foster cell proliferation (fibroblasts, adipocytes, and keratinocytes), leading to increased collagen deposits and overgrowth of subcutaneous adipose and connective tissues. Consequent processes, including thickening of the membranes of the lymphatic vessels and increased fibroblasts and inflammatory cells, lead to progressive subcutaneous fibrosis and increased fat deposition (Figure 9.2).

The accumulation of these fibrotic and adipose tissues is an important aspect of lymphoedema, which is often regarded merely as accumulation of fluids. They may be the reason that conservative (non-surgical) treatments are limited in their effectiveness in completely reducing swelling and returning the affected area to its usual dimensions.

Accumulation of surplus fluid and proteins may foster microbial growth, encouraging infections like cellulitis, which may be recurrent and cause further damage to the lymphatic capillaries. Lymphatic dysfunction also impairs local immune function, making the affected area vulnerable to infections.

These conditions – inflammation, fibrosis, infection, impaired immunity, deteriorating lymph vessels – all contribute to the progressive nature of lymphoedema, often combining to aggravate the lymphoedema and lead to deterioration of overall health.[8]

Risk factors for lymphoedema

Cancer itself may cause lymphoedema, therefore medical evaluation is advised when lymphoedema is suspected in people with or without a diagnosis of cancer. Other risk factors for cancer-related lymphoedema are listed in Table 9.1.

The case study of Linda at the end of this chapter illustrates how multiple risk factors can present in an individual.

Table 9.1: Risk factors for cancer treatment-related lymphoedema

Upper limb/trunk lymphoedema	Lower limb lymphoedema	Common to upper and lower body
• Surgery with axillary lymph node dissection, particularly if extensive breast or lymph node surgery • Radiotherapy to the breast, or to the axillary, internal mammary, or supraclavicular and infraclavicular lymph nodes • Scar formation, fibrosis, and radiodermatitis from post-operative axillary radiotherapy • Drain or wound complications or infection • Cording (axillary web syndrome)* • Seroma formation** • Taxane chemotherapy	• Surgery with inguinal lymph node dissection • Post-operative pelvic radiotherapy lymph node dissection • Recurrent soft tissue infection at the same site • Intrapelvic or intra-abdominal tumours that involve or directly compress lymphatic vessels • Immobilisation and prolonged limb dependency • Pendulous or large abdomen pressing down on inguinal nodes in sitting hinders lymphatic flow	• Obesity, especially a BMI > 25 • Advanced cancer • Congenital predisposition • Chronic skin disorders and inflammation • Trauma in the 'at-risk' limb (venepuncture, blood pressure measurement, injection)

*Cording (axillary web syndrome): the appearance of tender, painful cord-like structures below the skin; may be due to inflammation or thrombosis of lymph vessels.

**Seroma: an accumulation of fluid at or near a surgical wound.

Adapted from Lymphoedema Framework (2006) Best Practice for the Management of Lymphoedema.[9]

Onset of lymphoedema

Lymphoedema may occur at any time during and after cancer treatment. Several years may elapse from the end of cancer treatment to the onset of lymphoedema. Lymphoedema may also be present before symptoms become apparent, a stage known as pre-clinical lymphoedema.

While most cases of breast cancer-related lymphoedema (BCRL) are reported to develop within the first three years of cancer treatment, cases have developed 20 years or more after treatment.[10]

Time of onset may be related to the type of cancer treatment received, with axillary lymph node dissection (ALND) associated with early onset lymphoedema, and regional lymph node radiation associated with late onset lymphoedema.[10]

ESSENTIALS

Risk of lymphoedema and being 'at risk'
All patients who have had lymph node dissection for any type of solid tumour are at a **lifetime risk** of secondary lymphoedema.[3,7]

This includes these tumour types: breast, gynaecological, genitourinary, head and neck, melanoma.

Risk is also associated with radiotherapy and some chemotherapies. Risk does not diminish as time from treatment increases; studies report that risk may increase as time from treatment increases.[11]

Incidence
BCRL is the most widely studied form of lymphoedema, with most research and patient information directed at this cancer type. Even so, incidence is difficult to quantify, due to delayed onset of symptoms, lack of standardised diagnostic criteria, and misdiagnosis.

It is generally thought that one in five patients who undergo breast cancer surgery will develop arm lymphoedema at some stage in life.[12,13] The risks persist despite continual improvements in treatment techniques, such as sentinel lymph node biopsy (SLNB), to minimise damage to the lymphatic system.

Lymphoedema is associated with treatment for other cancers, including melanoma (16%), genitourinary cancers (10%), gynaecological cancers (20%), head and neck cancers (4%), and sarcomas (30%).[7]

Lymphoedema staging and characteristics
Lymphoedema is a progressive condition, meaning that without intervention, it can spread and develop complications. Early identification and treatment are vital, making the condition easier to treat, and more likely that patients will be able to self-manage with reduced reliance on healthcare professionals.[4]

Swelling is the focus of most clinical and research attention, with much discussion about the most appropriate measurement methods, also called volume measurement. Methods used range from simple tape measurement to the use of highly specialised technological equipment.[14]

The condition is complex, with many other troublesome features, the manifestation of which may depend on the stage and severity of lymphoedema. Staging (Table 9.2) demonstrates the progressive nature of lymphoedema and indicates why early diagnosis and treatment is essential to limit progression (Figures 9.3A and 9.3B).

Table 9.2: International Society of Lymphology (ISL) Staging[9]

ISL Stage	Characteristics
0	Subclinical. Swelling not evident, although lymph transport is impaired. This stage may exist for months or years before swelling is evident.
I	Early onset. Accumulation of tissue fluid that subsides with limb elevation. Oedema may be pitting (firm pressure for ten seconds of a finger or thumb on the area leaves an indentation when pressure ceases). Depth of indentation reflects severity (Figure 9.4).
II	Limb elevation alone rarely reduces swelling. Pitting is manifest.
II (late stage)	Tissue fibrosis is more evident. Pitting may or may not be present.
III	Tissue is hard (fibrotic). Pitting is absent. Skin changes develop, including thickening, hyperpigmentation, increased skin folds, fat deposits, papillomatosis, or warty overgrowths.

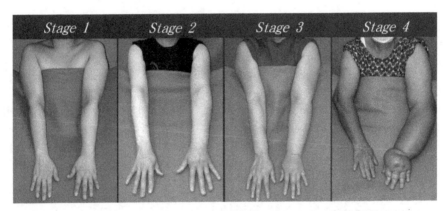

FIGURE 9.3A: ISL STAGES OF UPPER EXTREMITY LYMPHOEDEMA

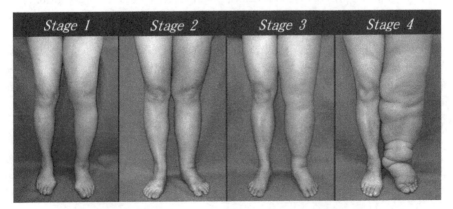

FIGURE 9.3B: ISL STAGES OF LOWER EXTREMITY LYMPHOEDEMA

Skin changes may range from skin dryness, to thickened but fragile tissue, to complex skin conditions (e.g. ulceration, lymphorrhoea), to lymphangiosarcoma (a rare form of lymphatic cancer). Patients are also at an increased risk of infection, particularly cellulitis.

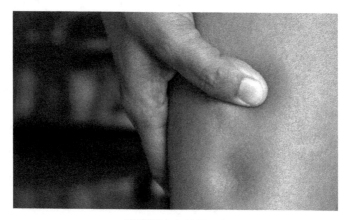

FIGURE 9.4: PITTING

Cellulitis

RED FLAG

Cellulitis is a potentially life-threatening complication for people with lymphoedema, whose compromised lymphatic system may not function adequately to fight infection. Up to 50% of people with lymphoedema experience one incident of cellulitis in their lifetime, and many experience recurrent cellulitis.[4]

Cellulitis is an acute, non-contagious infection of the skin and subcutaneous tissue. It generally develops quickly and is regarded as a medical emergency. Cellulitis can rapidly develop into sepsis with the potential for serious consequences such as gangrene, shock, or death.[4]

Practitioners should be aware of the:

* signs of cellulitis, for patients with or without a diagnosis of lymphoedema
* symptoms of sepsis and the need for rapid referral to specialist emergency care.

See Box 9.1 for signs of cellulitis.

Box 9.1: Signs of cellulitis[4,15]

It is important for practitioners to identify signs of cellulitis, which may occur even when there are no signs of lymphoedema. In mild cases, symptoms may be minimal or absent. Patients exhibiting any of the following signs should contact their medical team immediately:

- Flu-like symptoms (but not in all cases), including fever, shivers, muscular aches and pains, headache, nausea, vomiting.
- Areas of pre-existing swelling developing a rash or becoming red, hot, and tender to the touch. Swelling may dramatically increase, and pain may occur in the swollen area – or in the adjacent areas of lymph nodes (armpit or groin).

Cellulitis may develop when there is no pre-existing swelling or lymphoedema and symptoms may include:

- An area of red inflamed skin or darkening of the skin (Figures 9.5A and 9.5B can also be viewed in colour on the Singing Dragon Library).
- Fever.
- Numbness, tingling or other sensation in the hand, arm, leg, or foot.

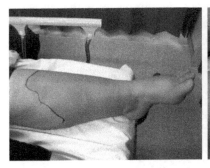 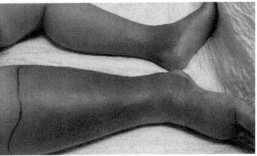

FIGURE 9.5A: CELLULITIS SHOWING SKIN COLOURATION IN LIGHT SKIN TONE

FIGURE 9.5B: CELLULITIS SHOWING SKIN COLOURATION IN DARK SKIN TONE

Treatment of cellulitis

Immediate treatment is essential to prevent the patient becoming very ill or developing sepsis, and to prevent further damage to the lymph system, which may in turn predispose the patient to further episodes of infection.

Antibiotics are the current recommended treatment, administered until all signs of inflammation have disappeared (usually 14 days, and up to one to two months or more). Patients under specialist lymphoedema care are likely to be aware of the signs and symptoms of cellulitis and know to obtain medical attention immediately. Many carry antibiotics to take at the first signs of cellulitis.

In severe cases, hospitalisation and intravenous antibiotics are necessary.[15] Patients experiencing two or more episodes of cellulitis in a year may be prescribed prophylactic antibiotics for a minimum of two years, or even for the remainder of their life if cellulitis recurs.

Cellulitis may also be a trigger for lymphoedema. At-risk patients with no previous history have developed lymphoedema following an episode of cellulitis. For this reason, all patients at risk of lymphoedema are advised to maintain skin integrity and reduce risk.

Biomedical management of lymphoedema

The evidence base for lymphoedema interventions is not always well developed, and often relies on clinical judgement and expert opinion. The most important messages are that:

- early intervention is key to optimal outcomes
- best practice involves a multidisciplinary approach.[3]

Surgical interventions

Surgical treatments, including liposuction, ablative surgery, and microsurgery, are gaining acceptance worldwide. These are currently appropriate for carefully selected patients and usually require combined physiotherapy or other compression techniques, as well as continued self-management, to maintain results.[3]

Conservative management of lymphoedema

Conservative (non-surgical) management involves a two-stage process.[2] These two stages, outlined below, apply to ISL Stages I–III (Table 9.2). Stage I conservative management is intensive care carried out by the medical professional. Stage II conservative management is a maintenance programme, carried out at home by the patient after discharge from Stage I.

People who are known to have pre-clinical lymphoedema (ISL Stage 0) may be provided with prophylactic care to prevent the onset of true lymphoedema. This comprises education on risk management and skin care, and may include compression to be worn during activities thought to overtax the lymphatic system.

Treatment, administered by appropriately trained practitioners, is individualised with attention paid to what is comfortable, acceptable, and possible for the patient. It is also affected by national standards and by access to medical equipment and supplies. Psychosocial support is a necessary component of lymphoedema treatment to improve quality of life.[2,3,9] It includes referral to appropriate professionals, such as social workers, counsellors, psychiatric professionals, nutritionists, and physical activity coaches.[16]

Stage I conservative management

Stage I is a course of intensive therapy, usually administered daily for two to four weeks. This benchmark of care for lymphoedema[3] is known variously as combined physical therapy (CPT), complex decongestive therapy (CDT), or complex decongestive phys-iotherapy (CDP).

The aim of Stage I is to reduce swelling, and, where required, to improve limb shape, subcutaneous tissue consistency, and skin condition. It comprises:

- skin care
- exercise
- specialist massage (manual lymphatic drainage (MLD))
- multi-layer lymphoedema bandaging (MLLB).

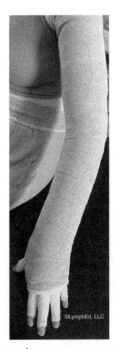

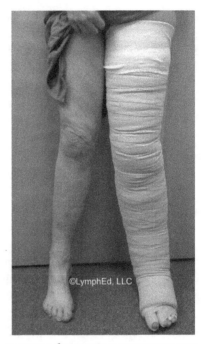

FIGURE 9.6A: ARM IN MULTI-LAYER LYMPHOEDEMA BANDAGING (MLLB)

FIGURE 9.6B: COMPARING UNAFFECTED LEG WITH AFFECTED LEG IN MULTI-LAYER LYMPHOEDEMA BANDAGING

Stage II conservative management – the 'four pillars'

Stage II follows directly on from Stage I, with the aim of conserving and optimising results achieved. It may be the initial treatment for some patients, or it may be concurrent with Stage I conservative management. It comprises the 'four pillars' of lymphoedema management:

1. Compression, meaning the wearing of specialist elasticated garments such as sleeves, gloves, and stockings (Figures 9.7A, 9.7B, 9.7C, 9.7D).
2. Skin care.
3. Continued remedial exercise.
4. Repeated light massage, usually self-administered (simple lymphatic drainage (SLD)) to encourage lymph drainage.[4]

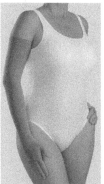

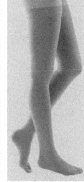

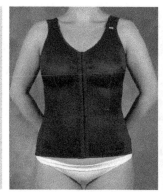

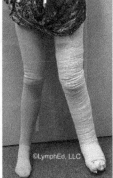

FIGURE 9.7A: COMPRESSION SLEEVE FOR ARM AND HAND

FIGURE 9.7B: COMPRESSION STOCKINGS

FIGURE 9.7C: COMPRESSION GARMENT FOR BREAST LYMPHOEDEMA

FIGURE 9.7D: COMPRESSION GARMENT (RIGHT LEG) AND MULTI-LAYER LYMPHOEDEMA BANDAGING (LEFT LEG)

Self-management

Self-management is an important aim of treatment, to give the patient long-term control of a chronic condition. In addition to the 'four pillars', it involves maintaining an appropriate body weight and self-monitoring for complications.

Self-management may be a daily, ongoing process for some people with lymphoedema. Effective in preventing progression of lymphoedema, it may be time consuming and burdensome for the individual, requiring continuous motivation to carry out the necessary steps.

Skin care

Maintaining skin integrity is an important factor for reducing risk in at-risk patients and essential for managing established lymphoedema, and aims to prevent complications such as cellulitis.

Skin integrity means that the skin is whole, intact, and undamaged. Compromised skin integrity is associated with complications such as skin tears and infections, which can cause pain and increased health complications leading to poor quality of life.[17] In general, people with or at risk of lymphoedema should keep their skin:

- clean and well dried after washing
- supple by moisturising daily.

Specifics about further skin care activities vary according to country or local practice. Professionals recognise that current advice is not evidence-based and there are concerns that it may cause patients stress. It is also recognised that most available research relates to BCRL, and care should be taken in extrapolating the advice to lymphoedema in other sites.[18,19]

In view of the lack of evidence-based guidelines, many specialist lymphoedema groups adopt a 'common sense approach', such as that set out in Box 9.2. Overall, the aim is to keep skin supple, healthy, and intact and avoid or limit situations that may introduce infection.

Box 9.2: Skin care guidelines[20]

- Moisturising: keep at-risk area clean and well moisturised to maintain skin integrity and reduce risk of cellulitis.
- Insect bites and sunburn: be aware of the risk from these and treat promptly should they occur.
- Hair removal: use of electrical shavers can reduce possible trauma from epilation.
- Injuries: take care to avoid or reduce likelihood of cuts, scratches, or bites.
- Wounds: seek medical advice if a wound does not seem to be healing.

For those at risk of upper limb lymphoedema:

- Use gloves to reduce potential for injury, for example when gardening or using a hot oven.
- If possible, use the contralateral limb for venepuncture/blood pressure monitoring (does not apply in emergencies).

For those at risk of lower limb lymphoedema:

- Avoid walking barefoot or wearing footwear that may cause blisters.

It is recommended to avoid medical interventions in an affected or at-risk limb except in life-compromising and life-saving situations. Sometime called non-accidental skin puncture (NASP) or venepuncture, these interventions include injections, IV access or fluid or drug therapy in an affected or at-risk limb. This advice also includes taking blood pressure.[21]

Lifestyle advice

Three key lifestyle considerations that expert opinion advises are applicable to people with or at risk of lymphoedema are to:

- maintain a healthy weight
- prevent and manage cellulitis
- be physically active.[20]

Maintain a healthy weight

Patients should be aware of the relationship of excess weight to the development and progression of lymphoedema and be supported in their efforts to maintain a healthy weight.

Weight gain and an elevated BMI (> 30), particularly pre-operatively, are among the strongest predictors for the development of BCRL and its progression to more advanced stages.[5,10,11] Weight loss has been shown to reduce arm volume in obese women with BCRL; however, weight loss alone is not a cure for lymphoedema.[3]

Correcting some dietary misconceptions

People with lymphoedema should be encouraged to adopt a healthy, balanced diet that includes all food groups. No special diet has been proven to be of benefit for most uncomplicated peripheral lymphoedema.[2,3] There are some popular misconceptions that would benefit from being corrected (Table 9.3).

Table 9.3: Misconceptions about diet for people with lymphoedema

Misconception	Correcting the misconception
Reducing protein intake will reduce lymphoedema. Lymphoedema is associated with the build-up of protein-rich fluid; thus, it is incorrectly assumed that reducing intake of proteins will reduce this fluid.	Protein-rich foods do not translate directly into protein-rich fluid. Furthermore, proteins are essential for growth and maintenance of many of the body's tissues as well as other body functions.[24]
Reducing fluid intake will reduce lymphoedema swelling.	Drinking insufficient fluids can cause dehydration, which can lead to an increase of transitional fluid to the tissues, thus adding to the overburdened lymphatic system. Patients should be encouraged to drink about 2 litres (8–10 glasses) of water per day, or more in hot weather or after exertion. Beverages with diuretic effects, such as coffee and alcohol, should be restricted.[24] Smoking and high sodium intake are also causes of dehydration.

Prevent and manage cellulitis

Cellulitis can be a trigger for lymphoedema in an at-risk limb and may exacerbate existing lymphoedema. Patients should be encouraged to develop a good skin care regime following guidance in Box 9.2.

Be physically active

Historically, breast cancer survivors were advised to avoid repetitive movements and carrying or lifting heavy items.

Moderate physical activity is now regarded as safe and desirable for people with lymphoedema.[22,23] Muscle contraction during exercise stimulates lymph flow through direct action on the lymphatic and venous vessels. This may help prevent lymphoedema in those at risk, and reduce the impact of the condition for those with established lymphoedema.[21]

Thus, patients should be encouraged to be active. For those unaccustomed to physical activity, any increase should be gradual. Wearing compression garments may be recommended for some forms of activity, and it is prudent for lymphoedema to be monitored by specialists. For all patients, regular activity should be a feature of daily life, as inactivity can result in limited range of movement and other complications.

Regular activity has further benefit on many conditions which affect cancer survivors, including heart problems, diabetes, obesity, and depression.

Symptoms associated with lymphoedema
Many symptoms are associated with lymphoedema, and may cause discomfort, disfigurement, disability, and distress. Breast cancer survivors with lymphoedema access healthcare services (including mental health services) more frequently than those without lymphoedema.[16] Individuals with lower body lymphoedema experience more frequent and severe symptoms than those with upper body lymphoedema, including more episodes of infection and related hospitalisations.[25]

Discomfort
As well as swelling and skin changes, people report heaviness of the limb(s), discomfort, skin tightness, pain, loss of normal sensation, and impaired function.

Wider effects include sleep disturbance, insomnia, fatigue, physical inactivity, and weight problems, as well as negative impacts on social and intimate interactions.

People with lower body lymphoedema may experience deteriorating health as swelling and discomfort in the legs, leading to inactivity. This may lead to weight gain, which further exacerbates the lymphoedema. Depression is frequently associated with this, and may be accompanied by comfort eating, resulting in a downward spiral of overall health.

Disfigurement
Inability to find clothes that fit and feeling 'ugly' contribute to poor body image. Many people dislike the compression garments used to manage the condition, feeling that they are unattractive, uncomfortable, and attract unwanted attention. Obesity is another important factor in lymphoedema, being both a result of lymphoedema (due to increased production of adipose tissue) and a risk factor for lymphoedema.

For some, these disfigurements are a constant reminder of cancer, causing distress.

Disability
The ability to carry out daily living activities, hobbies, and work tasks may be affected. There are also economic impacts. Treatment may be costly, patients may have to change jobs or stop working, income may decrease, and overall healthcare costs may increase.

Distress
Loss of confidence, social anxiety, and avoidance are common. Sexuality may also be affected, and relationships change.

Emotional disturbances include anxiety, feeling depressed, anger, and fear (often of the swelling progressing), as well as guilt feelings, grief, and inability to come to terms with the cancer diagnosis.

There may also be lack of motivation and disinterest in the activities required for self-management, which may be burdensome and time consuming.

Lymphoedema is more than just swelling

It is obvious that working with people with lymphoedema is about more than dealing with swelling, and good lymphoedema care focuses also on associated physiological and psychological symptoms.[3]

Acupuncture approaches to managing lymphoedema

There is little discussion in the biomedical literature about using acupuncture in lymphoedema management. One reviewer concluded that in spite of there being several studies reporting encouraging results for acupuncture as a preventative or therapeutic treatment for cancer patients with lymphoedema, 'the true risks and benefits of acupuncture are unknown given the methodological quality issues of the studies'.[26]

Other reviewers concur that the quality of research is compromised by small sample sizes, lack of controls, and no long-term outcomes, as well as little or no reporting of safety issues and side effects.[27,28] It is worth noting that these critiques apply equally to other lymphoedema-related interventions; a systematic review examining 26 studies that explored the use of adjunctive therapies for lymphoedema management concluded that none could be 'recommended for practice' based on the levels of evidence.[28]

Concerns about needling

As discussed, to maintain skin integrity it is recommended to avoid NASP or venepuncture in an affected or at-risk arm, except in a medical emergency.[9,21]

It follows that concerns about the safety of acupuncture needling in an affected or at-risk area are raised. Fortunately, acupuncture is not contraindicated in most international and many national guidelines for lymphoedema management. Best practice guidelines, and much information for patients, recommend avoiding acupuncture needling in the affected or at-risk area, for example, the limb on the affected (ipsilateral) side.[21]

Historically, some individuals have taken extreme positions, with some lymphoedema-specific websites advising that people with lymphoedema should avoid having acupuncture. On the other hand, many acupuncturists claim that needling directly into an affected area is safe and effective.

Even among the lymphoedema community, opinions differ concerning the risks of various medical interventions. Lymphoedema specialists debate the advice given to patients. One argument is that current recommendations are burdensome for patients, causing them unwarranted fear and limiting their daily activities.[18] The counter-argument is that caution is prudent to prevent or limit a chronic, progressive incurable condition.

Research to assess the safety of NASP is considered by many to be unethical as it may expose research participants to risk.[29,30] In the face of contradictory views and no rigorous evidence, what is the safe, effective approach for acupuncture?

There are regions or countries where acupuncture needling in an affected or at-risk area is accepted practice, particularly in China. As discussed, lymphoedema experts acknowledge the lack of robust evidence for guidelines for reducing risk of developing lymphoedema,[2,3] and an international panel of experts have developed a consensus 'common-sense approach'.[9] As research in the field of lymphoedema expands, many experts are beginning to investigate these guidelines, including the risk of NASP in an affected or at-risk area. However, until the evidence is clearly established, there is an argument for practising as safely as possible – to 'do no harm'.

What impact does adherence to this 'common-sense approach' of avoiding needling in the affected or at-risk area have on acupuncture treatment? Later in this chapter, I discuss my clinical and research experience of treating people with lymphoedema, in which I avoided using acupuncture in an at-risk or affected area and allowed a wide margin for safety.

East Asian medicine perspectives

Little is written in the English language about EAM approaches to lymphoedema. Contemporary Chinese medicine cancer textbooks mention lymphoedema, but with little discussion. Li notes that lymphoedema swelling may exacerbate pain.[31] Lahans discusses acupuncture safety for breast cancer patients treated with surgery and radiotherapy, and contraindicates needling in areas of lymphoedema, arguing that it increases risk of infection via the hole made by the needle.[32]

Aetiology in Chinese medicine

Authors of a systematic review categorise BCRL as 'edema' in traditional Chinese medicine caused by obstruction of the local meridians in the upper limbs, which impedes qi and Blood circulation, resulting in stagnant fluid overflowing into the skin.[33]

A Chinese study investigating the relationship between ultrasound imaging and TCM syndromes in limb lymphoedema lists three syndrome types:

- collateral obstruction due to cold dampness
- downward migration of damp heat
- phlegm stagnation and Blood stasis.

Importantly, this study focuses on tissue changes associated with lymphoedema, as opposed to fluid accumulation. The authors report that thickening of derma, hypodermis, and deep fascia was more pronounced in patients with phlegm stagnation and Blood stasis syndrome, and least in those with collateral obstruction due to cold dampness.[34]

Lymphoedema is a considerable health problem in China with 40–60,000 new cases of BCRL each year.[35] It is mostly treated with herbal medicine and application of heat. Thermotherapy, a form of microwave heating, is used in some countries for lymphoedema management, combined with skin care and external compression.[2] While warmth may benefit lymphoedema, heat can also exacerbate symptoms as vasodilation in the heated area can bring more fluid to the area than the dysfunctional lymphatic system can remove.

Research perspectives
The evidence base for EAM in lymphoedema management
Initial EAM research

Lymphoedema has attracted much interest throughout the EAM research community. The first important English language publication was by a Japanese team in 2002. It reported promising results in treating and preventing lymphoedema using acupuncture and moxibustion in 24 gynaecological cancer patients who had undergone pelvic lymph node dissection in a hospital setting.[36]

In their paper, Kanakura *et al.*[36] note that 'acupuncture points to improve lymphoedema have not been described in the literature'. Thus, the team chose their points using this rationale:

- SP-6 *Sanyinjiao* to 'enhance Spleen function and facilitate Blood circulation'
- BL-23 *Shenshu*, BL-67 *Zhiyin*, KID-1 *Yongquan* to 'regulate water and urine'
- ST-36 *Zusanli* to 'regulate a well-balanced condition of the whole body'
- REN-2 *Qugu*, REN-3 *Zhongji*, REN-12 *Zhongwan* for 'regulation of the systemic meridian vessels...[to improve lymph flow] leading to remission of lymphoedema and lymph cysts'.

Systematic reviews for EAM interventions for BCRL
Several studies have since been conducted around the world, including numerous recent studies in China. Access to Chinese language research papers has increased through the publication of several English language systematic reviews focusing on BCRL, with as many as five published in two years.[33,37-40]

These reviewers generally conclude that acupuncture and/or moxibustion appear to have a beneficial effect on BCRL. They also note that studies are low quality, compromised by poor design, small numbers of participants, and poor follow-up and safety reporting. While several reviewers interpret lack of adverse events reporting as confirmation that acupuncture is a safe intervention,[33,37,38,40] one review suggests that with such a 'small number of available studies, it is still difficult to suggest that [acupuncture] is safe for treating BCRL patients'.[39]

Research into acupuncture for BCRL
These systematic reviews report the points, modalities, and dosages used in the Chinese studies (Table 9.4), although details of rationale for the intervention, point selection, and needling techniques are not available in English. Studies published in English are also summarised below (Table 9.4).

Table 9.4: Points used in a selection of studies investigating acupuncture for BCRL*

Author (Publication date)	Chinese language publications			English language publications		
	Zhan et al. (2017)	Chen et al. (2018)	Zhao et al. (2019)	Alem & Gurgel (2008)[41]	Smith et al. (2014)[42]	Bao et al. (2018)[43]
Country	China	China	China	Brazil	Australia	USA
Study type	RCT	RCT	RCT	Case series	RCT	RCT
Participants (Control/Treatment)	75 (30/30)	60 (30/30)	72 (36/36)	29	20 (10/10)	82 (42/40)
Treatment frequency/duration	1x/day for 28 days (28 total)	1x/day for 28 days (28 total)	3x/week for 2 months (24 total)	1x/week for 6 months (24 total)	2x/week for 4 weeks, then 1x/week for 4 weeks (12 total)	2x/week for 6 weeks (12 total)
Arm needled	None	Ipsilateral	Ipsilateral	Contralateral	Contralateral	Both arms
Follow-up	None	None	None	None	None	3 months
Points chosen	ST-24 ST-26 REN-4 REN-6 REN-10 REN-12	**Acupoint massage plus 'Chinese medicine packet'** LU-2 LU-5 LI-1 TB-5 BL-13 GB-21	**Electro-acupuncture** LI-4 LI-11 LI-15 ST-25 ST-36 SP-9 SP-10 TB-5 REN-9 REN-12 **Auricular** CO17 *Sanjiao* CO18 *Endocrine* TG2p *Shenshangxian*	LU-5 LI-4 LI-15 ST-36 SP-6 SP-9 TB-5 TB-14 REN-2 REN-3 REN-12	3 points from these 3 groups **Group 1:** REN-2 REN-3 REN-12 **Group 2:** LU-5 LI-14 LI-15 TB-4 **Group 3:** ST-36 SP-6 SP-9 **Plus** points based on individual diagnosis	LU-5 LI-4 LI-15 ST-36 SP-6 TB-14 REN-3 REN-12

*Adapted from Jin et al. (2020)[38]

Commentary

What is striking in this summary are the high doses in terms of frequency and duration of treatment in the Chinese studies, with daily treatment over the course of a month. These treatment approaches are not usual practice outside the East Asian cultural sphere.

Otherwise, apart from Zhan *et al.*, the studies use similar points, including local and distal points. There is considerable variance on approaches to dealing with the affected arm. The English language studies discussed below provide some insight into the approaches chosen.

Summary of acupuncture approaches used in studies published in English
Improving range of movement for BCRL

In Brazil, Alem and Gurgel reported significant improvement after 24 acupuncture treatments in range of movement (ROM) of shoulder flexion and abduction in 29 women who had undergone breast surgery and presented with lymphoedema and/or restricted movement in the upper limb ipsilateral to surgery.[41]

Their stated rationale is 'TCM theory' and point selection is:

- REN-2, REN-3, REN-12 'to regulate the meridian of systemic vessels, and lead to increased lymphatic circulation and hence a reduction of lymphoedema and lymphatic cysts'
- LU-5, LI-4, LI-15, TB-5, TB-14 (all contralateral) 'for the sense of heaviness, limitation of movement and pain in the upper limbs'
- ST-36, SP-6, SP-9 'for oedema, gynaecological disturbances, and facilitating blood flow'.

Technique: Eleven stainless steel needles (0.25mm x 30mm) were inserted in the side of the body contralateral to the mastectomy site, from the upper limb down. Depth of needling varied according to location of point and patient's age, constitution, and response to manual stimulation. Needles were retained for 30 minutes; no additional stimulation was applied and there were no other co-interventions.

The first RCT exploring acupuncture for BCRL

Smith *et al.* in Australia conducted the first published randomised controlled trial (RCT) to determine the feasibility, acceptability, and safety of using acupuncture to treat BCRL.[42] Twenty women with stable unilateral intransient lymphoedema present for at least six months were randomised to either usual care or 12 acupuncture treatments over eight weeks.

The publication reported many methodological challenges, including defining and measuring lymphoedema. Although there was no change in extracellular fluid or patient-reported outcomes, the authors suggest that acupuncture may stabilise lymphoedema-related symptoms. This study avoided needling in the affected limb and the authors query whether needling the affected side would have a greater treatment effect.

Their stated rationale is 'TCM syndrome patterns' and the point selection is:

- Group 1: 'these are points traditionally associated with regulation of systemic vessels, increased lymphatic circulation and a reduction in lymphoedema'
- Group 2: 'on the unaffected side to address heaviness, limitation of movement and pain in the upper limbs'
- Group 3: 'other general points used to treat oedema in general'.

Technique: Serin stainless steel needles (0.20mm x 30mm), inserted to a depth dependent on skin thickness and subcutaneous fatty tissue at the site of the acupuncture point, were stimulated to achieve deqi and once again during treatment. Needles were retained for a minimum of 20 minutes. Needling in the affected arm was avoided; leg points were needled bilaterally.

Building a programme of research

Researchers at Memorial Sloan Kettering Cancer Centre (MSKCC) in the USA carried out pilot research evaluating 33 participants[44,45] followed by a waitlist controlled RCT recruiting 82 participants.[43]

Acupuncture needles were placed in the affected arm and elsewhere on the body, with treatment given twice weekly for six weeks. Mild bruising or minor pain was experienced by some participants at least once as well as one instance each of transient (four-day) exacerbation of lymphoedema and infection.

The researchers reported very promising outcomes from the pilot study, cited as a mean reduction in arm circumference of 0.90cm (n=33). Disappointingly, this was not realised in the RCT, which reported a mean reduction of only 0.38cm.

Their stated rationale for acupuncture point selection was 'determined on the basis of historical context, the published literature, and the consensus of our experienced group of MSKCC staff acupuncturists'.

Technique: Single-use filiform needles (32–36-gauge, 30–40mm length) penetrated 5–10mm into the skin and 'stimulated manually by gentle rotation with lift and thrust'. Deqi sensation was achieved at certain acupoints such as Ll-4 and ST-36. Each treatment lasted 30 minutes. All points apart from those on the torso were needled bilaterally.

Studies conducted in Korea

A systematic review of acupuncture as part of Korean medicine (KM) identified three publications focusing on lymphoedema, of which two were case studies reporting one patient each.[46]

The third paper, published in English, reports a pilot study of nine participants treated using *Saam* acupuncture, a style specific to traditional KM.[47] *Saam* acupuncture follows both Yin-Yang and Five Element theoretical frameworks, relying on supplementing deficiency and draining excess.

Treatment utilised 48 different sets of acupuncture points, drawing on 52 of the five shu points of the 12 meridians (located below the elbow and knee). Characteristics of this study include:

- Needling was avoided on *the entire body* on the affected side.

- A total of 4–8 needles per treatment were used, deqi was obtained, and the needles left in situ for about 30 minutes.
- Needling was supplemented by placing 'pellets' over the points for one hour after removing the needles.

The paper clearly reports adverse events, including two cases of lymphangitis (inflammation of the lymphatic vessels) which were not considered to be associated with acupuncture treatment as needles had not been placed in the affected arm. No other adverse events were reported either during the study or the four-week follow-up. The authors note that the size of both the affected and unaffected arms reduced but give no clear explanation of why this might happen.

Research into moxibustion for BCRL

Moxibustion as an intervention for lymphoedema has generated much research in China. In CM theory, moxibustion promotes qi and stimulates Blood circulation, which may reduce swelling. Animal studies suggest that moxibustion may reduce inflammatory cytokines, regulate lymph function, and improve blood circulation.[48]

Points and dose (frequency and duration of treatment) used in these Chinese studies are listed below (Table 9.5).

Commentary

As with the acupuncture studies in Table 9.4, frequency and duration of treatment are striking, varying from twice a week for four weeks to as frequently as daily for 42 days. The large numbers of points used is also interesting, particularly in the Zhao, Huang, and Jiang studies. As the majority of these are Chinese language publications, I am unable to discuss further details regarding rationale, technique, or the quality of safety reporting.

Adopting a different approach to acupuncture treatment of lymphoedema

Most research aims to reduce volume or circumference in BCRL, focusing primarily on fluid reduction, with little or no attention to other symptoms associated with lymphoedema.

In 2008–09, I obtained funding to conduct a feasibility study into using acupuncture and moxibustion to improve quality of life in cancer survivors with upper body lymphoedema, focusing on cancers of the breast and head and neck (see 'Case study: The feasibility of using acumoxa in the management of lymphoedema' later in this chapter).

While the main outcomes of this study were to improve quality of life rather than reduce the lymphoedema, I was interested in finding a credible approach to treatment with little established practice or evidence to guide me. At this time, Kanakura et al.[36] was the only published study; the Alem and Gurgel[41] research became available as my study was about to commence.

Table 9.5: Points used in a selection of Chinese RCTs investigating moxibustion for BCRL

Author (Publication date)	Zhao et al. (2012)	Huang et al. (2014)	Jiang et al. (2015)*	Yao et al. (2016)[48]	Yang et al. (2017)	Wang et al. (2019)[49]	Liu et al. (2019)	Lui et al. (2019)
Publication language	Chinese	Chinese	Chinese	English	Chinese	English	Chinese	Chinese
Participants (Control/ Treatment)	92 (46/46)	62 (31/31)	60 (30/30)	30 (15/15)	45 (23/22)	48 (24/24)	80 (40/40)	60 (30/30)
Treatment frequency/duration	5x/week for 9 weeks (45 total)	5x/week for 6 weeks (30 total)	5x/week for 8 weeks (40 total)	1x every 2 days for 30 days (15 total)	2x/week for 4 weeks (8 total)	1x every 2 days for 28 days (14 total)	1x/day for 42 days (42 total)	1x/day for 42 days (42 total)
Follow-up	4 weeks	None	None	4	4 months	None	None	None
Points chosen	LU-1 LU-7 LI-4 LI-11 LI-14 LI-15 ST-36 SP-9 SI-9 TB-5 TB-14 GB-21 LIV-3	LU-7 LI-4 LI-11 LI-14 LI-15 SP-9 SI-9 SJ-5 SJ-14 REN-9	LI-4 LI-11 ST-36 BL-17 GB-21 LIV-3 REN-6 DU-14	**Needling** LI-10 LI-11 LI-14 **Warm needling on** LI-15 TB-5 TB-1	LI-11 LI-14 SI-9 DU-3	LI-13 LI-14 SI-9 TB-5 BL-23 **Plus** ashi points	LI-11 LI-15 ST-36 SP-9 SJ-5 REN-9	**Warm needling** LU-7 LI-4 LI-11 LI-15 SP-9 TB-5 TB-14 GB-21 REN-9

*Specifies using 'thunder-fire moxibustion', a concentrated form of moxibustion treatment that utilises a mixture of herbs in the moxa stick to warm the meridians and dredge the collaterals, said to produce intense heat and therapeutic impact.[50]

Information about Chinese language studies taken from Jin et al. (2020)[38]

Searching for the root – the *biao*

Early research into the pathophysiology suggested that there was more to the development of lymphoedema than the initial 'insult' to the lymphatic system caused by surgery and radiotherapy.[51] Researchers into BCRL suggest that development of lymphoedema may be 'systemically driven' and not just dependent on 'changes in outflow resistance in the ipsilateral arm alone'.[5]

It seemed that to focus only on addressing the localised swelling confined treatment to the *ben* (or manifestation) of lymphoedema. While this is an important aspect of treatment, I was intrigued by the underlying cause, the *biao* (or root) of lymphoedema.

The role of the Directing Vessel (*Ren Mai*)

My instinct was to address both the *ben* and *biao*, the manifestation and the root of the condition. This led me to Maciocia's[52] extensive discussion of oedema, which aligns with the recent redefinition of lymphoedema, and shares a common characteristic of being a malfunction in the metabolism of fluids. Maciocia makes a case for the role of the *Ren Mai* in:

- promoting the transformation, transportation, and excretion of fluids
- activating the Triple Burner
- controlling fat tissue (*gao*) and membranes (*huang*).

Together, these three functions of the *Ren Mai* seemed to address the complexities of lymphoedema and might be the basis for an exploration of the condition in terms of CM theory.

Promoting transformation, transportation, and excretion of fluids

According to Maciocia, the patterns underlying oedema include:

- Lungs failing to diffuse and descend qi and transform fluids
- Spleen yang failing to transform and move fluids
- Kidney yang failing to move, transform, and excrete fluids.

Maciocia addresses these patterns using the opening and coupled points of the *Ren Mai* to descend the qi (LU-7 *Lieque*) and to stimulate the Kidneys (KID-6 *Zhaohai*). Supplementary points on the *Ren Mai* that promote the Triple Burner's function to metabolise fluids (see below) include:

- REN-17 *Shanzhong* to act on the upper burner and diffuse and descend Lung qi
- REN-12 *Zhongwan* to act on the middle burner and stimulate the Stomach and Spleen to transform and transport fluids
- REN-9 *Shuifen* to act on the middle burner and stimulate the Lungs, Spleen and Kidney to transform and transport fluids
- REN-5 *Shimen* (the front mu point of the Triple Burner) to promote transformation, transportation, and excretion of fluids in the lower burner.

This view of fluid metabolism may provide a useful basis for working with lymphoedema as a systemic condition, rather than a problem of localised swelling.

Activating the Triple Burner

The Triple Burner controls the ascending/descending and entering/exiting of qi in the 'qi mechanism'. This is the movement of qi to fulfil its various functions – to flow upward or downward according to the channel, to enter and exit the body's structures and organs, and to pass freely through all the cavities and organs:

> The Triple Burner makes the Original Qi separate and it controls the movement and passage of the three Qi through the five Yin and six Yang organs. (Chapter 66, *Classic of Difficulties*)

As the 'the official in charge of ditches' (Chapter 8, *Simple Questions*) the Triple Burner is responsible for the transformation, transportation, and excretion of fluids. Carrying out this function of fluid metabolism is closely intertwined with its function of controlling the transportation and penetration of qi: 'essentially the transformation and movement of fluids depend on Qi'.[52]

This complex process of transformation, transportation, and excretion of fluids, leading to the formation of body fluids in the three burners, seems to reflect the complex processes at work in the formation of lymphoedema, with its breakdown in the transformation and transportation of fluids that accumulate in the extracellular spaces. Since lymphoedema is not an inevitable consequence of surgical intervention, it might be argued that the development of lymphoedema relates to a breakdown in the qi mechanism.

Maciocia states the main points for activating the Triple Burner's function of moving qi are on the *Ren Mai* rather than the Triple Burner channel. In addition to the REN points listed above, REN-6 *Qihai* and REN-3 *Zhongji* are key points for moving qi in the lower burner.

Controlling fat tissue (gao) and membranes (huang)

The third aspect of Maciocia's discussion of the *Ren Mai* may apply to the tissue damage and fibrosis associated with lymphoedema. This relates to the *gao* and *huang*:

- *Gao*, meaning 'fat', may relate to adipose tissue.
- *Huang* refers to the membranes.

Together *gao* and *huang* 'represent a whole range of connective tissue including adipose tissue, superficial and deep fascia...[covering] the whole body with a layer immediately below the skin and an inner wrapper and anchoring the organs, muscles and bones'.[52]

REN-6 *Qihai* and REN-15 *Jiuwei* are the source points for membranes and fat tissue. Maciocia states that these points, as well as the entire *Ren Mai*, are related to the development of connective tissue. The focus of this action is the abdomen, with the *Ren Mai* giving access to the deeper fascia of the abdomen and thorax.

———

Maciocia's extensive discussion does not mention the lymphatic system. However, it may be possible that the influence of the *Ren Mai* on the deeper structures of the trunk also exerts an influence on the lymphatic structures in this area – especially the deep lymphatic system comprising the iliac, lumbar, and mediastinal lymph nodes, the cisterna chyli, and the left thoracic duct and the right lymphatic duct.

He notes the channels and the organs are 'linked, wrapped, padded and integrated by layers of Membrane (*huang*), the connective tissue of Western medicine' and 'Qi easily stagnates in the Membranes in the abdomen'. The Triple Burner is also implicated in the management of the membranes, as it is 'responsible for the movement of Qi in and out of the Membranes'.[52]

Is it possible that stagnation in the *huang* may in some way be related to an underlying pattern of stagnation in lymphoedema? If so, then treating the *Ren Mai* and the Triple Burner may have a fundamental role in the treatment, and perhaps even the prevention, of lymphoedema.

Putting it all together

This exploration of the role of the *Ren Mai* and Triple Burner in relation to lymphoedema is theoretical. It did inform my approach to treating the participants in my lymphoedema research; however, it was not possible to apply this in a systematic, rigorous way, as demonstrated in the extended case study of Ann in Chapter 14, Getting My Life Back.

Further exploration, in both clinical and research settings, is needed. However, this exploration of theory may be an important consideration for approaching lymphoedema as a systemic, as well as a local, problem. It attempts to address the *biao*, which may be as important a factor as focusing on the manifestation. Maxine's vignette illustrates the potential for this approach.

VIGNETTE: MAXINE AND THE EFFECT OF TREATING THE *BIAO*

Several months after participating in the lymphoedema study, Maxine (see Maxine's case study in Chapter 6, Cancer Related-Fatigue) fell, breaking the fall using her lymphoedema-affected arm. This caused swelling of her left arm, accompanied by dull, throbbing pain, which was worse at night and impaired Maxine's sleep. The lymphoedema nurse suggested the swelling would not diminish until the inflammation healed, and that Maxine should resume having acupuncture.

Maxine attended for acupuncture treatment six weeks after the fall. At her first treatment, I attempted to relieve the pain using local points for shoulder pain on the contralateral side. At her next treatment, Maxine reported that this had no effect.

Somewhat surprised, I decided to apply the protocol to 'promote transformation, transportation, and excretion of fluids', as follows:

- Open the *Ren Mai*, using LU-7 *Lieque* (needled on the right side, contralateral to the affected arm) and KID-6 *Zhaohai* (needled on the left side).
- Then, REN-12 *Zhongwan*, REN-7 *Yinjiao*, and REN-5 *Shimen*.
- TB-5 *Waiguan* on the right arm to alleviate pain in the left shoulder.[53]

All needles were inserted with even technique and retained for 20 minutes after deqi. During this time, I applied five cones of direct moxa to REN-17 *Shanzhong*. After 20 minutes, I removed the needles in the REN and Triple Burner points, ending with KID-6 and finally LU-7.

At her next treatment, Maxine reported the effect had been 'marvellous'. The pain disappeared, she slept well that night, and the swelling began to diminish the next day. Her only question was, 'Why didn't you do that at the first treatment?'

It is not possible, from this single case, to extrapolate how this approach would work in general for people with lymphoedema. Nevertheless, it is an example on which to build and develop further experience and evidence.

CASE STUDY: THE FEASIBILITY OF USING ACUMOXA IN THE MANAGEMENT OF LYMPHOEDEMA
Using acupuncture and moxibustion to improve wellbeing and quality of life in cancer survivors with upper body lymphoedema – a feasibility study[54–56]

In 2008–09 I conducted a feasibility study to explore using acupuncture and moxibustion (acu/moxa) as adjunctive treatment to usual lymphoedema care. The main aims were to:

- identify what symptoms people with upper body cancer treatment-related lymphoedema experienced
- explore whether acu/moxa treatment could alleviate those.

It was not an aim of the study to treat the lymphoedema. Reducing volume was not a primary aim, although we were interested to monitor any changes.

Needling restrictions
In designing this study, we conducted focus groups with patients and oncology healthcare professionals. Breast cancer patients stipulated that they did not want to be needled in the affected arm. Furthermore, the hospital's oncology healthcare professionals contra-indicated needling in the torso quadrant on the affected side as well as the affected arm of breast cancer patients.

'Torso quadrant' means anywhere on the torso above the waistline and lateral to the midline. Initially, the prospect of having one quarter of the body 'out of bounds' to needling was daunting. However, it provided an opportunity to explore acupuncture's potential while adhering to best practice guidelines (at that time) for lymphoedema care.

Methods and materials
The study recruited breast and head and neck cancer survivors with stable lymphoedema, who were in the maintenance phase of care with the hospital's lymphoedema service.

Participants received treatment once weekly, with an initial course of seven treatments followed by the option of another six treatments, for a potential total of 13 treatments.

Treatments were individualised and dynamic, changing to meet the individuals' needs as they progressed through treatment or presented with acute conditions. In most cases, we administered an Aggressive Energy Drain at the first treatment, and Internal Dragons at the second treatment. The rationale for this is discussed in Chapter 5, Toolkit.

Two acupuncturists delivered the treatments, drawing on CM and Five Elements theoretical frameworks.[54] Moxibustion (including direct moxa, stick moxa, and moxa on needles) was used as appropriate for the individual.

We avoided needling the:

- arm and torso quadrant on the affected side of breast cancer participants
- face, neck, and torso quadrant on the affected side of head and neck cancer participants.

We needled points on the Ren and Du channels. This meant that Aggressive Energy Drains used unilateral needling on the unaffected side of the body (rather than bilateral needling).

All participants received usual lymphoedema care in the hospital's lymphoedema clinic. They were referred to the study by the lymphoedema nurse who also monitored them at intervals throughout the study. This included taking volume measurements of breast cancer participants with arm lymphoedema to ensure the acu/moxa did not exacerbate the lymphoedema.

Validated questionnaires were used to measure outcomes, including the:

- Measure Yourself Medical Outcome Profile (MYMOP)
- Medical Outcomes Study Short Form (SF-36)
- Positive and Negative Affect Scale (PANAS).

Results

We recruited 35 participants (27 breast, eight head and neck cancer survivors), of whom 30 completed the full course of 13 treatments. Three chose to have seven treatments only. Two withdrew from the study, one because of cancer recurrence and the other because of demanding caring responsibilities.

Participants reported perceived changes in lymphoedema as well as quality of life, even though needling was restricted, and we were not treating lymphoedema per se. Additionally:

- breast cancer participants reported decreases in heaviness, pain, discomfort, and aching of the arm as well as perceived reductions in swelling
- head and neck cancer participants reported reduced musculoskeletal pain, increased mobility, and improved ability to carry out their self-management exercises.

Both groups reported improvements in many other symptoms, including anxiety, stress, feeling depressed, sleep disturbance, insomnia, as well as coping with major life events (such as bereavement). Increased energy levels were reported, and many patients said they were better able to cope with lymphoedema and their cancer diagnosis.

Adverse events

Participants were monitored until 12 weeks after their last treatment. Two incidents of cellulitis were reported; the lymphoedema nurse confirmed that these were not due to acu/moxa. Other adverse events included occasional bruising or bleeding at the needle site, light-headedness, and tiredness after treatment.

Changes in volume

Volume was measured three times – before treatment and after the 7th and 13th treatments – for breast cancer participants with arm lymphoedema. These measures showed great variability and fluctuations, with no consistent pattern. Some women improved steadily, for others swelling increased and then reduced, and others had swelling that reduced significantly before increasing again. Two participants had significant increases in volume. The lymphoedema nurse did not attribute this to acupuncture, as both women had a history of lack of concordance with their self-management plan.

While reduced volume at the end of 13 treatments was recorded for about half of the breast cancer participants, this study cannot claim that this is the result of acupuncture treatment. The swelling of lymphoedema is variable and subject to many factors, including weight (loss or gain), stress, physical activity, season, and concordance with self-management. At this stage, we must concede that acu/moxa treatment is just one of several variables that could have affected the reductions in swelling.

Conclusion

There are indicators that acu/moxa has the potential to reduce the symptom burden experienced by people with lymphoedema, and that benefits can be obtained while still adhering to best practice guidelines for needling. The detailed case study of Ann in Chapter 14 exemplifies the breadth and depth of effects that acu/moxa treatment can have, even with restricted needling.

Clinical perspectives

ESSENTIALS

In the absence of clear evidence as to the benefit or harm of applying acupuncture to an affected limb, current practice would advise caution and avoid needling limbs with or at risk of lymphoedema.[21]

In this section, I discuss options for treatment that respect this cautionary advice. Throughout this chapter and this book, I demonstrate that acupuncture treatment can be beneficial to cancer survivors, even when parts of the body are out of bounds to needling.

Developing a specific toolkit for cancer treatment-related lymphoedema

The prospect of avoiding needling areas of the body can seem daunting. Practitioners of Five Element acupuncture may find this particularly challenging when working with breast cancer survivors, and especially so when working with those with bilateral breast cancer.

In this section, I review some of the approaches introduced in Chapter 5, Toolkit, and discuss how they may increase the repertoire of available approaches when working with people living with or at risk of lymphoedema.

Utilising the richness and flexibility of the channels

The channel system that underpins acupuncture provides a rich treasury of possible strategies to draw on. The interconnectedness of the networks enables us to develop flexible, effective treatments when treating people with or at risk of lymphoedema.

This allows us to be adaptable in our approach, whether we are using acu/moxa to help manage the lymphoedema, or to address other health issues experienced by these survivors. It is not until we are challenged with restrictions on needling that we draw on what is already there in channel theory and in classical teaching.

The following suggestions are a selection of the many strategies possible, and this is not an exhaustive list. Some of these may be obvious, but when faced with the enormity of cancer-related symptoms, it is easy to overlook fundamental approaches. When treating people at risk of or with lymphoedema, I may draw on a selection of these approaches, combining the methods as appropriate for the individual.

Using distal points

Distal points are a mainstay of acupuncture treatment. It is not the purpose of this discussion to provide a full list of possible distal points to treat the range of conditions that cancer survivors present with. Rather, this is a reminder that these can function as effective alternatives when it is not possible to access local points. It is an opportunity to refresh our understanding of the intricacies of the meridian network and explore the functions of points we may not use habitually.

Selecting points below to treat above

Using points on the lower body to treat ailments on the upper body is a common tenet of acupuncture practice, and *The Yellow Emperor's Inner Classic* says, 'When the disease is above select [points] from below.'

This advice is especially helpful when access to points on the upper body is restricted. Points distal to the knees on the six primary channels of the leg can be used to treat disorders of the head, chest and upper back (upper jiao), as well as those of the abdomen, mid and lower back (middle and lower jiao).[53]

Points on the lower abdomen and lower back can also be useful to treat problems affecting the upper body.

Selecting points from above to treat below

The Yellow Emperor's Inner Classic also states, 'if the disease is below, select points above'. However, the range of points seems limited compared with those available when using points below to treat above. This highlights the challenges inherent in treating people whose lower body is affected, especially if the restriction is bilateral.

I conducted a small study using acu/moxa to improve wellbeing for people with lower limb lymphoedema, and had good results using upper body points only.[55] Working primarily to calm the shen in highly anxious people with chronic (non-cancer related) lymphoedema improved a number of aspects of quality of life, including sleep, pain, self-confidence, and motivation to self-manage their condition.

Deadman *et al.*[53] cite points that may have potential for people with lower limb lymphoedema, including:

- ST-4 *Dican* for swelling of the leg
- DU-16 *Fengfu* for numbness of the legs
- LU-5 *Chize* for knee problems.

Selecting points according to channel connections

Points on the Stomach or Bladder channels can be used to regulate the spirit, as their divergent channels pass through the Heart. This strategy can be useful for managing distress, especially in patients with bilateral upper body risk, where needling the Heart and Pericardium channels may be contraindicated.

Cross (contralateral) needling

Many practitioners needle bilaterally or select points on the affected side of the body. It is also possible to select points on one side of the body to treat disorders on the opposite side (contralateral needling). The *Spiritual Pivot* advises, 'if the left is affected, the right is treated, and if the right affected, the left is needled'.

Contralateral needling is useful when treating people with lymphoedema, especially head and neck cancer survivors. Local points on the Stomach channel (such as ST-3 *Juliao*, ST-4 *Dican*, ST-5 *Daying*, ST-6 *Jiache*, ST-7 *Xiaguan*) are useful for alleviating pain, numbness, swelling, mouth dryness, and functional disorders.[54] I needle the relevant points on the contralateral side, combining them with distal points on the Stomach channel, as well as opening the Yang Linking Vessel (discussed below).

Cross needling is also useful for patients with unilateral arm lymphoedema. Needling the points on the relevant channels on the contralateral arm can be effective. In some cases, I have taught patients how to locate specific points so that they can self-manage with acupressure. Contralateral needling can also be effective for lymphoedema in the breast, as illustrated in Miriam's vignette (below).

VIGNETTE: MIRIAM AND A CASE OF BREAST AND TRUNK LYMPHOEDEMA

Miriam, aged 44, had lymphoedema in the left breast and trunk following a radical mastectomy. She experienced breast pain, discomfort, swelling, shoulder pain, restricted movement, and a sensation of a 'sausage stuffed under her armpit'.

To address the pain of the lateral costal area, shoulder, and arm, as well as swelling of the axilla and restricted arm movement, I used:[53]

- points on the Gall Bladder channel including GB-22 *Yuanye*, GB-23 *Zhejin*, GB-24 *Riyue*, GB-25 *Jingmen*, GB-26 *Daimai*, selected according to presentation of symptoms at each appointment. These were needled on the contralateral side
- selected distal points, needled on the affected side including GB-41 *Zulinqi* and LIV-3 *Taichong*, which affect both the breast and the lateral costal region.

Miriam responded well to this approach. By treatment 6, she perceived that the swelling had reduced and reported that she no longer experienced any pain. Miriam also said that as well as reducing her physical discomfort, acupuncture helped relieve her anxieties about the swelling.

Using empirical points

Of the empirical points, I have found ST-38 *Tiaokou* useful for treating shoulder pain, particularly for breast cancer survivors, as shown in Grace's vignette (below). Deadman *et al.*[53] advise that this point should be needled on the affected side with the patient sitting, and once qi is obtained, manipulate the needle with the patients moving their shoulder. However, I have had success needling ST-38 *Tiaokou* without manipulation, and with the patient lying down.

VIGNETTE: GRACE AND A CASE OF TREATING SHOULDER PAIN WITH EMPIRICAL POINTS

Grace, aged 63, was attending for acupuncture to support her through treatment for recurrence of breast cancer. Her initial cancer treatment involved removal of 19 lymph nodes on the left side.

Planning for her second course of radiotherapy aggravated an old shoulder injury that had not troubled her for many years. She experienced severe pain, which was worse when sitting and lying and better with movement. This kept her awake at night, with consequent damage to her energy and morale. As using local points on the same side was not possible, I chose to use ST-38 *Tiaokou*, an empirical point for treating shoulder disorders.[53]

Tender on palpation, Grace initially found needling ST-38 extremely painful, so I removed the needle and warmed the point using stick moxa for several minutes. I supplemented this by needling:

- GB-34 *Yanglingquan* as a supplementary distal point to treat stiffness and tightness of the shoulder joint and sinews

- ear points Shoulder, Master Shoulder, Point Zero, Thalamus Point, *Shenmen*, and Triple Warmer.[56] All needling of distal and ear points was on the affected (left) side.

When Grace attended the following week, she said she had felt so poorly after treatment that she was on the point of discontinuing acupuncture. However, the next day she awoke feeling fine, and the following day her shoulder was '80% better'. As she could now lie down without discomfort, her sleep improved, and she was able to resume her hobbies of knitting and gardening. The shoulder still ached, and I repeated the treatment. As ST-38 *Tiaokou* on the left side was still extremely sensitive, I needled it on the right side instead. This treatment administered weekly eliminated the pain and enabled Grace to lie in the required position daily during the course of radiotherapy treatment.

ST-38 *Tiaokou* played a further key role during a subsequent course of radiotherapy, when Grace was treated for tumour spread to the right side. Again, radiotherapy triggered pain, this time in the right shoulder, disrupting her sleep and making radiotherapy treatment painful. This time, the point was less sensitive, and Grace was able to tolerate needling of ST-38 on the right (affected) side.

Using the eight extraordinary vessels

In Chapter 5, Toolkit, I discuss the use of two extraordinary vessels, the Directing Vessel (*Ren Mai*) and Yang Linking Vessel (*Yang Wei Mei*). These are not the only extraordinary vessels that are useful when treating cancer survivors; they are simply the ones I have used most extensively in treating lymphoedema-related problems. Other extraordinary vessels should be considered, as appropriate to the individual patient's presentation. The point of discussing them in relation to lymphoedema is that they allow another way of accessing areas of the body where it is prudent to avoid needling.

This may pose a challenge to those practitioners who, like myself, follow Maciocia's gender-specific procedure.[52] This involves using the opening and coupled points unilaterally and crossed over, called 'host–guest'.

This means that for a man, the opening point on the left is needled first, followed by the coupled point on the right. For a woman, the opening point on the right is used, along with the coupled point on the left. Obviously, this works so long as needling in the left arm and right leg of a man, and the right arm and left leg of a woman is not contraindicated. So, can we still access the extraordinary vessels when patients have or are at risk of lymphoedema?

In my work to date, I have followed Maciocia's gender-specific approach when possible. When it has not been possible, I have simply reversed the points, that is, needling the opening point on the left side and the coupled point on the right side for women with breast cancer on their right side.

Using the Ren and Du channels

In designing the research discussed above, we asked lymphoedema experts about the safety of needling the Ren and Du channels, the channels on the midline of the torso and back. They could not advise us about this.

The specialist lymphoedema nurse reasoned that the Ren and Du channels equated to 'watersheds' in manual lymphatic drainage, and that it might be safe to needle points along these channels.

We followed this approach in the research, using REN points on the upper body (as well as those on the lower body), especially REN-9 *Shuifen*, REN-12 *Zhongwan*, REN-14 *Juque*, REN-15 *Jiuwei*, and REN-17 *Shanzhong* (it is my personal preference to moxa this point, usually with direct moxa, rather than needle it) on both breast and head and neck cancer participants, as appropriate to the individual. REN-24 *Chengjiang* was also needled to address xerostomia experienced by some head and neck cancer participants.

As it transpired, we used few points on the Du channel, apart from DU-20 *Baihui* and DU-4 *Mingmen*, although this was not due to deliberate avoidance.

We did not observe any adverse reactions to this approach, although some breast cancer participants did not like removing clothing to allow access to points along the Ren channel.

Using microsystems

Microsystems are an obvious choice in situations when body points are not accessible. Ear, scalp, tongue, hand, foot, wrist, and ankle microsystems offer the practitioner a wealth of choice. The NADA five-point ear acupuncture, discussed in Chapter 5, Toolkit, neatly side-steps issues of avoiding at-risk and affected arms of breast cancer participants in research into using acupuncture to manage hot flushes (see Chapter 8, Cancer Treatment-Related Hot Flushes and Night Sweats).

Microsystems can be used on their own, in combination with other microsystems, or in combination with body points. I frequently use the NADA protocol with body points when working with breast cancer survivors. Hand acupuncture, whether Korean or Japanese, would be applicable to patients with lower body lymphoedema. The application of these systems is ready to be explored more fully.

Adapting existing protocols

Many existing point combinations calling for bilateral needling can be adapted for use with cancer survivors with or at risk of lymphoedema. As discussed in Chapter 5, Toolkit, Four Gates (bilateral LI-4 *Hegu* and LIV-3 *Taichong*) can be adapted to Three Gates (unilateral LI-4 and bilateral LIV-3) for breast cancer patients.

Other bilateral protocols can be adapted. In the research cited above, we adapted the Five Element protocols for clearing Aggressive Energy and External Dragons. For the former, we needled the back shu points unilaterally for breast cancer patients; in the latter, we needled BL-11 *Dazhu* unilaterally for all patients with upper body lymphoedema. In all cases, we observed responses that were equivalent to what we would have anticipated with bilateral needling.[54]

Treating the person, not the condition

When faced by the disfigurement, distress, and disability caused by lymphoedema, it is easy to focus on treating the swelling. Lymphoedema is a chronic condition, and the evidence to say exactly what role acupuncture can play in its resolution remains inconclusive.

By shifting the focus from the lymphoedema to the individual, acupuncturists can facilitate improvements in overall health. In our research, focusing on improving wellbeing resulted in participants reporting diminished symptoms (including lymphoedema-specific problems), increased energy and vitality, motivation for self-care, and improved ability to cope, as illustrated in Figure 9.8.

These are important changes for people with a chronic condition (lymphoedema), especially when that condition is a consequence of another chronic condition (cancer). The links between improvements in wellbeing and reduced volume still need to be proven; however, there are indications that this may be possible.

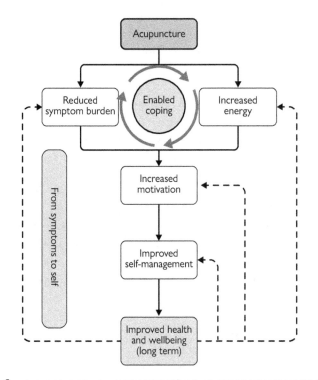

FIGURE 9.8: ACUPUNCTURE AS A CATALYST FOR LONG-TERM HEALTH IMPROVEMENT
SHOWING ENABLED COPING AND MOVING FROM SYMPTOM TO SELF

Some additional comments on needling

Some acupuncturists maintain it is safe to use acupuncture in an at-risk or affected area, because acupuncture is not a form of venepuncture and does not puncture veins. They conclude that the guidelines for acupuncture needling are not relevant.

My experience of working with cancer survivors is that there is a higher propensity for these patients to bruise or bleed at the needle site, a possible result of the cancer treatments weakening the Spleen's ability to hold the Blood. In this vulnerable population, acupuncture may unintentionally traumatise the area, causing undesired results.

Furthermore, there is a rationale to support working with, rather than contrary to, advice given to the patient by their oncology team. As we have seen, breast cancer patients are advised to avoid many procedures on the affected or at-risk area. Contradicting their medical advice can create confusion, and possibly lack of trust, in their acupuncturist. Fortunately for acupuncturists, it is possible to be adaptable and flexible, while remaining effective.

Moxibution, cupping and *gua sha*
Practitioners often ask about using moxibustion, cupping, and *gua sha* on an at-risk or affected area. We have seen that there is much research into using moxibustion and less for *gua sha* and cupping.

It may be prudent to avoid *gua sha* and cupping. *Gua sha*, and cupping to a lesser extent, risks damaging fragile skin. Furthermore, these modalities, like deep massage, may damage tissues and exacerbate oedema by increasing capillary filtration.[9]

Further roles for acupuncturists in lymphoedema management
I have suggested several strategies that acupuncturists can adopt when treating cancer survivors with or at risk of lymphoedema. The role that acupuncturists can play in lymphoedema management extends beyond acupuncture treatment; they can act as important agents in early identification of this condition and in patient education.

ESSENTIALS

It is important to recognise the signs of lymphoedema early and refer patients to appropriate professionals.

In addition, all healthcare providers should be aware of the associated psychological symptoms, such as psychological distress, sleep problems, negative self-image, and lack of confidence.[3]

Diagnosing lymphoedema
It is not the acupuncturist's role to diagnose lymphoedema unless they have specialist lymphoedema training. It is important that this is done by a medical professional, ideally specialising in lymphoedema.

If an acupuncturist suspects lymphoedema, they should refer the patient to the relevant specialist lymphoedema care facilities available, or to the patient's general practitioner or specialist cancer professionals (such as a breast care nurse).

Early identification
Early identification and referral to specialised treatment is key to limiting the potentially damaging effects of lymphoedema. Monitoring changes, especially those that may seem minor, can make a major contribution to lymphoedema care. There are five essential things that acupuncturists can do to help improve overall lymphoedema care, listed below.

ESSENTIALS

- Know who is at risk.
- Identify early.
- Support self-management.
- Reduce the symptom burden.
- Observe safe practice guidelines.

Know who is at risk

Knowing who is at risk is essential for monitoring for early signs of lymphoedema as well as for safe practice.

If the patient has had cancer treatment, it is necessary to ascertain what treatments they have had, to determine the level of risk (Table 9.1). Additionally, knowing whether there is any family history of swelling may be a useful indicator of genetic predisposition to lymphoedema.

Identify early

Early identification minimises progression of lymphoedema. While the condition is at subclinical and early stages (ISL 0 and I), lymphoedema is largely fluid and is amenable to treatment with simple compression. Treatment at these early stages increases the possibility of reversing any changes that have already happened as well as preventing further ones from developing.

At Stage II and above, chronic inflammation of the tissue leads to fibrosis and adipose tissue, making the condition more complex and irreversible without proper treatment.

Acupuncturists can play an important role in the containment of lymphoedema by recognising early signs and symptoms (Box 9.3) and then making appropriate referrals. The close attention we pay to changes in symptoms, however slight, positions us to help identify lymphoedema in its early stages.

Box 9.3: Early signs and symptoms of lymphoedema

- Clothing or jewellery (e.g. sleeve, shoe, or ring) becoming tighter.
- Feeling of heaviness, tightness, fullness, or stiffness.
- Aching.
- Observable swelling (for 'at-risk' patients, this is a sign even if it goes down at night).
- Skin changes – thickening or peau d'orange (orange peel skin) particularly in the breast or abdominal apron (accumulation of fat that hangs down like an apron).

If a patient presents with swelling, these questions may be relevant:

- How long have you had this swelling?
- Do you know what triggered the swelling?
- Do you have any family member with this swelling?
- Does this swelling change? Does it go down on elevation or overnight? Does it improve with exercise?
- Do you have any other symptoms like heaviness, pain, numbness, or tingling?
- Has a physician addressed your swelling?

Support self-management

Self-care, an essential part of managing lymphoedema, may be burdensome for some individuals. Acupuncturists can play an important role in encouraging cancer survivors to carry out their self-management routines. These vary according to patient, so it is useful to ascertain each person's maintenance plan. It may be necessary to encourage patients to:

- wear their compression garments as prescribed
- carry out skin care activities, such as frequent moisturising
- exercise appropriately
- carry out routine simple lymphatic drainage.

It is helpful to support patients in following the guidelines for minimising the risk of developing lymphoedema (Box 9.4). These actions are also important for reducing the risk of deterioration in patients with existing lymphoedema.

It is especially important to encourage patients to maintain a reasonable weight.

Box 9.4: Common-sense approach to minimising risk of developing lymphoedema[9]

- Take good care of skin and nails.
- Maintain optimal body weight.
- Avoid injury to area at risk.
- Avoid tight underwear, clothing, jewellery, watches.
- Avoid exposure to extreme cold or heat.
- Use high-factor sunscreen and insect repellent.
- Use mosquito nets in lymphatic filariasis endemic areas.
- Wear prophylactic compression garments, if prescribed.
- Undertake exercise/movement and limb elevation.
- Wear comfortable, supportive footwear.

Reduce the symptom burden

Cancer survivors with or at risk of lymphoedema experience many associated symptoms on physical, mental, and emotional levels. Acupuncture treatment can address many of these symptoms, leading to improved wellbeing, quality of life, and ability to cope with chronic health issues. These symptoms include, but are not limited to:

- pain, discomfort
- depression, anxiety
- sleep problems
- physical disability
- obesity
- body image problems
- sexual dysfunction
- adjustment to cancer diagnosis
- relationship problems.

It can be useful to avoid focusing exclusively on volume reduction (swelling). Studies have shown that, contrary to what we might expect, volume does not always relate to quality of life. Many patients with high volumes live comfortably with their condition, while others with minimal swelling experience distress.

Furthermore, swelling can vary according to several factors, including activity levels, weight changes, stress, and seasonal changes.

Observe safe practice guidelines
In this chapter, I have discussed the possible risks of needling an affected or at-risk area, and reasons why it is prudent to avoid this. I have also presented several strategies to overcome restrictions on needling.

To treat within safe practice guidelines may require creativity in finding alternative solutions. This might involve thinking 'outside the box' of our usual practice and exploring new techniques. Practising EAM should teach us that there is never one single way to approach a problem; the richness of acupuncture offers the possibilities of many solutions to a problem.

Patient perspectives

CASE STUDY: LINDA AND MONITORING FOR EARLY ONSET LYMPHOEDEMA
Introduction
Linda's case study provides an example of early stage lymphoedema, tracing its development over a course of acupuncture treatment. It highlights how cancer survivors may choose to disconnect from facing up to the risk of developing this condition.

Background
Linda, aged 66, was diagnosed with breast cancer eight months before coming for acupuncture treatment for hot flushes and night sweats (HFNS). Surgery had been performed three times to excise a lump in the upper left breast, and to identify and

remove one lymph node with metastatic carcinoma. This was followed by radiotherapy, completed two months before Linda commenced acupuncture, and hormonal treatment with Arimidex®.

At her first acupuncture appointment, we discussed avoiding needling in the left arm, her arm at risk for lymphoedema, due to the surgeries, lymph node removal, and radiotherapy.

Her HFNS responded well to treatment, and I addressed other symptoms as they presented. I worked with Linda extensively on aspects of lifestyle, advising a balance of daily rest, exercise, and healthy eating. Linda enjoyed the profound relaxation that she experienced during acupuncture treatment. After an initial period of weekly treatment, she attended at four- and then six-week intervals, partly because she travelled extensively.

Diagnosed shortly after remarrying, Linda found that her preoccupation with cancer treatment had marred newlywed happiness. On finishing active cancer treatment, she embarked on a programme of health improvements, including a bladder operation and extensive dental work. Linda and her husband also took several holidays abroad. She seemed desperate to put the experience of cancer behind her.

Linda's risk factors for lymphoedema

Linda had several risk factors for lymphoedema, and I was concerned to monitor her arm for any signs of early onset. In addition to surgery with axillary lymph node dissection and radiotherapy, she experienced post-operative complications including haematoma, seroma, and tissue fibrosis.

Arm discomfort

At her eighth treatment (three months after commencing acupuncture), she reported that her left arm had become uncomfortable during the previous week. Linda was reluctant to follow my advice to contact her breast care nurse, as she did not want to bother her. At her quarterly follow-up, her oncologist identified cording (axillary web syndrome), another risk factor for lymphoedema. Exercise and self-treatment with low-level laser for six months were prescribed.

Rash

Shortly after, Linda reported a rash on her finger around her wedding ring. Again, she did not wish to bother the breast nurse with something apparently trivial. Concerned that there was no apparent cause for the rash, which did not heal, I mentioned it in a follow-up letter to her oncologist. I also suggested Linda stop wearing her wedding ring, as the metal might be an irritant. Reluctantly, she did this, and the rash soon disappeared.

Cellulitis?

At her 15th treatment (ten months into her acupuncture treatment, and one year since the end of her cancer treatment), Linda reported that her left hand had turned red and begun to swell on the evening of her previous acupuncture treatment. She contacted her doctor, and attended Accident and Emergency, where she received immediate treatment with antibiotics.

I was grateful that I had adhered to safe practice by not needling the at-risk arm, so that acupuncture could not be seen to be the cause of this acute infection. While neither Linda nor the doctor mentioned the word 'cellulitis', the rapid action to prescribe immediate antibiotic treatment suggested that this was cellulitis.

Avoidance

At this point, I questioned Linda carefully about the information she had received about lymphoedema and cellulitis. She admitted that she had ignored the leaflets provided by her oncology team. Prior to and during her cancer treatment, she was too focused on the cancer and its treatments to read the leaflets. Following her treatment, she was keen to put the experience behind her. Consequently, the leaflets languished in a box.

I strongly advised Linda to read the leaflets; it was increasingly apparent to me that she was a high risk for lymphoedema. Two acupuncture sessions (and two months) later, Linda was still adamant that 14 months after the end of her cancer treatment, she wanted to forget about the experience and had no desire to read the lymphoedema information.

Two months later, Linda completed the six-month course of laser treatment. On stopping the treatment, she reported the return of the tight sensation under her arm, and again I encouraged her to see her breast care nurse.

Acting

Linda did eventually act; two months later she reported that she had seen her breast care nurse, who referred her to the lymphoedema service. She was prescribed a compression sleeve to wear continuously for two months. It was good that Linda was now getting appropriate care for the arm; it had taken time and much persuasion to get her there.

Linda continues to wear a compression sleeve and her swollen arm still requires specialist care. Lymphoedema was caught at a reasonably early stage – it might have been treated earlier if Linda had been able to cope with the information she had been given.

Summary

Linda's eagerness to put her cancer experience behind her put her at risk of developing a serious consequence of cancer treatment. Her case demonstrates the importance of knowing the risk factors of lymphoedema, and of recognising early signs and symptoms. It also demonstrates how important avoiding needling an at-risk area can be.

Video link

To meet a patient with lymphoedema and hear what they have to say about their acupuncture experience, watch this brief video about acupuncture and lymphoedema: www.youtube.com/watch?v=oZgzrFwuiBY&t=30s

CHAPTER SUMMARY
Acupuncturists have a unique set of skills that can be used to improve quality of life for people with lymphoedema.
Acupuncturists can:

- be an integral part of the multidisciplinary approach to the management of cancer treatment-related lymphoedema
- be effective even if needling is contraindicated in areas of the body
- be in the forefront for early identification of lymphoedema
- support self-management
- reduce associated symptom burden.

References

1. Ganz PA The quality of life after breast cancer – solving the problem of lymphedema. N. Engl. J. Med. 1999;340(5):383–385.
2. Executive Committee of the International Society of Lymphology The diagnosis and treatment of peripheral lymphedema: 2020 Consensus Document of the International Society of Lymphology. Lymphology 2020;53(1):3–19.
3. Neligan PC, Masia J, Piller NB Lymphedema: complete medical and surgical management. Stuttgart: Georg Thieme Verlag; 2016.
4. British Lymphology Society Lymph facts: what is lymphoedema? UK: British Lymphology Society; 2020. Available from: www.thebls.com/documents-library/lymph-facts-what-is-lymphoedema
5. Mortimer PS, Rockson SG New developments in clinical aspects of lymphatic disease. J. Clin. Invest. 2014;124(3):915–921.
6. British Lymphology Society Lymph facts: who has a predisposition to lymphoedema and why? UK: British Lymphology Society; 2020. Available from: www.thebls.com/documents-library/lymph-facts-who-has-a-predisposition-to-lymphoedema-and-why
7. Cormier JN, Askew RL, Mungovan KS, et al. Lymphedema beyond breast cancer: a systematic review and meta-analysis of cancer-related secondary lymphedema. Cancer 2010;116(22):5138–5149.
8. Rockson S Lymphedema. Am. J. Med. 2001;110:288–295.
9. Lymphoedema Framework Best practice for the management of lymphoedema. International consensus. London: MEP Ltd; 2006.
10. McDuff SGR, Mina AI, Brunelle CL, et al. Timing of lymphedema after treatment for breast cancer: when are patients most at risk? Int. J. Radiat. Oncol. Biol. Phys. 2019;103(1):62–70.
11. Togawa K, Ma H, Sullivan-Halley J, et al. Risk factors for self-reported arm lymphedema among female breast cancer survivors: a prospective cohort study. Breast Cancer Res. 2014;16(4):414.
12. National Cancer Action Team Lymphoedema – a consequence of cancer and its treatment; 2012.
13. DiSipio T, Rye S, Newman B, et al. Incidence of unilateral arm lymphoedema after breast cancer: a systematic review and meta-analysis. Lancet Oncol. 2013;14(6):500–515.
14. Pappalardo M, Starnoni M, Franceschini G, et al. Breast cancer-related lymphedema: recent updates on diagnosis, severity and available treatments. J. P. Med. 2021;11(5):402.
15. British Lymphology Society, Lymphoedema Support Network Consensus document on the management of cellulitis in lymphoedema (revised December 2016). UK: British Lymphology Society; 2016. Available from: www. thebls.com/documents-library/consensus-document-on-the-management-of-cellulitis-in-lymphoedema
16. Ridner S The psyco-social impact of lymphedema. Lymphat. Res. Biol. 2009;7(2):109–112.
17. Wounds UK Best practice statement: Maintaining skin integrity. London: Wounds UK; 2018. Available from: www.wounds-uk.com/resources/details/maintaining-skin-integrity
18. Asdourian MS, Skolny MN, Brunelle C, et al. Precautions for breast cancer-related lymphoedema: risk from air travel, ipsilateral arm blood pressure measurements, skin puncture, extreme temperatures, and cellulitis. Lancet Oncol. 2016;17(9):e392–405.
19. Dessources K, Aviki E, Leitao MM, Jr. Lower extremity lymphedema in patients with gynecologic malignancies. Int. J. Gynecol. Cancer 2020;30(2):252–260.

20. British Lymphology Society Lymph facts: what information, advice and support should be provided for those-at-risk-of-lymphoedema? UK: British Lymphology Society; 2020. Available from: www.thebls.com/documents-library/lymph-facts-what-information-advice-and-support-should-be-provided-for-those-at-risk-of-lymphoedema

21. Rockson SG Lymphedema. Vasc. Med. 2016;21(1):77–81.

22. Shaitelman SF, Cromwell KD, Rasmussen JC, et al. Recent progress in the treatment and prevention of cancer-related lymphedema. CA. Cancer J. Clin. 2015;65(1):55–81.

23. British Lymphology Society Lymph facts: Activity and Exercise. UK: British Lymphology Society; 2020. Available from: https://www.thebls.com/documents-library/lymph-facts-activity-and-exercise

24. Lee T Navigating lymphoedema: a guide for cancer survivors. Australia: Teresa Lee; 2020.

25. Ridner SH, Deng J, Fu MR, et al. Symptom burden and infections occurrence among individuals with extremity lymphedema. Lymphology 2012;45:113–123.

26. Wanchai A, Armer JM, Stewart BR Complementary and alternative medicine and lymphedema. Semin. Oncol. Nurs. 2013;29(1):41–49.

27. Chao LF, Zhang AL, Liu HE, et al. The efficacy of acupoint stimulation for the management of therapy-related adverse events in patients with breast cancer: a systematic review. Breast Cancer Res. Treat. 2009;118(2):255–267.

28. Rodrick JR, Poage E, Wanchai A, et al. Complementary, alternative, and other noncomplete decongestive therapy treatment methods in the management of lymphedema: a systematic search and review. PM R 2014;6(3):250–274; quiz 274.

29. Nudelman J Debunking lymphedema risk-reduction behaviors: risky conclusions. Lymphat. Res. Biol. 2016;14(3):124–126.

30. Cheng CT, Deitch JM, Haines IE, et al. Do medical procedures in the arm increase the risk of lymph-oedema after axillary surgery? A review. ANZ J. Surg. 2014;84(7-8):510–514.

31. Li P Management of cancer with Chinese medicine. London: Donica Publishing Ltd; 2003.

32. Lahans T Integrating conventional and Chinese medicine in cancer care: a clinical guide. Philadelphia: Churchill Livingstone; 2007.

33. Hou W, Pei L, Song Y, et al. Acupuncture therapy for breast cancer-related lymphedema: A systematic review and meta-analysis. J. Obstet. Gynaecol. Res. 2019;45(12):2307–2317.

34. Liu M, Zhang Y, Song F-c, et al. Relationship between ultrasound imaging and traditional Chinese medicine syndrome in limb lymphedema. Journal of Chinese Integrative Medicine 2009;7(5):481–521.

35. Liu NF Lymphedema in China – experiences and prospects. Lymphology 2007;40:153–156.

36. Kanakura Y, Niwa K, Kometani K, et al. Effectiveness of acupuncture and moxibustion treatment for lymphedema following intrapelvic lymph node dissection: a preliminary report. Am. J. Chin. Med. 2002;30(1):37–43.

37. Chien TJ, Liu CY, Fang CJ The effect of acupuncture in breast cancer-related lymphoedema (BCRL): a systematic review and meta-analysis. Integr. Cancer Ther. 2019;18:1534735419866910.

38. Jin H, Xiang Y, Feng Y, et al. Effectiveness and safety of acupuncture moxibustion therapy used in breast cancer-related lymphedema: a systematic review and meta-analysis. Evid. Based. Complement. Alternat. Med. 2020:3237451.

39. Yu S, Zhu L, Xie P, et al. Effects of acupuncture on breast cancer-related lymphoedema: A systematic review and meta-analysis. Explore (NY) 2020;16(2):97–102.

40. Zhang X, Wang X, Zhang B, et al. Effects of acupuncture on breast cancer-related lymphoedema: a systematic review and meta-analysis of randomised controlled trials. Acupunct. Med. 2019;37(1):16–24.

41. Alem M, Gurgel MSC Acupuncture in the rehabilitation of women after breast cancer – a case series. Acupunct. Med. 2008;26(2):86–93.

42. Smith C, Pirotta M, Kilbreath S A feasibility study to examine the role of acupuncture to reduce symptoms of lymphoedema after breast cancer: a randomised controlled trial. Acupunct. Med. 2014;32(5):387–393.

43. Bao T, Zhi I, Vertosick E, et al. Acupuncture for breast cancer-related lymphedema: a randomized controlled trial. Breast Cancer Res. Treat. 2018;170(1):77–87.

44. Cassileth BR, Van Zee KJ, Chan Y, et al. A safety and efficacy pilot study of acupuncture for the treatment of chronic lymphoedema. Acupunct. Med. 2011;29:166–167.

45. Cassileth BR, van Zee KJ, Yeung KS, et al. Acupuncture in the treatment of upper-limb lymphedema: results of a pilot study. Cancer 2013;119(13):2455–2461.

46. Kim TH, Kang JW, Lee MS Current evidence of acupuncture for symptoms related to breast cancer survivors: A PRISMA-compliant systematic review of clinical studies in Korea. Medicine (Baltimore). 2018;97(32):e11793.

47. Jeong Y, Kwon H, Park Y, et al. Treatment of lymphedema with Saam acupuncture in patients with breast cancer: a pilot study. Med. Acupunct. 2015;27(3):206–215.

48. Yao C, Xu Y, Chen L, *et al*. Effects of warm acupuncture on breast cancer-related chronic lymphedema: a randomized controlled trial. Curr. Oncol. 2016;23(1):e27–34.
49. Wang C, Yang M, Fan Y, *et al.* Moxibustion as a therapy for breast cancer-related lymphedema in female adults: a preliminary randomized controlled trial. Integr. Cancer Ther. 2019;18:1534735419866919.
50. Huang R, Huang Y, Huang R, *et al.* Thunder-fire moxibustion for cervical spondylosis: a systematic review and meta-analysis. Evid. Based. Complement. Alternat. Med. 2020;2020:5816717.
51. Mortimer PS The pathophysiology of lymphedema. Cancer (Suppl.) 1998;83(12):2798–2802.
52. Maciocia G The channels of acupuncture: clinical use of the secondary channels and eight extraordinary vessels. Edinburgh: Churchill Livingstone; 2006.
53. Deadman P, Al-Khafaji M, Baker K A manual of acupuncture. Hove: The Journal of Chinese Medicine; 2007.
54. de Valois B, Peckham R Treating the person and not the disease: acupuncture in the management of cancer treatment-related lymphoedema. Eur. J. Orient. Med. 2011;6(6):37–49.
55. de Valois B Acupuncture and moxibustion in the management of non-cancer-related lower limb lymphoedema. Eur. J. Orient. Med. 2013;7(4):13–21.
56. Oleson T Auriculotherapy manual: Chinese and Western systems of ear acupuncture. 2nd ed. Los Angeles: Health Care Alternatives; 1998.

Chapter 10

Chronic Post-Cancer Treatment Pain (CPCTP)

Introduction

The prevalence of cancer treatment-related pain, and the potential for acupuncture to alleviate this, is expressed in the following quotations:

> All modalities of cancer treatment – surgery, chemotherapy, radiation therapy (FT), transplants and immunotherapy – can be painful. (Glare *et al.*)[1]

> [Acupuncture] relieved the pain in my shoulders, cutting my pain killers from eight a day to two. (Alan, a head and neck cancer survivor)[2]

One of the most distressing and disabling symptoms experienced by patients and survivors, cancer-related pain is a major healthcare challenge.[3] Moderate to severe pain is reported by 40% of patients with early or intermediate stage cancer, and by 90% of those with advanced cancer.[4]

Chronic pain is not limited to individuals living with early, advanced, or metastatic cancer.[5] It may affect disease-free survivors, and is mainly the consequence of cancer treatments – surgery, radiotherapy, and systemic anti-cancer therapy – rather than the disease itself. Pain may persist after cancer treatment has finished, or emerge months or years later.[3]

Chronic post-cancer treatment pain is thought to affect around 30–50% of cancer survivors.[3] Associated with fatigue, anxiety, depression, and sleep disturbance in a symptom cluster, each of these symptoms can further impact pain, increasing its severity. Together, they negatively impact quality of life.

Management of chronic pain relies on multidisciplinary approaches to address its complexity. This encompasses medical management of pain, as well as interventions to address social, emotional, and spiritual issues. Expertise may be needed from a variety of specialists including social workers, psychologists, occupational and physical therapists, and spiritual advisors.[6]

Acupuncture can play an important role in this multidisciplinary approach. It can help to reduce the symptom burden, improve comfort and function, and has the potential to address emotional and spiritual issues implicated in pain.

Importantly, in the era of the opioid crisis, acupuncture offers a non-pharmacological treatment option for pain management. Its potential to reduce (and sometimes eliminate) the need for pharmaceuticals minimises the side effects and risks of these medications. This capacity makes acupuncture a valuable resource for helping to manage chronic post-cancer treatment pain and can make an important contribution to improving survivors' quality of life.

Pain is a vast subject, even pain related to cancer. To clarify, the focus of this chapter is chronic post-cancer treatment pain (later referred to as CPCTP) and applies to cancer survivors who:

- have completed primary or first line treatment given with curative intent, typically for early-stage cancer and who appear to be disease-free
- experience pain that is attributed to cancer treatment, and that has persisted beyond the usual time expected for tissue damaged by treatment to recover.[1]

For information about other aspects of pain, such as the biomedical mechanisms, the reader should consult the many information sources available on this subject.

RED FLAG

Any new pain, particularly if it is severe and uncontrolled, should be assessed promptly by the appropriate healthcare professional.

Pain can be a sign of cancer recurrence. New pain reported by cancer survivors should be investigated thoroughly to ensure it is not a sign of disease progression or second cancers.[7,8]

Classification of chronic cancer-related pain

TERMINOLOGY

While 'cancer pain' is widely used, the International Association for the Study of Pain (IASP)[7] notes it is a poorly defined term, which may not adequately describe or differentiate the types of pain associated with the different stages of the cancer trajectory.

IASP's detailed classification of the types of 'cancer pain' is presented in Box 10.1 and illustrated in Figure 10.1. It clearly articulates the difference between:

- pain caused by the cancer itself (chronic cancer pain) and
- pain resulting from cancer treatments (chronic post-cancer treatment pain).

Many other terms are used in the medical literature. For example, 'post-cancer pain syndrome' encompasses long-lasting and late onset pain resulting from cancer treatment as well as its related cluster of symptoms, including fatigue, anxiety, depression, and sleep disturbance.[3] Other terms are also applied and are used throughout this chapter, as many papers were published prior to the IASP definition, or authors choose to use other terms.

Box 10.1: IASP classification of chronic cancer-related pain for the International Classification of Diseases (ICD)[7]

Chronic cancer-related pain: An overall term defining 'chronic pain caused by primary cancer itself (chronic cancer pain) or its treatment (chronic post-cancer treatment pain). It is distinct from pain caused by comorbid disease.'

Chronic cancer pain: One of two main sub-classifications, this refers to 'chronic pain caused by the primary cancer or metastases' consisting of inflammatory and neuropathic mechanisms that are a direct effect of tissue response to the primary tumour or metastases. Further sub-classifications are:

- chronic visceral cancer pain
- chronic bone cancer pain
- chronic neuropathic cancer pain
- other chronic cancer pain.

Chronic post-cancer treatment pain: The second main sub-classification, this refers to chronic pain caused by cancer treatments, typically surgery, chemotherapy, and radiotherapy. Further sub-classifications under this heading are:

- *Chronic post-cancer medicine pain* – 'chronic pain caused by any disease-modifying anti-cancer medicine, including systemic chemotherapy, hormonal treatment, and biological therapies'. This has a further sub-classification, *chronic painful chemotherapy-induced polyneuropathy*, which is 'chronic peripheral neuropathic pain caused by oral or intravenous chemotherapy given to treat the primary tumour or metastases'.
- *Chronic post-radiotherapy pain* – 'chronic pain caused by delayed local damage to the nervous system, bones, or other soft tissues in the field of radiotherapy given to treat the primary tumour or metastases'. This has a further sub-classification, *chronic painful radiation-induced neuropathy*, which is chronic pain caused by delayed local damage to the nervous system in the field of radiotherapy given to treat the primary tumour or metastases.
- *Chronic post-cancer surgery pain* – this is chronic pain associated with surgery to remove cancer or the metastases and encompasses 'chronic pain after biopsy or from a chest or abdominal insertion for pleural effusion or peritoneal ascites'.
- *Other chronic post-cancer treatment pain* – refers to chronic pain caused by cancer treatment that is not related to the previous categories.

IASP notes that it is possible for chronic cancer pain and chronic post-treatment cancer pain to be concurrent, as well as chronic pain from non-cancer-related comorbidities.

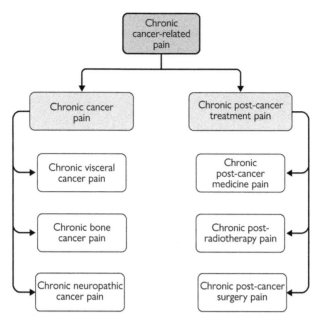

FIGURE IO.I: IASP CLASSIFICATION OF CHRONIC CANCER-RELATED PAIN[7]

Incidence and prevalence of CPCTP

An estimated 33–40% of cancer survivors who have completed curative treatment experience chronic pain, equating to 6.6–8 million individuals in the USA alone.[1,7] This number is expected to rise over the coming years as the number of cancer survivors increases.

A seminal study of over 30,000 people in the USA found that 34% of cancer survivors reported ongoing pain compared with 18% of those without a history of cancer.[9] In that study, 81.6% of the 1904 cancer survivors surveyed were two or more years post cancer diagnosis, of whom 33.1% were over II years post diagnosis. The study found that recurring pain did not decrease significantly as time from treatment increased, suggesting that persistent pain may indeed persist for many years after treatment.

Biomedical perspectives
Aetiology

Cancer treatments contribute to a range of consequences, and pain is generally categorised as:

- **Neuropathic:** caused by a lesion or disease of the somatosensory nervous system.[10]
- **Nociceptive:** caused by ongoing tissue damage, either somatic (such as bone pain) or visceral (such as gut or hepatic pain).[11]

Neuropathic pain is the most common type of pain in cancer survivors. Resulting from injury to the peripheral or central nervous system caused by surgery, radiotherapy, and/or systemic anti-cancer therapy (Box 10.2), it is challenging to treat because of its severity, persistence, and resistance to simple analgesics.[3,5,8,12]

Box 10.2: Common CPCTP syndromes[1]
Neuropathic pain:

- Persistent pain post cancer surgery
- Chemotherapy-induced peripheral neuropathy (CIPN)
- Chronic pain post radiotherapy

Nociceptive pain:

- Musculoskeletal pain post surgery or radiotherapy
- Aromatase inhibitor-associated musculoskeletal syndrome (AIMSS)
- Rheumatic and musculoskeletal pain associated with checkpoint inhibitors
- Joint and fascia manifestations of chronic graft versus host disease

---

Pain as part of a symptom cluster
CPCTP should be viewed in the context of a symptom cluster that includes:

- depression
- fatigue
- insomnia
- tiredness
- memory difficulties.

Any of these symptoms may exacerbate or be exacerbated by pain, causing serious negative impacts on survivors' quality of life.

Problems associated with normal ageing also contribute to the complexity of pain. As survivors live longer, chronic non-cancer pain of ageing (e.g. osteoarthritis) and other comorbidities may present alongside CPCTP. While older survivors are more likely to experience comorbidities which contribute to their burden of pain, younger survivors may experience more psychosocial distress which exacerbates symptom frequency and severity.[7,9]

Treatment-related pain is generally expected to diminish over time, as injured tissues heal and regenerate.[3,12,13] However, pain may be severe and long lasting for some survivors. For example, above-average pain has been reported for over 30% of breast cancer survivors ten years after treatment.[3,9,13]

Types of pain by treatment and by cancer
Factors influencing the physical aspects of CPCTP include:

- type and stage of cancer
- type(s) of cancer treatment received
- time since completing treatment
- comorbid conditions
- age, gender, and cultural background
- decade in which treatment was administered (treatments have improved over time).

Physical pain is also impacted by stress and psychological pain.

Effective pain management during acute stages, including appropriate patient information to help patients understand the cause of pain, is thought to reduce the incidence of chronic pain in cancer survivors.[6]

The following discussion of CPCTP is organised by cancer treatment modality: surgery, radiotherapy, and systemic anti-cancer treatments. Within each treatment modality, common pain syndromes associated with specific cancers are discussed. CPCTP is not limited to these cancer types or interventions; however, these pain syndromes are common in the medical literature about pain in survivorship.

CPCTP syndromes related to surgery

Chronic pain is a potential consequence of any surgery;[6] in the general population nearly 20% of subjects studied experienced moderate to severe pain more than three months following surgery.[14] Among cancer survivors, high prevalence rates of what is also called persistent post-surgical pain (PPSP) are associated with certain procedures (Box 10.3). The most common include:

- thoracotomy 30–50%
- limb amputation 30–85%
- hernia repair 20–60%
- breast surgery 15–55%.[15]

Box 10.3: CPCTP syndromes related to surgery[12]

- Intercostal neuralgia
- Lymphoedema
- Neuroma pain
- Pain related to breast implants/reconstruction
- Phantom limb pain
- Post-mastectomy pain
- Post-surgical neck dissection pain
- Post-thoracotomy pain (surgery that cuts into the chest cavity)

The multiple risk factors for persistent post-surgical pain (Table 10.1) illustrate the complexity of this condition and the need for multimodal management, including psychological interventions.

Table 10.1: Risk factors for the development of persistent post-surgical pain[15]

Patient factors	Surgical factors	Other factors
Anxiety	Longer duration of procedure	Chemotherapy
Depression	Nerve retraction or destruction	Post-operative pain
Genetic factors	Open surgical procedure	Radiotherapy
Pain catastrophising*	Drain use	Surgery in low-volume centres
Pre-existing pain		
Raised BMI		
Young age (older age risk for phantom pain)		

*The tendency to focus on and exaggerate the threat of pain and to feel helpless in the context of pain.

Breast surgery

Chronic pain is a common consequence, reported to occur in approximately 15–60% of women undergoing breast surgery.[15,16] Even modern less invasive surgical techniques such as lumpectomy and axillary dissection and/or reconstruction may be associated with as much or more pain than standard modified radical mastectomy,[6,12] with studies reporting higher prevalence associated with axillary lymph node dissection (ALND).[16] Chronic pain is also associated with graft sites in reconstructive surgery, where tissue is taken from the abdomen and back, and with breast prosthesis implants.

Pain can present in the arm, neck, shoulder, axilla, chest wall, or breast; loss of shoulder function is common. Types of pain include:

- allodynia – pain from a stimulus that does not usually provoke pain, such as temperature
- hyperalgesia – increased sensitivity to pain
- paraesthesia – tingling, tickling, pricking, burning sensations
- phantom breast pain
- scar pain.

Post-operative pain is expected to diminish gradually in the year following surgery. For a proportion of women, it may not resolve even after considerable time, with studies reporting pain up to and beyond eight years post treatment.[16,17] Phantom breast pain and arm pain may be of longer duration.

Factors implicated in chronic pain after breast surgery include poor post-operative pain control, extent of axillary dissection, radiation therapy, and overall psychological state. The decade in which treatment was given is also a factor, as surgical procedures have improved over time.[6,16]

Head and neck cancer

Surgically induced pain may result from damage to local muscle, bone, or nerve tissues. Commonly injured nerves include the accessory nerve, the cranial nerve XI (which innervates the trapezius muscle), and/or the superficial cervical plexus.

Consequences include loss of sensation, decreased range of motion, reduced shoulder abduction, shoulder pain, neck pain, and myofascial pain. While studies report severe chronic pain in the first year post surgery,[6,8] many individuals experience ongoing pain for many years post treatment (see Bob's case study below).

Head and neck cancer survivors may also experience chronic pain at sites of tissue removal for reconstruction procedures (graft sites), typically in the arm or leg.

Post-amputation pain

Amputation occurs in many cancers, including bone cancers, soft tissue sarcomas, and breast cancer (mastectomy). Post-amputation pain may be classified as:

- phantom pain or sensation – pain or other unpleasant feelings experienced in the part of the body that has been amputated
- stump pain – pain localised to the actual area of the amputation.[8]

Nearly all amputees experience phantom sensation, while pain is reported for 7–72% of cases.[6] Sensations include:

- perceptions of a specific position, shape, or movement of the phantom limb
- feelings of warmth or cold
- paraesthesia (itching, tingling, or electrical sensations).[8]

Pain felt in the phantom limb may subside in the first year following amputation. If it persists beyond this, it may become a lifelong problem.

CPCTP syndromes related to radiotherapy

Chronic pain related to radiotherapy is usually a late effect of treatment, which may arise months or years post treatment. Onset varies and has been reported from six months to 34 years after treatment.[6,8,12] While incidence is declining as radiotherapy techniques become more targeted, post-radiotherapy pain affects around 2% of breast cancer survivors and up to 15% of head and neck cancer survivors.[1] Most cancer patients receiving radiotherapy will also have experienced other cancer treatments, making it difficult to determine the exact cause of persistent pain.[12,15,16]

Radiation can damage areas of the nervous system, leading to dysfunction of the associated nerve structures. In general, radiation damage is thought not to resolve over time. Serious cases may result in loss of muscle function or paralysis. Associated pain is characterised by stabbing or burning sensations in the area of the distribution of the affected nerve structures.[8] Box 10.4 lists common post-radiotherapy pain conditions identified for cancer survivors.

> ### Box 10.4: CPCTP syndromes related to radiotherapy[1,12,15]
>
> - Chest pain/tightness
> - Cystitis
> - Enteritis/proctitis
> - Erectile dysfunction and other changes in sexual function
> - Fibrosis of the skin or myofascia
> - Fistula formation
> - Mucositis
> - Myelopathy
> - Osteoradionecrosis
> - Pelvic insufficiency fractures
> - Peripheral nerve entrapment
> - Plexopathies
> - Adhesions in the radiation field (usually gastrointestinal or abdominal)

Breast cancer

Radiation is a risk factor for pain of the breast and arm in women treated for breast cancer, possibly due to connective tissue fibrosis and neural damage.

Radiation-induced brachial plexopathy (RIBP) is a rare severe late consequence thought to affect 1–5% of women after radiotherapy. A progressive, painful paralysis of the shoulder, it may present from six months to over 20 years after treatment. Early symptoms include abnormal sensation (dysesthesia) and pain or weakness, progressing to pain and weakness of the limb leading to a flaccid arm.[6,15] The incidence of RIBP has reduced over time due to changes in radiotherapy dose, including reduction in total radiation dose and dose per fraction.[15]

Lung cancer

RIBP is more common after treatment for apical lung cancer (usually non-small-cell lung cancers), with an incidence of 12% at three years.[1]

Pelvic cancers

Chronic radiation enteritis (inflammation of the small intestine) occurs in 5–20% of patients undergoing pelvic or abdominal radiotherapy, although incidence rates of 50% are associated with high-dose radiation. Cramping, bloating, diarrhoea, fistula, or damage to the mucosa can accompany intermittent or constant pain.[8]

Chronic proctitis (inflammation of the rectum) is a consequence of pelvic radiotherapy, affecting 2–5% of survivors of prostate, cervical, and endometrial cancers and 12% of rectal cancer survivors. Symptoms include pain on defecation, diarrhoea, rectal pain, urgency, bleeding, feeling of incomplete defecation (tenesmus), mucous discharge, constipation, and stricture formation.[8]

Radiation myelopathy is injury to the spinal cord caused by ionising radiotherapy. Early symptoms and signs include paraesthesia (tingling, tickling, pricking, or burning sensations in the skin) and muscle weakness in the legs, progressing to gait disturbance or hemiplegia. It may be accompanied by pain or abnormal sensation at or below the level of injury.[6]

Prostate cancer

Chronic pelvic pain and painful urination are associated with brachytherapy. Pain may be localised to the prostate or diffused throughout the urinary tract or pelvis, and be present during urination or exacerbated by urination.[6]

Changes in sexual function include erectile dysfunction, painful erections, and orgasm-associated pain.[1]

Head and neck cancers

Osteoradionecrosis of the jaw, an area of exposed irradiated bone that fails to heal over a period of three to six months, is a serious late complication of head and neck squamous cell carcinoma treated with radiotherapy.[18] Changes in the metabolic homeostasis following radiation progress to a state of hypoxia and hypovascularity, which lead to tissue breakdown causing disabling pain and non-healing wounds. Reported incidence ranges from 3% to 15%, and the mean duration of its development is 22–47 months after completing radiotherapy.[19]

Further discussion of CPCTP in head and neck cancer survivors can be found in Bob's case study (below) and in Chapter 7, Dry Mouth.

CPCTP syndromes related to systemic anti-cancer therapies

Chemotherapy

Chemotherapy-induced peripheral neuropathy (CIPN)

Of CPCTP syndromes related to chemotherapy (Box 10.5), CIPN is the most common. Associated with numerous cytotoxic drugs (e.g. taxanes, platinums, vinca alkaloids, epothilones, eribulin, and bortezomib),[20] it is characterised by symmetrical, distal, painful neuropathy described as tingling, burning, or numbness.[12]

Box 10.5: CPCTP related to chemotherapy[12]

- Arthralgia/myalgia
- Chemotherapy-induced peripheral neuropathy (CIPN)
- Muscle cramps
- Osteonecrosis
- Osteoporosis

CIPN is usually acute, occurring during chemotherapy cycles, and decreases over time. However, some chemotherapy agents are associated with a phenomenon called 'coasting'

(Table 10.2), which is the worsening of symptoms weeks or months after the last dose of chemotherapy.

For some patients, CIPN may remain debilitating for years.[20] The literature reports persistent CIPN symptoms in 11–80% of breast cancer survivors at one to three years after chemotherapy. Evaluation of long-term consequences found that 42% of breast cancer patients receiving doxetaxel experienced CIPN two years after chemotherapy, as did 84% of colorectal cancer patients treated with oxaliplatin.[21] Chronic CIPN is also associated with the proteasome inhibitor bortezomib (lasting three to six months, or longer), thalidomide, and lenalidomide (persisting for a year or longer).[12]

Table 10.2: Chemotherapy agents associated with 'coasting'[12]

Chemotherapy class	Agents	Notes
Vinca alkaloids	Vincristine, vinblastine, vinorelbine, vindesine	May resolve within 3 months; more likely to persist with vincristine.
Platinum compounds	Cisplatin, carboplatin, oxaliplatin	Coasting is common
Taxanes	Paclitaxel, docetaxel	Coasting is common.

Hormonal therapies
Aromatase inhibitor-associated musculoskeletal syndrome (AIMSS)
Of CPCTP syndromes related to hormonal therapies, arthralgia (or AIMSS) is reported by 40–50% of post-menopausal women taking AIs for oestrogen receptor positive breast cancer.[12,22] Joint pain and stiffness affects the hands, arms, knees, ankles, hips, and back; it is worse in the morning and may improve with movement.

Onset of AIMSS usually occurs within the first three months of hormone therapy. Continuation of symptoms significantly affects quality of life, causing many women to stop taking AIs. A study of pharmacy records showed that adherence to therapy dropped to 62–79% after three years.[12] This has potential consequences for survival, as it increases the risk of cancer recurrence.

Box 10.6: CPCTP related to hormonal therapies[12]

- Arthralgia/myalgia
- Muscle cramps/spasms
- Carpal tunnel syndrome
- Trigger finger
- Osteoporosis

Pain and the emotions

Feelings of loss and grief about change in body shape and image may exacerbate physical pain.

Radiotherapy is experienced by some patients (e.g. breast and pelvic cancer survivors) as dehumanising. Disrobing and allowing radiotherapists to place them into vulnerable positions for treatment may cause psychological pain and anxiety, especially in those with a history of sexual abuse. Head and neck cancer patients are fitted with masks that are bolted to the treatment tables; this can be traumatic and contribute to emotional suffering, which in turn may contribute to physical pain.

Summary of CPCTP

This discussion illustrates some of the many types of pain that are a consequence of cancer treatments, which can persist and affect survivors' quality of life.

It also highlights the complexity of pain management. Any pain is complex to manage and treat; cancer survivors may experience multiple types of pain if they have undergone multiple types of cancer treatment. The picture may be further complicated by emotional trauma, by pain from comorbidities, and the pain associated with ageing.

ESSENTIALS

Finding a 'silver bullet' intervention that will prevent or even manage CPCTP is highly improbable. Complex approaches, comprising a number of concurrent interventions, are thought to provide better outcomes.[15]

Biomedical management of CPCTP

Expert guidelines for managing pain are continually reviewed and updated by specialist oncology organisations, including the:

- American Society of Clinical Oncology (ASCO)
- European Society for Medical Oncology (ESMO)
- Society of Integrative Oncology (SIO).

Many guidelines for managing chronic pain in adult cancer survivors recommend that:

- treatment aims to improve function as well as relieve pain
- goals are tailored to the individual.[5,12]

A multidisciplinary approach is considered helpful, especially when chronic pain is accompanied by comorbidities such as depression, sleep problems, or fatigue.[1,23] Multidisciplinary programmes focusing on improving comfort and function may offer a combination of multiple therapies, including:

- pharmacological approaches
- physical therapy

- physical activity
- psychosocial interventions
- integrative or complementary and alternative medicine.[12]

Assessing pain

Assessing pain is an essential aspect of pain management; 'pain cannot be treated if it cannot be assessed'.[24] As pain is a subjective experience, patient self-report is regarded as the most reliable indicator of the presence and intensity of pain. Validated pain measures used for adults (Figure 10.2) include the:

- Visual Analogue Scale (VAS)
- Verbal Rating Scale
- Numeric Rating Scale (NRS).

Many variations of these are possible, such as picture-based scales for people with learning disabilities.

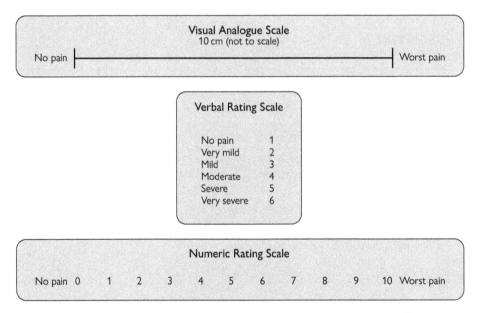

FIGURE 10.2: VALIDATED, FREQUENTLY USED PAIN ASSESSMENT TOOLS[11]

The NRS is commonly recommended as a measure of pain intensity and may also be used to measure other aspects of pain such as distress or interference. Easy to administer and score (Box 10.7), it is reliable for older patients or those with poor literacy. It is regarded as more reliable than the VAS. As its scale has more points, it is better for expressing change than the Verbal Rating Scale.[25]

Box 10.7: Using the Numeric Rating Scale

To use the NRS, the respondent selects a whole number (0–10) that best reflects the intensity (or other quality, as requested) of their pain, with the spectrum ranging from 0 = no pain to 10 = extreme pain/worst possible pain. It is often categorised as:

- no pain = 0
- mild pain = 1–3
- moderate pain = 4–6
- severe pain = 7–10.

Unidimensional measures, which typically focus on pain intensity, are useful for measuring a single aspect of pain. However, it is recommended that pain is assessed in a wider context that considers the physical, psychological, social, and spiritual aspects of pain, as well as determining the patient's own goals for comfort and function.[15] It is recommended that goal setting for pain should focus on reducing pain to a level that allows for an acceptable quality of life to the patient.[26]

Pharmacological approaches

Management of cancer-related pain has been based on the World Health Organization (WHO) three-step analgesic ladder (Figure 10.3), which progresses from:

- non-opioids (aspirin and paracetamol) to
- mild opioids (codeine) to
- strong opioids (morphine) for progressively severe pain.

Additional drugs (adjuvants) are recommended to calm fear and anxiety.[27]

Opioids

The relevance of the World Health Organization analgesic ladder for use with survivors who have completed treatment or are in remission is a topic of debate in the medical literature, particularly in relation to the long-term use of opioids.[1,15] In the age of the opioid crisis, concerns about addiction and abuse are paramount, although there are conflicting data available about opioid addiction in people with cancer. (Ironically, this can lead to under prescribing, leaving survivors with chronic pain and poor quality of life.)

Other concerns focus on the persistent adverse events associated with opioid use (Table 10.3). There are also theories about the impact opioids may have on immune function and potential cancer recurrence, although these are yet to be substantiated.[15]

Opioids are indicated when moderate to severe cancer treatment-related pain does not respond to non-opioid approaches. When their use is necessary, long-term opioids are recommended to be used cautiously and with careful monitoring.[1,15]

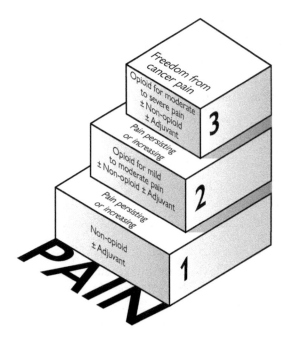

FIGURE 10.3: WORLD HEALTH ORGANIZATION ANALGESIC LADDER

Adjuvant analgesics

Adjuvant analgesics (Table 10.3) are medications with other primary indications that possess analgesic properties under certain circumstances. Used in all steps of the WHO ladder, they may be prescribed as first-line or monotherapy. Recommended before opioids for management of cancer treatment-related pain, their use has been linked to improvement in cancer-related pain, anxiety and depression, and lower opioid doses.[1]

Table 10.3: Pharmacological treatment of chronic pain in cancer survivors[1,22,28]

Category	Drug	Some adverse effects/cautions
Opioids	Morphine is the most frequently used. Buprenorphine, codeine fentanyl, hydrocodone, hydromorphone, methadone, oxycodone, oxymorphone, tapentadol, tramadol	**Cardiovascular:** hypotension. **Central nervous system:** sedation, dizziness, delirium, hallucinations, impaired cognitive status, sleep disturbance. **Gastrointestinal:** Constipation, nausea, vomiting. **Autonomic nervous system:** dry mouth (xerostomia), bladder dysfunction, urinary retention. **Respiratory:** respiratory depression (rare). **Dermatologic:** pruritus. **Miscellaneous:** hyperalgesia, opioid endocrinopathy/hypogonadism, hypoglycaemia. Risk of abuse or addiction; concerns about long-term side effects.[28]
Adjuvant analgesics		
Acetaminophen	Paracetamol	To be used with care or avoided in patients who are elderly or have renal, hepatic, or cardiac disease.

Non-steroidal anti-inflammatory drugs (NSAIDs)	Celecoxib, diclofenac, ibuprofen, ketoprofen, ketorolac, naproxen	Gastrointestinal irritation, ulcer formation, and dyspepsia, with other side effects of concern being cardiotoxicity, nephrotoxicity, hepatotoxicity, and hematologic effects.[28]
Antidepressants	Tricyclic antidepressants (TCAs): amitriptyline, desipramine, nortriptyline	Anticholinergic* effects, that result in drowsiness, dry mouth, orthostatic hypotension, weight gain. Significant drug interactions are a concern. Used with caution in elderly patients and those with seizure disorders, and pre-existing cardiac disease.
	SNRIs: duloxetine, venlafaxine	**Duloxetine:** Constipation, dry mouth, fatigue, headache, nausea. **Venlafaxine:** headache, hypertension, nausea, somnolence, vomiting.
Anticonvulsants	Gabapentin, pregabalin	Ataxia, dizziness, dry mouth, nausea, peripheral oedema, sedation.
Corticosteroids	Dexamethasone, methylprednisolone, prednisone	**Short term:** hyperglycemia, immunosuppression, insomnia, psychiatric disorders. **Long term:** myopathy, peptic ulceration, osteoporosis, Cushing syndrome.
Topical agents	Lignocaine transdermal patches and capsaicin cream for post-surgical pain; amitriptyline cream or high-dose capsaicin 8% patch for CIPN. Also, products such as Voltarol® gel, Deep Heat®, ibuprofen gel	Skin reaction (rare).

*Anticholergenics affect the parasympathetic nerve system, responsible for involuntary movement of muscles throughout the body. A wide range of physical and mental effects is possible, and may include blurred vision, constipation, dry mouth, decreased saliva, decreased sweating, difficulty urinating, drowsiness, hallucinations, confusion, delirium, memory impairment, sedation.

Non-pharmacological therapies

Guidelines for pain management include encouraging survivors to participate actively in their pain management, with an emphasis on self-activation and non-pharmacological therapies. Focusing on outcomes such as improved function, sleep, social activities, mood, and coping skills are also recommended as helpful strategies in pain management.[3]

Many non-pharmacological approaches are considered helpful in pain management, ranging from neurostimulatory interventions to psychological therapy to integrative medicine (complementary and alternative medicines) (Table 10.4).[3,12,22] Spiritual care should also be addressed.[29] In many countries or localities, access to or reimbursement for such interventions is limited and treatment may remain primarily biomedical.

These interventions address multiple factors that contribute to pain levels rather than being targeted directly at pain reduction per se. For example, there is strong evidence that depression and anxiety are associated with increased pain in cancer survivors generally, while high levels of pre-operative anxiety, depression, distress, and catastroph-ising were observed to be associated with post-surgical pain in early stage breast cancer patients up to and beyond a year post surgery.[1]

Many experts remain sceptical about the role of complementary and alternative medicines. Nevertheless, they are recommended as potentially helpful interventions in expert guidelines[23] and in reviews of management of CPCTP, especially as they are seen as useful for relieving the emotional distress commonly associated with pain.[1]

Table 10.4: Non-pharmacological approaches to management of chronic cancer pain[1,12]

Treatment approach	Examples
Exercise	Regular exercise routines, strength training, weight-bearing exercise, aerobic exercise.
Education	Pain management (including the need to report pain and the importance of taking pain medication); coping skills (cognitive and behavioural).
Integrative interventions (complementary and alternative medicines)	Acupuncture, acupressure, biofeedback, foot massage, guided imagery, hypnosis, light-touch massage, Swedish massage.
Interventional approaches (neuromodulation)	Nerve blocks, trigger point injections, spinal cord stimulators, implanted intrathecal pumps, transcutaneous electrical nerve stimulation (TENS).
Other interventions	Applications of heat by hot pack, paraffin wax, heat pads, compresses, ultrasound, moist heat, laser. Applications of cold by ice, cryotherapy.
Physical therapy and rehabilitation	Progressive resistance training; techniques such as myofascial release, visceral therapy, neuromuscular re-education, craniosacral manipulation, kinesiology taping, orthotics.
Psychological interventions	Acceptance-based training, active coping training, behavioural activation, cognitive behavioural therapy (CBT), cognitive restructuring, distraction training, mindfulness-based stress reduction,[30] stress management, psychosocial support.
Spiritual care	Physicians, hospital chaplains, and support groups may provide support to address spiritual concerns of patients.[29]

Acupuncture in the management of chronic cancer pain

Acupuncture is often recommended as a treatment modality in the management of cancer pain.[5,12,22] Recently published guidelines from the Society of Integrative Oncology (SIO) and the American Society of Clinical Oncology (ASCO) recommend acupuncture for several types of cancer-related pain, including AIMSS.[31]

Glare *et al.* regard acupuncture as a useful therapy that can complement other treat-ments and enhance the quality of care of survivors with CPCTP, stating that it 'can assist cancer survivors with post-surgical pain and postradiation syndromes, even pain that has persisted for years'.[1,12]

Benefits extend beyond relief of pain; side effects of pharmaceuticals are minimised or avoided, as are the risk of dependence, addiction, or withdrawal. Acupuncture treatment can improve or restore physical function and address emotional aspects of pain, as well as other symptoms in the associated cluster, including anxiety, depression, and insomnia.

East Asian medicine perspectives
Pain in the theory of Chinese medicine
In *Management of Cancer with Chinese Medicine*, Li Peiwen states that according to Chinese medicine theory, the basic cause of pain is obstruction of qi and Blood in the *zang-fu* organs, channels, and network vessels: 'where there is obstruction, there is pain'.[32] The pathology can be due to:

- **Excess patterns:** invasion and accumulation of pathogenic factors inhibits movement of qi and Blood in the channels and network vessels. This obstruction causes pain: 'Where free flow is obstructed, there is pain.'[32]
- **Deficiency patterns:** pain may be caused by deficiency of qi, Blood, yin, yang; or by the *zang-fu* (organs), channels, and network vessels being deprived of moisture, nourishment, or warmth: 'Where nourishment is insufficient, there is pain.'[32]

Acupuncture can be useful for:

- eliminating or reducing factors that cause stagnation of qi and Blood and impede their movement
- treating the pathology by dredging the channels and network vessels to restore the free flow of qi and Blood
- treating the symptoms by quieting the Heart and shifting the spirit, as a means of distracting the patient's attention from the pain.

Post-amputation pain
While much of Li Peiwen's discussion focuses on pain caused by cancer itself or experienced during active treatment, he provides useful advice for addressing post-amputation pain (Table 10.5) and stump pain (Table 10.6).[32]

Table 10.5: A protocol for addressing post-amputation pain

Treatment principles	Dredge the Liver and regulate qi; free the network vessels to alleviate pain.
Main points	Bilateral (as possible): LI-4 *Hegu* SP-6 *Sanyinjiao* LIV-3 *Taichong* Points specific to the amputation (see below) should be needled unilaterally on the side contralateral to the amputation.

For amputation of the:					
Fingers	**Forearm**	**Upper arm**	**Toes**	**Below knee joint**	**Below hip joint**
Select the corresponding jing-well point(s): LI-1 LU-11 HE-9 SI-1 PC-9 or TB-1	Add: LI-10 TB-5	Add: LI-14 LI-15	Select the corresponding jing-well point(s): ST-45 SP-1 BL-67 KID-1 GB-44 or LIV-1	Add: GB-34 GB-39	Add: ST-31 ST-32

Technique	Use reducing method with strong stimulation. Retain needles for 20–30 minutes.

Table 10.6: A protocol for stump pain

Treatment principles	Regulate and harmonise qi and Blood.
Main points	Select the relevant shu transport points 2 cun above the stump on each of the 6 channels (3 yin and 3 yang). The most likely combinations are:

Arm Jing-river points		Arm He-sea points		Leg Jing-river points		Leg He-sea points	
Yin	Yang	Yin	Yang	Yin	Yang	Yin	Yang
LU-8	LI-5	LU-5	LI-11	SP-5	ST-41	SP-9	ST-36
HE-4	SI-5	HE-3	SI-8	KID-7	BL-60	KID-10	BL-40
P-5	TB-6	P-3	TB-10	LIV-5	GB-38	LIV-9	GB-34

Alternative points	If transport points are not available, select one local point on each of the 6 channels (3 yin and 3 yang).
Technique	Insert needles obliquely upward at a 45° angle to the skin surface.
Moxibustion	Do not apply moxa for the first 2 months after amputation. If pain is present after 2 months, apply moxa and acupuncture.

Research perspectives
Systematic reviews of using acupuncture to manage CPCTP
Research into using acupuncture to manage cancer-related pain focuses mainly on pain experienced during active treatment or associated with late-stage and advanced cancer. When it does exist, evidence for acupuncture relating specifically to CPCTP may not be separated out from pain associated with other stages.

Systematic reviews of acupuncture and cancer-related pain
This is especially true in the case of systematic reviews of cancer pain.

For example, in a systematic review of acupuncture and acupressure for improving cancer pain, the 17 randomised controlled trials (RCTs) included cancer patients from across the cancer trajectory.[33] The authors conclude that there is a moderate level of evidence for the positive effect of acupuncture on reducing pain intensity, and acupuncture may be associated with reduced opioid use when added to analgesic therapy. Relatively few adverse events were reported. Acupuncture was associated with greater pain reduction compared with sham control, a result which differs from many previous systematic reviews.

By contrast, one earlier systematic review distinguished between tumour-related and treatment-related pain. Although it found acupuncture to be effective for relieving pain associated with malignancy and surgery, the authors concluded that there was insufficient evidence to support the beneficial effects of acupuncture for chemotherapy, radiotherapy, or hormone treatment-induced pain.[34]

Systematic reviews of acupuncture and chemotherapy-induced peripheral neuropathy (CIPN)
Of numerous systematic reviews of acupuncture for CIPN, one includes studies investigating survivors post treatment. Analysing results of 386 cancer survivors participating in six high-quality RCTs, it found significant improvements in pain scores and quality of life associated with acupuncture treatment.[35]

Systematic reviews of acupuncture and aromatase inhibitor-induced arthralgia
A systematic review of seven RCTs involving 603 survivors with AIMSS reported significant improvements compared with control groups. Measured using the Brief Pain Inventory (BPI) score, these included improvements in the pain-related interference score, pain severity score, and worst pain score compared with drugs and no treatment.[36] No severe adverse events were reported in the studies. The authors conclude that acupuncture is a safe and effective treatment for the painful consequences of aromatase inhibitors. Many of the studies included in this review are presented below (Table 10.7, Table 10.8, and Table 10.13).

Research investigating acupuncture to manage CPCTP
Selected details of studies including or focusing specifically on CPCTP syndromes are presented below according to the type of pain investigated. Within each pain category,

details are presented in two tables: the first summarises the points used and the second summarises study design and outcomes. The pain categories are as follows:

- Aromatase inhibitor associated musculoskeletal syndrome (AIMSS) or arthralgia (Table 10.7, Table 10.8, and Table 10.13).
- Chemotherapy-induced peripheral neuropathy (CIPN) (Table 10.9 and Table 10.10).
- Miscellaneous (Table 10.11, Table 10.12, and Table 10.13). Commentary on the studies overall.

These illustrate a wide range of approaches to standardisation of treatment protocols, ranging from fixed or standardised approaches that do not vary in their point selection to semi-individualised and highly individualised approaches. Benefits of standardised protocols versus individualised are also explored. Of special interest is 'manualisation', discussed separately later in the chapter.

The Mao studies[51,52] also seek to address pain as part of a symptom cluster, and include options to address general aching, anxiety, depression, fatigue, and sleep.

Overall, outcomes are positive and promising, although there is very little long-term follow-up. There are some other points of interest:

Modalities: A wide range of acupuncture modalities is used. Electro-acupuncture is popular, as are forms of auriculotherapy (including indwelling 'implants'). Moxibustion is not used in these studies.

Dose: Numbers of needles or points used varies greatly, ranging from Molassiotis's care to observe an 'equal dose' of four points bilaterally for all participants, to Pfister's range of a minimum of eight points to a maximum of 26 points (39 needles) per treatment.

Number of treatments given varies from 2 to 18, although over half of the studies settle for 10–12 treatments. Frequency of treatment is mostly once or twice a week; the range is Schroeder's once a month (supplemented with ear implants) to Jeong's more intensive three treatments a week.

Adverse events: Reporting of adverse events is quite good in these studies. Treatments overall were well tolerated with mostly mild adverse events that were easily resolved. Participants in Mao's study for musculoskeletal pain found battlefield acupuncture sufficiently painful to cause them to withdraw from the study.

Lymphoedema: Jeong and Molassiotis are the only studies to avoid needling a limb at risk of or affected by lymphoedema. In their arthralgia studies, Mao and Oh both report needling the at-risk or affected limb with no associated adverse events.

However, neither study reports assessing impact on lymphoedema as an outcome, and due to the small numbers of participants (67 and 32 respectively), it cannot be assumed that there is no risk associated with needling the affected arm.

Table 10.7: Five RCTs using acupuncture to manage aromatase inhibitor (AI)-related arthralgia: Acupuncture points used

Author (Publication date)	Crew et al.[37] (2010)	Bao et al.[38] (2013)	Oh et al.[39] (2013)		Mao et al.[40] (2014)	Hershman et al.[41] (2015)
Protocol	Semi-individualised	Fixed	Fixed		Manualised	Semi-individualised
Points used	Ear acupuncture (Unilateral, alternate ears at each treatment) Shenmen Sympathetic Kidney Liver Upper Lung **Standardised** LI-4 ST-41 KID-3 TB-5 GB-34 GB-41 *Individualised (up to 3 of the most painful areas)* **Knee** ST-34 SP-9 SP-10 **Fingers** LI-3 SI-3 SI-5 **Lumbar** BL-23 DU-3 DU-8 **Shoulder** LI-15 SI-10 TB-14 **Hip** GB-30 GB-39 **Wrist** LI-5 TB-4	Bilateral: LI-4 ST-36 BL-65 KID-3 P-6 GB-34 REN-4 REN-6 REN-12	*Day 1* Bilateral: LI-4 (U) LI-11(U) ST-40 (L) GB-34(L) On both days: LIV-3 (L) DU-20 M-HN-1 *Shishencong* M-UE-22 *Baxie* **Electrical stimulation** Negative pole: LI-4 TB-5 Positive pole: LI-11 GB-21 Pulse width 0.5–0.7ms at alternating frequencies of 2–10 Hz to maximum comfortable intensity for 20 minutes.	*Day 2* Bilateral: ST-36(L) SP-6 (L) TB-5 (U) GB-21(U)	See 'Manualisation' below	As per Crew et al. (2010) – see previous column. Also described in detail in Greenlee et al. (2015).[42]

Table 10.8: Five RCTs using acupuncture to manage aromatase inhibitor (AI)-related arthralgia: Summary of study design and outcomes

Author (Publication date)	Crew et al.[37] (2010)	Bao et al.[38] (2013)	Oh et al.[39] (2013)	Mao et al.[40] (2014)	Hershman et al.[41] (2015)
Country	USA	USA	Australia	USA	USA
Study design	RCT based on prior pilot study[43]	RCT	RCT	RCT based on prior feasibility study[44]	RCT
Tumour type	Breast	Breast	Breast	Breast	Breast
Cancer treatment stage	Postmenopausal women with Stage I–III cancer receiving AI therapy ≥ 3 months	Postmenopausal women with Stage 0–III cancer receiving AI therapy ≥ 1 month	Postmenopausal women with Stage I–IIIa cancer receiving AI therapy ≥ 6 months	Women with history of Stage I–III cancer experiencing joint pain attributed to AI therapy for ≥ 3 months	Pre- or post-menopausal women with Stage I–III breast cancer receiving AI* therapy for ≥ 30 days
Participants	51	51	32	67	226
Comparison (Comparison/Acu)	Sham acu (18/20)	Sham acu (24/23)	Sham acu vs electroacu (15/14)	Sham vs waitlist vs acu (22/23/22)	Sham vs waitlist vs acu (59/57/110)
Treatment frequency/duration	2x/week for 6 weeks (12 total)	1x/week for 8 weeks (8 total)	2x/week for 6 weeks (12 total)	2x/week for 2 weeks, then 1/week for 6 weeks (10 total)	2x/week for 6 weeks, then 1/week for 6 weeks (18 total)
Follow-up after end of tx (EOT)	None	4 weeks after EOT (12 weeks)	6 weeks after EOT (12 weeks)	4 weeks after EOT (12 weeks)	At intervals up to 52 weeks from baseline
Rationale	TCM and NADA	Clinical experience	Previous studies	TCM theory that regards joint pain as part of Bi Syndrome	Expert acupuncturists plus previous studies
Protocol	Semi-individualised	Fixed	Fixed	Manualised	Semi-individualised
Points used	See Table 10.7				

Adverse events	3 participants found acupuncture moderately painful (including 1 in the sham group). No other adverse events were reported.	No significant side effects were observed.	'No certain side effects'. Authors suggest needling in area at risk or affected by lymphoedema 'is safe when acu is performed by a qualified acupuncturist'.	18 acu-related adverse events reported by 8 participants; all mild and spontaneously resolved; 6 related to deqi sensation. Pain similarly reported in electroacu (n=5) and sham (n=4) groups.	Grade 1 bruising, the most common adverse event, experienced by participants in the acu group (47%) and the sham group (25%). In both groups: 1 episode each of grade 2 presyncope.
Summary of results	At EOT, true acu group showed significant improvement in joint pain, stiffness, functional ability, and physical wellbeing. No significant benefits observed in sham group.	Sham and true acu groups showed significant improvement in AI-associated musculoskeletal symptoms. No significant difference between groups at EOT. 12-week follow-up, true acu group symptoms less severe blood tests: significant reduction of IL-17 (p≤.009) in both groups; no modulation observed in estradiol, ß-endorphin, or other proinflammatory cytokine concentrations in either group.	No significant differences between sham and real acupuncture observed. 'Positive trends in stiffness and physical function at week 12 in favour of EA.' The authors hypothesise that individualisation may have improved outcomes.	Compared with waitlist controls, electroacu produced significant and clinically important reductions in pain severity (p=.0004), pain-related interference (p=.0006), and functional outcomes in upper and lower extremities. These were observed at EOT persisting to week 12 follow-up. No adverse events were associated with needling in an arm at risk of or affected by lymphoedema.	Significant reduction in joint pain reported for true acu group at 6 weeks compared with sham and waitlist controls, although clinical importance uncertain. Addition of maintenance acu (1x/week for 6 weeks) showed significant improvement at 12 weeks in average pain, worst pain, pain interference, pain severity, or worst stiffness for true acu compared with waitlist, and only with average pain compared with sham.

Table 10.9: Four studies using acupuncture to manage chemotherapy-induced peripheral neuropathy (CIPN): Acupuncture points used

Author (Publication date)	Schroeder et al. (2011)[45]	Jeong et al. (2018)[46]	Molassiotis et al. (2019)[47]	Bao et al. (2021)[48]
Protocol	Standardised	Standardised	Semi-individualised	Semi-individualised
Points used	**Bilateral:** ST-34 EX-LE-12 *Qiduan** x 5 EX-LE-8 *Bafeng* x 4 (20 needles per session)	**Upper extremity:** Bilateral** LI-4 LI-11 M-UE-9 *Baxie* x 4 **Lower extremity:** Bilateral ST-36 LIV-3 M-LE-8 *Bafeng* x 4 (18 points in total) The extremity on the side affected by cancer was not needled to avoid risk of infection or exacerbating lymphoedema.	**If upper limbs involved:** LI-4 LI-11 And 1 of the following: P-7 TB-5 Ex-UE-9 *Baxie* **If lower limbs involved:** ST-36 SP-6 And 1 of the following: ST-41 LIV-3 Ex-LE-10 *Bafeng* *For participants with low pain threshold, only:* TB-5 (upper limb) ST-41 (lower limb) Flexibility of point selection was allowed to avoid limb at risk of lymphoedema. An equal 'dose' of points was used for all patients (4 points bilaterally).	**Bilateral ear points:** *Shenmen* Point Zero Plus one additional auricular point where an electrodermal signal is detected **Plus** Bilateral body points: LI-4 ST-40 SI-3 P-6 GB-42 LIV-3 *Bafeng* 2 *Bafeng* 3 Electrostimulation (bilateral) 2–5Hz 20 mins from LIV-3 (-) to GB-42 (+). Needling to elicit deqi at LI-4, ST-40, and SI-3. Acupuncturists have the option of not inserting needles in extremities that have no symptoms.

*EX-LE-12 *Qiduan* – located at the tip of each toe.

Table 10.10: Four studies using acupuncture to manage chemotherapy-induced peripheral neuropathy (CIPN): Summary of study design and outcomes

Author (Publication date)	Schroeder et al. (2011)[45]	Jeong et al. (2018)[46]	Molassiotis et al. (2019)[47]	Bao et al. (2021)[8]
Country	Portugal	Korea	Hong Kong	USA
Study design	Controlled 'pilot study'	Single arm pilot	RCT	RCT
Tumour type	Various, including breast, colon, bronchial, lymphoma, pleural mesothelioma	Breast	Various, including breast, gynaecological, colorectal, or head and neck cancer, and multiple myeloma	Breast, colorectal
Cancer treatment stage	Post chemotherapy	Post chemotherapy	During or post chemotherapy (90% participants were post chemotherapy)	≥ 3 months since completion of neurotoxic chemotherapy
Chemotherapy	Various	Anthracycline followed by taxane-based regimen	Various	Various
Extremities	Lower	Upper and lower	Upper and lower	Upper and lower
Participants	11	10	87	75
Comparison (Comparison/Acu)	Best medical care (5/6)	N/A	Standard care (43/44)	Sham vs usual care vs acu (23/21/24)
Treatment frequency/duration	1x/week for 10 weeks (10 total)	3x/week for 4 weeks (12 total)	2x/week for 8 weeks (16 total)	2x/week for 2 weeks then weekly for 6 weeks (10 total)
Follow-up after end of tx (EOT)	3 months after EOT	4 weeks after EOT	6 and 12 weeks after EOT	4 weeks after EOT
Rationale	TCM	Traditional Korean Medicine (TKM)	TCM diagnosis 'blood and qi stagnation and accumulation of dampness'	Clinical experience and prior research
Protocol	Standardised	Standardised	Semi-individualised	Semi-individualised

cont.

Author (Publication date)	Schroeder et al. (2011)[45]	Jeong et al. (2018)[46]	Molassiotis et al. (2019)[47]	Bao et al. (2021)[48]
Points used	See Table 10.9			
Adverse events	Not reported in the paper.	No serious adverse events were reported.	No adverse events were reported after checking therapists' records.	'Adverse events were few and mild.'
Summary of results	Mean time since end of chemotherapy tx was just over 10.5 months for both groups (range 1–21 months). Primary outcome: nerve conduction studies (NCS) of the sural nerve. Five participants in acu group showed improvement in NCS; in control group, 1 improved, 3 stayed the same, 1 worsened. Authors speculate that acupuncture increases blood flow in the limbs, potentially contributing to nerve repair.	Primary outcome = severity of CIPN, assessed by the Neuropathic Pain Symptom Inventory (NPSI) and NCS showed significant improvement at EOT (p=.003), persisting for 4 weeks after EOT. Secondary measure = quality of life, assessed using the SF-36, showed significant improvements in several domains.	Authors' summary: 'Significant changes at 8 weeks were detected in relation to primary outcome (pain), the clinical neurological assessment, quality of life domains, and symptom distress (all p<.05). Improvements in pain interference, neurotoxicity-related symptoms, and functional aspects of quality of life were sustained in the 14-week assessment (p<.05), as were physical and functional wellbeing at the 20-week assessment (p<.05).' Conclusion: acu effective for treating CIPN and improving quality of life, with 'longer term effects evident'.	Significant improvement in CIPN symptoms, especially: CIPN pain compared with UC at 8 weeks. Numeric Rating Scale (NRS) measured pain compared with sham at 12 weeks.

Table 10.11: Three RCTs using acupuncture to manage miscellaneous CPCTP syndromes: Acupuncture points used

Author (Publication date)	Alimi et al.[49] (2003)	Pfister et al.[50] (2010)	Mao et al.[51] (2021)
Protocol	Individualised	Semi-individualised	EA = individualised according to manual AA = standardised
Points used	For auricular acupuncture: Individualised ear points, identified using electrical detection of the electrodermal activity of ear reflex points.[52] Sterile steel implants were inserted in an average of 7 auricular points (range 5–18). Patients recorded when needles fell out and reported this at a return visit one month after treatment.	**Standardised** Bilateral: Ear point *Shenmen* LI-4 *Hegu* SP-6 *Sanyinjiao* DU-20 *Baihui* M-UE-24 *Luozhen* **Individualised** 'Zone distal points (front, middle, and back) chosen according to the primary zone(s) of pain; local ashi tender points with the greatest sensitivity to palpation pressure.' Plus: LI-2 *Erjian* for patients with dry mouth (bilateral) 'The total number of acupoints (needles) used ranged from a minimum of eight points (14 needles) to a maximum of 26 points (39 needles).'	For points, see 'Manualisation' below **Methods for each group:** *Auricular acupuncture (AA)* Specialised (ASP) needle placed in *cingulate gyrus* earpoint in one ear. Patient asked to walk for 1 minute, then rate severity. If severity > 1/10, *cingulate gyrus* needled in the other ear. Process repeated for the following earpoints: *thalamus* *omega 2* *point zero* *Shenmen* Acupuncturists stopped placing needles if: 1) pain severity decreased to 0 or 1 out of 10; 2) patient declined further needling; 3) vasovagal response was observed. Up to 10 needles inserted, remained in situ 3–4 days. Patients trained to remove them safely. *Electro-acupuncture (EA)* METHOD: Choice of: ≥ 4 local points around body area patient finds most painful (4 points connected to TENS unit at 2 Hz, increase to appropriate level, set for 30 minutes). **Plus** ≥ 4 distal points to address general constitutional symptoms. Total number of points 10–20.

Table 10.12: Three RCTs using acupuncture to manage miscellaneous CPCTP syndromes: Summary of study design and outcomes

Author (Publication date)	Alimi et al.[49] (2003)	Pfister et al.[50] (2010)	Mao et al.[51] (2021)
Country	France	USA	USA
Study design	RCT	RCT	RCT
Pain syndrome	Chronic peripheral or central neuropathic pain	Chronic pain or dysfunction	Musculoskeletal pain
Tumour type	Various, including breast, head and neck, lung, and others	Head and neck	Various, including breast, prostate, lymphoma, and others
Cancer treatment stage	After treatment of cancer	≥ 3 months post surgery and radiotherapy	Prior cancer diagnosis and no current evidence of disease
Participants	90	58	360
Comparison (Comparison/Acu)	Placebo auricular acu vs placebo auricular seed vs auricular acupuncture (30/31/29)	Usual care vs acupuncture (30/28)	Usual care (UC) vs auricular acupuncture (AA) vs electro-acupuncture (EA) (72/143/145)
Treatment frequency/duration	2 treatments, 1 month apart (2 total)	1x/week for 4 weeks (4 total) Plus additional 5th treatment post assessment	1x/week for 10 weeks (10 total)
Follow-up after end of tx (EOT)	1 month	2 weeks after EOT (day 42)	2, 6, and 14 weeks after EOT (weeks 13, 16, and 24)
Rationale	Auricular acupuncture using electrodermal response at ear points	TCM	EA based on classical acupuncture textbooks and consultation with experts in China and USA AA = 'battlefield acupuncture'
Protocol	Individualised	Semi-individualised	EA = individualised according to manual (see 'Manualisation' below) AA = standardised

Points used	See Table 10.11
Adverse events	No infection at treated ear points reported by patients or recorded by clinicians. No other adverse events reported.	No serious adverse events attributed to acupuncture. 27 minor adverse events recorded, mainly temporarily increased pain, minor bruising or bleeding, and 'constitutional symptoms'.	Adverse events mild to moderate in both groups. EA group: bruising reported by 10.4% of participants. AA group: ear pain reported by 18.9% of participants. EA group: 1 participant (0.7%) discontinued treatment due to an adverse event, compared with 15 (10.5%) in AA group.
Summary of results	'The main outcome was pain assessed at 2 months...pain intensity decreased by 36% at 2 months from baseline...'	'Significant reductions in pain, dysfunction ...were observed. ...data support the potential role of acupuncture in addressing post-neck dissection pain and dysfunction.'	Compared with UC, EA reduced pain severity by 1.9 (p<.001) and 1.6 (p<.001) points at 12 weeks. No significant difference in pain reduction between EA and AA. In AA, 1/10 participants unable to tolerate the intervention and dropped out. Overall, acu produced benefit over UC, including reduced pain severity, analgesic use, and improvements in physical function and quality of life.

Manualisation

Manualisation involves designing treatment protocols to satisfy the research requirement for standardisation and replicability (the ability to repeat or replicate the study), while allowing flexibility to tailor the intervention to the individual participant.[53] This approach is especially appropriate when addressing pain, given the variety of locations in which pain manifests. It also allows the acupuncturist to use their clinical judgement within a research context.

Mao *et al.*'s studies demonstrate a sophisticated approach to manualisation in studies for arthralgia[39] and musculoskeletal pain.[40,51] Design details and outcomes for these studies are summarised above (Table 10.8 and Table 10.12); points in the manualisation are summarised below (Table 10.13).

Table 10.13: Points used in manualisation of two RCTs by Mao *et al.*

Note:

As the athralgia and the musculoskeletal (MSK) pain studies share many points, I have presented them in the same table. Columns headed 'MSK' list points used in the musculoskeletal pain study that are additional to those listed in the arthralgia study.

*MN-LE-16 *Xiyan* is the only point used in the arthralgia study (for knee pain) not also used in the MSK study.

Upper extremity		Lower extremity		General	
Arthralgia	*MSK*	*Arthralgia*	*MSK*	*Arthralgia*	*MSK*
Shoulder:	**Shoulder:**	**Hip:**	**Hip:**	**Aching:**	**Aching:**
LI-15	SI-3	BL-37	GB-40	SP-9	Four Gates:
SI-9	**Hand/finger:**	GB-30	Foot/toe:	SP-21	LI-4 and LIV-3
SI-10	LI-4	GB-39	LIV-3	SI-3	**Anxiety:**
TB-14	**Neck pain:**	**Knee:**	**Low back**	BL-17	M-HN-3
Scapula:	GB-20	ST-34	**pain:**	BL-62	Yintang
SI-11	GB-21	ST-35	BL-23	**Anxiety:**	**Fatigue:**
SI-12	DU-14	SP-9	BL-25	P-6	REN-6
SI-14	M-BW-35	GB-34	BL-40	LIV-3	**Sleep:**
BL-43	Huatuojiaji	GB-35	BL-57	**Fatigue:**	HE-7
Elbow:	M-UE-24	MN-LE-16	BL-60	ST-36	N-HN-54
LU-5	Luozhen	Xiyan*	M-BW-35	SP-6	Anmian
LI-4		**Leg:**	Huatuojiaji		**Depression:**
LI-11		BL-57			BL-18
TB-5		BL-58			LIV-3
TB-10		**Ankle:**			DU-20
Hand/finger:		ST-41			
LI-3		SP-5			
SI-3		BL-60			
M-UE-22		KID-3			
Baxie		GB-40			
		Foot/toe:			
		SP-4			
		BL-65			
		M-LE-8			
		Bafeng			

The evidence base for using moxibustion for pain management

Studies investigating using moxibustion to manage cancer treatment-related pain focus on survivors undergoing active treatment for advanced, late-stage cancer. There appear to be no studies focusing on CPCTP.

Clinical perspectives

Developing a toolkit for CPCTP

Drawing on the multiple functions of points to address the pain symptom cluster

Acupuncture can be a safe, effective intervention for addressing CPCTP. It can simultaneously address physical pain and encompass other symptoms in the pain cluster, often by drawing on the multiple functions of points. For example, PC-6 *Neiguan* is indicated for pain of the arm, elbow, head, and neck and also to calm the shen and address insomnia.[54]

In addition to using local and distal points to address pain, I like to use a 'general analgesic', such as Four Gates (LI-4 *Hegu* and LIV-3 *Taichong*). This relieves pain, harmonises qi, calms the shen, and relieves anxiety. See the cases studies of Bob (below) and Rosa (see Chapters 4 and 5).

Treating multiple types of pain in the same session

Drawing on the multiple functions of points is also helpful when survivors present with multiple types of pain, including comorbidities. These can often be addressed in the same session, without needing to use large numbers of needles. Again, Four Gates is useful.

Five Element approaches

Five Element acupuncture can be very good for addressing pain; I find clearing blocks especially beneficial. With its focus on treating the CF and addressing the levels of body, mind, and spirit, Five Element acupuncture has the potential to encompass many aspects of the pain symptom cluster, including emotional and spiritual aspects of pain.

Moxibustion and heat

I use moxibustion and heat lamps extensively when working with survivors with CPCTP. As always, the points and procedures vary according to many factors, including the Chinese medicine diagnosis, the patient's preferences, and the working environment (ability to use moxa, access to heat lamps and heat pads).

Commonly used to warm channels and painful areas, moxa can also address the emotional and spiritual components of pain (see 'Treating the spirit' in Chapter 5, Toolkit).

Using the extraordinary vessels

The extraordinary vessels are also useful in pain management. The Yang Linking Vessel is invaluable for addressing pain experienced by head and neck cancer survivors, as illustrated in JR's case study in Chapter 5, Toolkit.

Using microsystems

Microsystems such as ear acupuncture and the NADA protocol can be used independently or combined with body acupuncture. Ear seeds can give the patient a sense of control, and can be placed to target areas of pain or address other symptoms in the pain cluster.

Other systems

Many styles of acupuncture promote themselves as pain management systems and can be included in a practitioner's toolkit.

Lifestyle advice

Acupuncturists can play a vital role in helping cancer survivors to understand and manage pain.

ESSENTIALS

Prevention is key to pain management.

Patients may require less pain medication if pain is prevented. Sometimes, patients put off taking analgesics until they are in pain again. This leads to inconsistent and incomplete pain relief, and higher doses may be needed once a person is in pain.

Patients should understand this, and the importance of taking pain medication:

- at the first signs of pain
- before preparing to do an activity that causes discomfort.

If patients understand this, they may choose to take a smaller dose at onset or in anticipation of pain.

Keeping a pain diary can help to identify triggers and what helps the pain. They also enable the person to be in more in control. An example pain diary can be found at Macmillan Cancer Support's website.[*]

Cancer organisations may issue information booklets on managing pain that are useful to patients and their practitioners.

Sometimes, survivors are reluctant to seek medical advice for their pain, often because they don't wish to burden busy healthcare professionals. Acupuncturists can encourage them to seek appropriate medical advice for pain and pain management, as well as to ensure there is no recurrence or new cancer.

Evidence for the effectiveness of physical activity for reducing pain is inconclusive. Chinese medicine theory is that physical activity relieves stagnation of qi and Blood; these syndromes are at the root of pain syndromes. Acupuncturists should encourage physical activity as appropriate to the individual's capacity and preferences (see Chapter 13, Reducing Risk of Recurrence and Subsequent Primary Cancers).

---

[*]   www.macmillan.org.uk/dfsmedia/1a6f23537f7f4519bb0cf14c45b2a629/1506-10061

ESSENTIALS

Pain is complex and can be difficult to treat. Acupuncturists should feel comfortable with being part of a multidisciplinary approach to pain management and feel able to refer patients to other health professionals.

Patient perspectives

CASE STUDY: BOB AND CHRONIC CANCER PAIN

Bob's case illustrates the challenges of managing pain in cancer survivors with chronic and complex issues. For other discussions of pain management, see the studies of:

- Rosa in Chapter 4, Offering Complex Patients a Simple Piece of Heaven, which presents cancer treatment-related consequences, the problems of ageing, and post-surgical pain syndrome for non-cancer-related comorbidities.
- JR in Chapter 5, Toolkit, which presents another view of CPCTP in a head and neck cancer survivor.
- Ann in Chapter 14, Getting My Life Back, which chronicles both chronic pain from breast cancer treatment-related lymphoedema and acute non-cancer-related pain.

Introduction

Bob was a head and neck cancer survivor, whose lymphoedema specialist nurse referred him to the study of using acupuncture to improve wellbeing and quality of life for people with lymphoedema (see Chapter 9, Cancer Treatment-Related Lymphoedema). As a study participant, he consented to the use of his anonymised data in written reports.

Background

Bob, aged 56, was diagnosed three years previously with squamous cell carcinoma of the left floor of the mouth with spread to the local lymph nodes (T2N2M0). Surgical interventions included removal of the primary tumour and lymph nodes in the neck, with reconstructive surgery using tissue from the left forearm (a 'flap').

Bone death (osteoradionecrosis, see 'Head and neck cancers', earlier in this chapter) was a consequence of post-operative radiotherapy to the left neck and mandible. For Bob, the resulting discomfort was sufficient to warrant further surgery; his jaw was removed and replaced with one fashioned from bone taken from his fibula (called a 'bone flap'). Lymphoedema developed and was managed by the lymphoedema specialist clinic. A year after this surgery, Bob still experienced pain of the jaw and neck, with tightness and restricted movement of the shoulder. The lymphoedema nurse referred him for acupuncture.

Selected case history details

Chronic cancer pain

Pain management was a key issue for Bob, who was working with his palliative care consultant to reduce medications. For two and a half years, he had been taking:

- co-codamol (two to three three times a day)
- diclofenac (50mg)
- pregabalin (150mg)
- fentanyl patches (100mcg/hour)
- oramorph (40ml/day).

Lansoprazole was prescribed to protect his stomach lining, and Bob occasionally took laxatives.

Movement and pressure triggered 'stabbing' pain in Bob's neck, radiating to his shoulder, trapezius, and scapula. This was 'like an electrical shooting pain from the neck down' and had been constant since the first surgery three years previously. When tired, Bob's leg ached along the fibula where tissue for the bone flap had been removed.

Associated and other painful conditions
An infection from recent dental work caused mouth pain, and was controlled with antibiotics and mouthwash.

Questioning the systems
Sleep: Broken. Going to bed at midnight, would sleep for one to two hours, then wake for an hour, until 8 or 9am. Stayed in bed on a 'bad day'; these happened regularly every two weeks, although recently this reduced to once in three weeks. On 'bad days', which lasted up to three days, Bob felt unwell and had no energy – 'can't even move across the room'. There were no identifiable triggers.

Appetite: Poor; Bob forced himself to eat. Aiming to eat three meals a day, he usually managed two meals plus a snack. He had lost 2 stone (28lb or 12.7kg).

Drink: Drank two litres of water a day; consumed one to two pints of beer, but not every day. Salivary glands on the left were damaged by surgery; remaining glands produced either excess or insufficient saliva. However, dry mouth was not a problem.

Bowels: Constipation, a side effect of medications, was remedied with laxatives.

Urination: None.

Temperature: More sensitive to cold than he had been formerly; hands and feet especially cold.

Headaches: 'Blinders', one to two per week, with pain all over his head. Managed with pain medication.

Health history: Surgery in childhood for depression of the sternum, a congenital condition. Emphysema as an adult. Smoking history: 30–40 cigarettes/day for over 40 years; now smoked fewer than ten per day and wanted to stop.

Physical examination: Tongue: Dry, peeled, red, with purple distended sublingual veins. **Pulses:** Left side almost impalpable; I wondered if this was because of the scarring from the tissue removal for the flap; right side strong, almost even, with the middle position slightly stronger.

Diagnosis: I found it difficult to settle on a diagnosis, either CM or CF. While he was pleasant and charming, it was as if a wall of glass surrounded Bob. It seemed difficult to contact the 'man inside'. This odd sensation may have been due to the opioids. Seven Dragons are indicated when it is not possible to 'reach' the person, and although our encounters were pleasant, I felt unable to 'reach' Bob. The history of traumatic events (cancer diagnosis and treatments), repeated surgeries, and intensive medication also supported using Dragons.

Treatment approach

Bob's priorities for treatment were to:

- relieve the pain in his neck and shoulder
- relieve the pain in his foot and leg.

DIY was an activity he wanted to have the energy to do.

Bob's complex health conditions posed considerable challenges for treatment planning. He had a history of poor attendance at appointments; the thick file of hospital notes contained numerous letters documenting non-attendance for appointments. It required considerable flexibility on my part to keep him on a reasonably regular schedule of treatments. Even so, he would forget appointments, cancel at short notice, or arrive extremely late. Despite this, we managed nine treatments over 12 weeks. See Chapter 5, Toolkit, for details of the approaches used.

Bob's initial treatments

Table 10.14: Bob's treatments 1–4

Abbreviation: Tx treatment

Tx	Treatment principles	Points	Notes
1	Clear block to treatment: Aggressive Energy (AE) Drain[1]	BL-13 *Feishu* BL-14 *Jueyinshu* BL-15 *Xinshu* BL-18 *Ganshu* BL-20 *Pishu* BL-23 *Shenshu* Plus 3 check needles	Bilateral superficial needling.

cont.

Tx	Treatment principles	Points	Notes
2	Clear block to treatment: Internal Dragons (IDs)[2]	Master point 0.25 cun below REN-15 Jiuwei ST-25 Tianshu ST-32 Futu ST-41 Jiexi	All points bilateral except Master point.
3, 4	Clear block to treatment: External Dragons (EDs)[2]	DU-20 Baihui BL-11 Dazhu BL-23 Shenshu BL-61 Pucan	All points bilateral except DU-20.
	Support spirit (using yuan source points of fire)[3]	SI-4 Wangu HE-7 Shenmen	Bilateral, no retention.

Tx 1: As per the study protocol, the first treatment was an AE Drain. No erythema appeared, nor could I detect a pulse change. Nevertheless, at the next session, Bob said he felt 'buoyant' afterwards, and this lasted a 'couple of hours'. He also enjoyed a night of 'uninterrupted' sleep after treatment, which was unusual for him. There was no discernible change to the pain.

Tx 2: As discussed above, Seven Dragons was indicated; however, administering Internal Dragons (IDs) posed challenges. Intensive scarring on Bob's torso made needling REN-15 master difficult, so I needled as near to the point as the scarring allowed. During the treatment, Bob reported feeling sensations of warmth in his feet, particularly on the left. I also discerned pulse changes on the left.

Tx 3: Bob said he felt good after the IDs the previous week, but experienced stomach pains for an hour afterward. He was uncertain whether this caused by treatment or indigestion. Again, he slept well on the night of treatment, although overall his sleep pattern was unchanged. Bob felt he got more from the first treatment (AE Drain).

Life was challenging for Bob. As well as feeling run down, 'every phone call' seemed to be bad news. He attended a funeral the previous week; this week, a relative died in an accident.

At this session, I administered External Dragons (EDs), with Bob lying prone on the couch. This was very uncomfortable for Bob, who moved around considerably after needle insertion, trying to get comfortable. Eventually, I positioned him on his side, and he managed to relax.

Tx 4: Despite the challenges of the previous session, Bob reported positive results. He did not need medication after the session and was able to forgo dosage twice that afternoon and evening. Sleep was 'a lot better', he found it easier to get up in the morning, and his energy was improving. Doing DIY on his house was a treatment objective, and he was now finding this easier.

Because of the challenges of administering EDs at treatment 3, I chose to repeat this, hoping to further improve the outcome. Positioned on a chair, Bob leaned forward, using the treatment couch for support. This was more comfortable, and I administered EDs without incident.

Bob's subsequent treatments

Table 10.15: Bob's treatments 5–9

Abbreviation: Tx treatment

Tx	Treatment principles	Points	Notes
5	Address pain (generally)	Four Gates: Ll-4 *Hegu* and LIV-3 *Taichong*	All points bilateral with retention.
	Address pain in mouth	ST-44 *Neiting*	
6	Address pain generally and in mouth	As per Tx 5	
	Address shoulder pain	Sl-11 *Tianzong* Ahshi points on left shoulder blade	Left side only.
7	Harmonise Liver qi to: relieve muscle cramp improve mood	BL-18 *Ganshu* BL-47 *Hunmen* GB-34 *Yanglingquan* DU-3 *Yaoyangguan*	All points bilateral except DU-3.
8	Address muscle cramps and pain	Four Gates: Ll-4 *Hegu* and LIV-3 *Taichong*	All points bilateral.
		BL-17 *Geshu* BL-43 *Gaohuangshu*	
9	Relieve stress	Four Gates: Ll-4 *Hegu* and LIV-3 *Taichong*	All points bilateral.
	Address pain of shoulder, neck, back	Stick moxa over affected area on left side	

Tx 5: Bob cancelled the next appointment as he was feeling unwell. When I saw him two weeks later, he said nausea had started on his return home after treatment 4. He felt better after resting for a couple of hours.

Nevertheless, sleep continued to improve, and his recovery from his 'bad days' took one day, instead of the usual two to three days. He was back on the usual schedule of painkillers – his mouth was very sore and dental surgery was scheduled for the next week.

At this treatment, I administered Four Gates as pain relief, adding ST-44 to relieve mouth pain. Bob felt the effects immediately, saying he could 'feel energy buzz through his system'. At the end of the session, he felt very relaxed and said the pain had reduced.

Tx 6: Bob reported that Four Gates had alleviated his mouth pain and improved shoulder pain as well. Sleep was 'really excellent'. This was a relief, as he had not slept well for 'a couple of years', and this had been getting worse. Dental surgery two days before was painful and only partially successful; more work was scheduled for the next month.

Shoulder pain had flared the day after surgery but had subsided. I repeated Four Gates, adding points to address the shoulder.

Tx 7: We reviewed progress. Bob felt treatment had been 'really beneficial'. After nearly three years of sleeplessness, he was sleeping nights. He had experienced no pain in his neck and shoulder during the previous week.

He was now bothered by spasm and cramp in his leg muscles. He began to talk about his emotions; he was feeling down because of the recent spate of bereavements. He was due to move to the country in a few weeks' time; however, he wished to continue treatment until he relocated.

Tx 8: Bob saw my colleague Rachel Peckham, as I was absent. He arrived half an hour late for his appointment because he felt unwell on waking. His shoulder had been good since the previous treatment, and the muscle cramping had improved.

Tx 9: I saw Bob two weeks later. He had moved house, and the associated stress caused his shoulder pain to flare. I supplemented Four Gates with stick moxa over the affected area. He did not attend for his tenth treatment and did not contact us to arrange further treatment.

Short- and long-term feedback

After his seventh treatment, Bob wrote:

> After having two major operations and numerous minor procedures I have had to take a lot of medication and this treatment has helped me reduce my dosage, which in itself is a major improvement. Also, after having had three years of sleepless nights I am finding I am able to sleep mostly uninterrupted which I find beneficial in all aspects of my day-to-day life. Overall, I feel that my quality of life has *most definitely* improved and that this treatment has helped me immeasurably.

Summary

I admit I was surprised at how well Bob responded, given his intransigent pain and complex presentation. The acupuncture treatments were quite simple and used minimal local points, and yet they improved key aspects of the pain symptom cluster (pain and sleep). This was despite Bob's erratic appointment keeping and the ongoing traumas of his dental work and bereavement.

CHAPTER SUMMARY

- Pain is an issue for many cancer survivors post treatment and may emerge or continue months or years after treatment.
- It is vital to observe the red flags for pain and refer patients for investigation.
- CPCTP is a complex, multifactorial condition that is challenging to manage and treat. It requires multiple concurrent interventions and multidisciplinary care.
- It should be viewed as part of a symptom cluster that includes anxiety, depression, and insomnia.
- Acupuncture may alleviate and sometimes eliminate pain and contribute to improved function. It may also simultaneously address other symptoms in the symptom cluster.
- Acupuncture is a valuable addition to the repertoire of interventions to treat pain, especially as it may reduce or eliminate the need for pharmacological interventions, thus minimising or preventing side effects and potential addiction issues.

References

1. Glare P, Aubrey K, Gulati A, *et al.* Pharmacologic management of persistent pain in cancer survivors. Drugs 2022;82(3):275-291.
2. de Valois B, Peckham R Treating the person and not the disease: acupuncture in the management of cancer treatment-related lymphoedema. Eur. J. Orient. Med. 2011;6(6):37-49.
3. Aaronson NK, Mattioli V, Minton O, *et al.* Beyond treatment: psychosocial and behavioural issues in cancer survivorship research and practice. Eur. J. Cancer Supplement 2014;12(1):54-64.
4. Chang V, Sekine R Pain. In: Feuerstein M, editor. Handbook of cancer surviorship. New York: Springer; 2007. pp. 151-172.
5. Levy MH, Chwisteck M, Mehta RS Management of chronic pain in cancer survivors. Cancer J. 2008;14(6):401-409.
6. Burton AW, Fanciullo GJ, Beasley R, *et al.* Chronic pain in the cancer survivor: a new frontier. Pain Medicine 2007;8(2):189-198.
7. Bennett MI, Kaasa S, Barke A, *et al.* The IASP classification of chronic pain for ICD-11: chronic cancer-related pain. Pain 2019;160(1):38-44.
8. Polomano R, Ashburn M, Farrar J Pain syndromes in cancer survivors. In: Bruera E, editor. Cancer pain: assessment and management. New York: Cambridge University Press; 2010. pp. 145-162.
9. Mao J, Armstrong K, Bowman M, *et al.* Symptom burden among cancer survivors: impact of age and comorbidity. J. A. Board Fam. Med. 2007;20(5):434-443.
10. International Association for the Study of Pain Terminology. 2021. Available from: www.iasp-pain.org/resources/terminology
11. Fallon M, Giusti R, Aielli F, *et al.* Management of cancer pain in adult patients: ESMO Clinical Practice Guidelines. Ann. Oncol. 2018;29(Suppl. 4):iv166-iv191.
12. Glare P, Davies P, Finaly E, *et al.* Pain in cancer survivors. J. Clin. Oncol. 2014;32(16):1739-1747.
13. Mast ME Survivors of breast cancer: illness uncertainty, positive reappraisal, and emotional distress. Oncol. Nurs. Forum 1998;25(3):555-562.
14. Johansen A, Romundstad L, Nielsen CS, *et al.* Persistent postsurgical pain in a general population: prevalence and predictors in the Tromsø study. Pain 2012;153(7):1390-1396.
15. Brown MRD, Farquhar-Smith P, Magee DJ Pain in the cancer survivor. Cancer Treat. Res. 2021;182:57-84.
16. Wang K, Yee C, Tam S, *et al.* Prevalence of pain in patients with breast cancer post-treatment: A systematic review. Breast 2018;42:113-127.
17. Sheridan D, Foo I, O'Shea H, *et al.* Long-term follow-up of pain and emotional characteristics of women after surgery for breast cancer. J. Pain Symptom Manage. 2012;44(4):608-614.

18. Kubota H, Miyawaki D, Mukumoto N, *et al.* Risk factors for osteoradionecrosis of the jaw in patients with head and neck squamous cell carcinoma. Radiat. Oncol. 2021;16(1):1.

19. Mayland E, Sweeny L A review of advanced head and neck osteoradionecrosis. Plast. Aesthet. Res. 2021;8(62). Available from: http://dx.doi.org/10.20517/2347-9264.2021.38

20. Loprinzi CL, Lacchetti C, Bleeker J, *et al.* Prevention and management of chemotherapy-induced peripheral neuropathy in survivors of adult cancers: ASCO Guideline Update. J. Clin. Oncol. 2020;38(28):3325–3348.

21. Maihöfner C, Diel I, Tesch H, *et al.* Chemotherapy-induced peripheral neuropathy (CIPN): current therapies and topical treatment option with high-concentration capsaicin. Support. Care Cancer 2021;29(8):4223–4238.

22. Pachman D, Barton D, Swetz K, *et al.* Troublesome symptoms in cancer survivors: fatigue, insomnia, neuropathy, and pain. J. Clin. Oncol. 2012;30:3687–3696.

23. Paice JA, Portenoy R, Lacchetti C, *et al.* Management of Chronic Pain in Survivors of Adult Cancers: American Society of Clinical Oncology Clinical Practice Guideline. J. Clin. Oncol. 2016;34(27):3325–3345.

24. Karcioglu O, Topacoglu H, Dikme O, *et al.* A systematic review of the pain scales in adults: which to use? Am. J. Emerg. Med. 2018;36(4):707–714.

25. Faculty of Pain Medicine British Pain Society Outcome measures. London: Faculty of Pain Medicine; 2019. Available from: www.fpm.ac.uk/sites/fpm/files/documents/2019-07/Outcome%20measures%20 2019.pdf

26. WHO Guidelines for the Pharmacological and Radiotherapeutic Management of Cancer Pain in Adults and Adolescents. Geneva: World Health Organization; 2018. 5, Cancer Pain Management – Guiding Principles. Available from: https://www.ncbi.nlm.nih.gov/books/NBK537483

27. Anekar AA, Cascella M. WHO Analgesic Ladder; Updated 15 May 2022. In: StatPearls [Internet]. Treasure Island (FL): StatPearls Publishing; 2022 Jan. Available from: www.ncbi.nlm.nih.gov/books/NBK554435

28. PDQ° Supportive and Palliative Care Editorial Board PDQ Cancer Pain – Health professional version. Bethesda, MD: National Cancer Institute; Updated 18 March 2022. Available from: www.cancer.gov/ about-cancer/treatment/side-effects/pain/pain-hp-pdq

29. PDQ° Supportive and Palliative Care Editorial Board PDQ Spirituality in Cancer Care. Bethesda, MD: National Cancer Institute; 2022. Available from: www.cancer.gov/about-cancer/coping/day-to-day/ faith-and-spirituality/spirituality-hp-pdq

30. Zeidan F, Emerson NM, Farris SR, *et al.* Mindfulness meditation-based pain relief employs different neural mechanisms than placebo and sham mindfulness meditation-induced analgesia. J. Neurosci. 2015;35(46):15307–15325.

31. Mao JJ, Ismaila N, Bao T, *et al.* Integrative Medicine for Pain Management in Oncology: Society for Integrative Oncology-ASCO Guideline. J. Clin. Oncol. 2022;40(34):3998–4024.

32. Li P Management of cancer with Chinese medicine. London: Donica Publishing Ltd; 2003.

33. He Y, Guo X, May BH, *et al.* Clinical evidence for association of acupuncture and acupressure with improved cancer pain: A systematic review and meta-analysis. JAMA Oncol. 2020;6(2):271–278.

34. Chiu HY, Hsieh YJ, Tsai PS Systematic review and meta-analysis of acupuncture to reduce cancer-related pain. Eur. J. Cancer Care (Engl). 2017;26(2).

35. Chien TJ, Liu CY, Fang CJ, *et al.* The efficacy of acupuncture in chemotherapy-induced peripheral neuropathy: systematic review and meta-analysis. Integr. Cancer Ther. 2019;18:1534735419886662.

36. Liu X, Lu J, Wang G, *et al.* Acupuncture for arthralgia induced by aromatase inhibitors in patients with breast cancer: A systematic review and meta-analysis. Integr. Cancer Ther. 2021;20:15347354209808II.

37. Crew K, Capodice JL, Greenlee H, *et al.* Randomized, blinded, sham-controlled trial of acupuncture for the management of aromatase inhibitor-associated joint symptoms in women with early-stage breast cancer. J. Clin. Oncol. 2010;28(7):1154–1160.

38. Bao T, Cai L, Snyder C, *et al.* Patient-reported outcomes in women with breast cancer enrolled in a dual-center, double-blind, randomized controlled trial assessing the effect of acupuncture in reducing aromatase inhibitor-induced musculoskeletal symptoms. Cancer 2014;120(3):381–389.

39. Oh B, Kimble B, Costa DS, *et al.* Acupuncture for treatment of arthralgia secondary to aromatase inhibitor therapy in women with early breast cancer: pilot study. Acupunct. Med. 2013;31(3):264–271.

40. Mao JJ, Xie SX, Farrar JT, *et al.* A randomised trial of electro-acupuncture for arthralgia related to aromatase inhibitor use. Eur. J. Cancer 2014;50(2):267–276.

41. Hershman DL, Unger JM, Greenlee H, *et al.* Effect of acupuncture vs sham acupuncture or waitlist control on joint pain related to aromatase inhibitors among women with early-stage breast cancer: a randomized clinical trial. JAMA 2018;320(2):167–176.

42. Greenlee H, Crew KD, Capodice J, *et al.* Methods to standardize a multicenter acupuncture trial protocol to reduce aromatase inhibitor-related joint symptoms in breast cancer patients. J. Acupunct. Meridian Stud. 2015;8(3):152–158.

———

43. Crew K, Capodice JL, Greenlee H, *et al.* Pilot study of acupuncture for the treatment of joint symptoms related to adjuvant aromatase inhibitor therapy in postmenopausal breast cancer patients. J. Cancer Surviv. 2007;1:283–291.
44. Mao JJ, Bruner DW, Stricker C, *et al.* Feasibility trial of electroacupuncture for aromatase inhibitor—related arthralgia in breast cancer survivors. Integr. Cancer Ther. 2009;8(2):123–129.
45. Schroeder S, Meyer-Hamme G, Epplée S Acupuncture for chemotherapy-induced peripheral neuropathy (CIPN): a pilot study using neurography. Acupunct. Med. 2012;30(1):4–7.
46. Jeong YJ, Kwak MA, Seo JC, *et al.* Acupuncture for the treatment of taxane-induced peripheral neuropathy in breast cancer patients: a pilot trial. Evid. Based. Complement. Alternat. Med. 2018;2018:5367014.
47. Molassiotis A, Suen LKP, Cheng HL, *et al.* A randomized assessor-blinded wait-list-controlled trial to assess the effectiveness of acupuncture in the management of chemotherapy-induced peripheral neuropathy. Integr. Cancer Ther. 2019;18:1534735419836501.
48. Bao T, Patil S, Chen C, *et al.* Effect of acupuncture vs sham procedure on chemotherapy-induced peripheral neuropathy symptoms: a randomized clinical trial. JAMA Netw. Open 2020;3(3):e200681.
49. Alimi D, Rubino C, Pichard-Léandri E, *et al.* Analgesic effect of auricular acupuncture for cancer pain: a randomized, blinded, controlled trial. J. Clin. Oncol. 2003;21(22):4120–4126.
50. Pfister DG, Cassileth BR, Deng GE, *et al.* Acupuncture for pain and dysfunction after neck dissection: results of a randomized controlled trial. J. Clin. Oncol. 2010;28(15):2565–2570.
51. Mao JJ, Liou KT, Baser RE, *et al.* Effectiveness of electroacupuncture or auricular acupuncture vs usual care for chronic musculoskeletal pain among cancer survivors: the PEACE randomized clinical trial. JAMA Oncol. 2021;7(5):720–727.
52. Oleson T Auriculotherapy manual: Chinese and Western systems of ear acupuncture. 3rd ed. Edinburgh: Churchill Livingstone; 2003.
53. Schnyer RN, Allen JJ Bridging the gap in complementary and alternative medicine research: manualization as a means of promoting standardization and flexibility of treatment in clinical trials of acupuncture. J. Altern. Complement. Med. 2002;8(5):623–634.
54. Deadman P, Al-Khafaji M, Baker K A manual of acupuncture. Hove: The Journal of Chinese Medicine; 2007.

Part III

MILESTONES AND BEYOND

Chapter 11

Survivorship: Navigating the Milestones

Introduction

The challenges of life post-cancer treatment are encapsulated in these quotations:

> The aftermath of treatment is often worse than the disease itself. (Dr Natalie Doyle)[1]

> I am really grateful that 'they' seem to have cured the cancer but...there is always a shadow hanging over everything in the future and an 'in case' or 'maybe' is always present. That I should 'regard myself as a woman who has *had* cancer' does not really remove this anxiety. (Emily, a cancer survivor)

Congratulations! Cancer treatment has finished. Life can now get back to normal.

This is the expectation and hope of individuals at the end of primary treatment. Fortunately, many cancer survivors enjoy long-term disease-free survival and good quality of life after treatment. Several studies have reported high or improved quality of life many years post treatment for survivors of a range of tumour types, including breast cancer and non-Hodgkin lymphoma.[2-4] A study of older adult, long-term survivors of breast, prostate, and colorectal cancers concluded that 'most survivors report fairly few continuing symptoms, few functional difficulties, and low levels of distress...[and] do not experience serious psychological problems.'[5]

Experiencing cancer can have many positive impacts. A cancer diagnosis may be a catalyst for personal growth, an opportunity for redefining oneself, for taking stock of what is important and for changing priorities. Survivors may discover a deeper appreciation of life, improved relationships, changes in religious belief and spirituality, along with changed health behaviours (such as improvements in diet and exercise), and improved self-esteem. Post-traumatic growth refers to the process of searching for or discovering the benefits or positive outcomes of experiencing trauma such as cancer and its related life changes.[1,2,6,7]

No less significantly, feeling that nothing has changed, or simply returning to 'life as normal', may also be considered a positive outcome of having cancer.[1]

While many cancer survivors find it possible to return to life as it was before diagnosis, or to find a more profound experience of life, others struggle with the aftermath of diagnosis and treatment. Colorectal cancer survivors, for example, are reported to have high levels of limiting comorbidities up to and beyond five years following cancer surgery, including anxiety and depression.[8,9] The prevalence of depression among these survivors has been found to exceed that in the general population, even five years after surgery.[10]

Thus, it may be an unexpected and cruel blow when life does not return to what it was before the intrusion of the cancer treatment, and research reveals complex and contradictory results.[11] While one third of non-Hodgkin lymphoma survivors reported improved quality of life, nearly 40% of participants in the same study experienced low or worsening quality of life.[4]

A large UK study found that while many cancer survivors report good health, ongoing poor health and disability were reported by 10–20% of those without another chronic condition, and 25–30% of those with a chronic condition in addition to cancer.[12] The study also reported that survivors make greater use of health services to address ongoing health problems, including poor general health, poor physical wellbeing, and pain. Issues are not limited to physical symptoms, and changes may be emotional, social, and financial.

This chapter discusses some of the challenges experienced by survivors as they navigate through the years following primary treatment. It is structured using the milestones of one, five, and ten years post diagnosis used in oncology. These are key points that survivors may be likely to notice, as they are often marked by a step-change in treatment and follow-up.

In this chapter, challenges arising around these milestones are illustrated using extended case studies of survivors who had acupuncture. First, I begin with a discussion of fear of recurrence, a phenomenon common to almost all stages of the survivorship pathway.

Fear of recurrence

TERMINOLOGY

Fear of recurrence (FOR), sometimes referred to in the medical literature as fear of cancer recurrence (FCR), is defined as 'the fear that cancer could return or progress in the same place or in another part of the body'.[13]

One of the most reported problems experienced by cancer survivors, fear of recurrence may occur any time across the cancer trajectory. It may be especially powerful at the end of primary treatment when individuals may be uncertain about treatment outcomes (Figure 11.1), and remains a significant concern even ten years after diagnosis.[13,14]

A survey in England showed that one year post diagnosis, 47% of cancer survivors surveyed feared their cancer would return, and 27% were afraid of dying.[15,16] While these fears reduced over time, they were still comparatively high five years post diagnosis at 42.5% and 22% respectively.

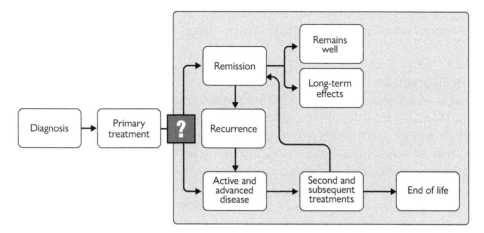

FIGURE II.I: THE SURVIVORSHIP PATHWAY AND FEAR OF RECURRENCE: WHAT NOW?

While fear of recurrence might be expected shortly after diagnosis and treatment, this fear persists and has significant effects for many years.[17] For some, it becomes chronic and remains a lifelong concern.[13] Detrimental to quality of life and psychosocial wellbeing, it is implicated in anxiety and depression experienced by long-term survivors.[14,17] It may increase vigilance (hypervigilance) in monitoring for signs of recurrence, or stimulate avoidance behaviour, leading to missing medical appointments or ignoring symptoms. It may be distressing, disabling, and lead to an inability to plan for the future.[13,18,19]

Fear of recurrence may be a fluctuating rather than constant state. It may be triggered by the appearance of new or unusual symptoms or by specific situations such as:

- imminent follow-up care appointments or medical check-ups
- routine tests ('scanxiety' is a term coined to describe anxiety or distress associated with having scans[20])
- news items about cancer in the media
- cancer diagnoses of friends or family
- relapse or death of a fellow survivor
- reminders of the cancer experience (such as sight of the cancer treatment centre).

Anniversaries of cancer diagnosis and specific stages of treatment may also provoke fear of recurrence. The case studies of Rose and Claire (later in this chapter) illustrate the powerful effect these triggers can have on the wellbeing of long-term survivors.

Acupuncturists should be aware of the potential for their patients to experience fear of recurrence, even many years after diagnosis, and be aware of possible triggers. Many patients, especially long-term survivors, may feel embarrassed about fear of recurrence, thinking they should have overcome such feelings.

It is helpful to acknowledge a patient's fear of recurrence, reassuring them that this is a normal response to a potentially life-threatening experience. When possible, I encourage them to give voice to their fears and encourage them to identify triggers.

This can help the person cope with and manage fear of recurrence and can be supported by acupuncture treatment appropriate to that individual.

The milestones
Lost in transition – adjusting to life immediately post treatment

The transition from active treatment to follow-up may be associated with distress. This is partly due to the loss of frequent medical monitoring and support, including relationships with medical staff, as well as a shift towards individual responsibility for self-management. Feelings of abandonment, vulnerability, and the loss of a 'safety net' are common at this time.[21]

Two breast cancer survivors participating in a focus group articulated their experiences of the aftermath of cancer treatment:

> I'd lost me, I'd got so used to everybody saying 'do this, do that' because when you're diagnosed you're put on this train, they lock the doors and they don't let you off, you know. And then suddenly you arrive at the station and they say 'go away for three months'. (003 BC)[22]

> Because you just go through so much, the [cancer] treatment is so awful, and then you have all these added bits on the end, you know. So it makes you feel really down and really depressed. (013 BC)

Navigating the change from patient to survivor is challenging, and many people feel 'lost' in this transition.[23] The boundaries of this transition may also be blurred, as primary treatment is followed by adjuvant treatments (e.g. hormonal treatments or biological targeted therapies such as Herceptin®) that continue for many years. One cancer survivor eloquently expressed this lack of clarity:

> I am not sure whether I've 'had' cancer, or I 'have' cancer. When does it become the past tense?[24]

The general perception from medical and social perspectives is that the physical cancer has been treated. This leaves the survivor to put their life back together. Family, friends, and the workplace may regard the struggle as over and expect the survivor to resume life as it was before cancer. This is a time when the survivor may need more, rather than less, support from healthcare and societal networks.

Thus, survivors may seek support from acupuncture at this time of transition. This can be a challenging time for both patient and practitioner. While many survivors find acupuncture treatment beneficial, others may struggle to incorporate it into their lives at a very difficult time.

In choosing a case study to illustrate the transitional phase, I have selected one that exemplifies the complex pressures prevalent during this time, and how these can overwhelm the potential benefits of acupuncture treatment.

CASE STUDY: SUSAN AND NAVIGATING POST TREATMENT

Introduction

Susan gave her consent to this case study, which encapsulates the complexity of competing pressures as survivors strive to return to normal following the disruption to their lives caused by cancer diagnosis and treatment. For Susan, this was a cocktail comprising:

- the consequences of cancer treatment (hot flushes, fatigue, emotional trauma)
- the pressure to return to work and resume previous activities
- living with existing chronic comorbidities (depression, overweight)
- the diagnosis of new comorbidities (diabetes)
- the demands of family life, including parenting a child who also had a chronic, life-threatening condition
- deaths of close family members.

The added pressures on an already demanding lifestyle burdened Susan's energy, making it difficult for her to cope as she made the transition to life post treatment.

Background

Susan, aged 55, started having acupuncture three weeks after finishing radiotherapy for early-stage breast cancer. Table 11.1 details her cancer diagnosis and treatment. On diagnosis, she discontinued hormone replacement therapy (HRT), which she had taken for several years to manage natural menopause. To manage the resultant hot flushes and night sweats (HFNS), her oncologist suggested she try acupuncture.

Table 11.1: Susan's history of cancer diagnosis and treatment

From diagnosis to post treatment	
May	Diagnosis T1N1M0 ductal carcinoma left breast; discontinued HRT
June	Wide local excision and sentinel lymph node biopsy
July	Re-excision to remove residual ductal carcinoma in situ (DCIS)
Oct	Commenced radiotherapy
Nov	Radiotherapy completed *Started acupuncture treatment*
Dec	Commenced adjuvant hormonal treatment (anastrozole) for five years *Stopped acupuncture treatment*

Susan enjoyed a successful career at the top of a competitive, demanding sector. Her only child had a debilitating health condition and experienced a life-threatening acute episode while Susan was undergoing cancer treatment.

She arrived for her first acupuncture appointment looking tired and frazzled. Her complexion was dull and pale. It was difficult to establish rapport, and Susan appeared uncomfortable with establishing eye contact. She seemed simultaneously to be seeking and resisting help. (One consequence of this 'push–pull' energy was on my note-taking, and I missed recording some details of the traditional diagnosis.)

Main complaints

HFNS were Susan's main complaint. On my request, she commenced keeping a diary of HFNS incidents (see Chapter 8, Cancer Treatment-Related Hot Flushes and Night Sweats, and the online Appendices) three days before attending her first treatment. Users of this diary are asked to note every HFNS and rate the severity of each incident as 1) mild, 2) moderate, or 3) severe. Users provide their own definitions of severity.

In this short period, Susan recorded an average of 13 HFNS per day, ranging from 8 to 17, with an average severity score of 22 per day, ranging from 15 to 30. Susan's definitions were:

1. mild = 'warm'
2. moderate = 'wet'
3. severe = 'very wet, hair, elbows, forehead'.

Susan was especially concerned about the HFNS. She was due to begin a course of adjuvant anastrozole in the next month, and her oncologist had advised that this could increase her HFNS. Clonidine had been prescribed three months earlier to manage the HFNS resulting from stopping HRT, but this was not providing sufficient relief.

Fatigue was also a problem. Susan had taken some months off work (the exact period is not captured in my notes). This had not been restful, as she was occupied with her child's grave health condition. Now, she frequently 'came over tired', especially in the afternoons and was tired on waking in the morning.

Her priorities for treatment were to reduce the HFNS and fatigue.

Questioning the systems

Sleep: Susan described herself as a good sleeper. However, she went to bed at irregular times; if she went early, she did not sleep through. She tended to fall asleep at midnight, and wake at 7am. Sleep was disturbed by going to the toilet during the night, night sweats between 3 and 5am, and her husband's sleep apnoea. She sometimes had disturbing dreams, generally about being locked into something; she could wake herself to stop these. She did not feel refreshed on waking.

Appetite: Susan's eating habits had changed recently. A former Weight Watcher, she knew about healthy eating and weight management. Recently she had 'gone off proper balanced meals'; she and her child were treating themselves with cake, ice-cream, chocolate, and biscuits, although Susan was limiting these treats to two per day. Whereas she used to cook the evening meal, often using Weight Watchers recipes, she now relied on pre-prepared foods. Weight had been and continued to be an issue for Susan; she did not disclose details of her present weight.

Drink: Susan drank a lot of fridge cold water, a glass of orange juice in the morning, and two cups of coffee during the day. She was not drinking alcohol at present.

Bowels: Susan had a movement every day. Stool consistency was variable, sometimes 'reasonably solid' but she tended to 'looseness'. She experienced considerable bowel symptoms including stomach pains, bloating, and flatulence, and she wondered if she had irritable bowel syndrome (IBS).

Urination: Susan had an overactive bladder, which was managed by prescribed tolterodine tartrate.

Sweating and temperature: See 'Main complaints'.

Pain: Since surgery, she experienced pain in the left breast.

Gynaecological history: A natural pregnancy had ended in miscarriage. The second of two rounds of IVF was successful, and she gave birth at the age of 41.

Head and body: Details not recorded.

Personal health history: Susan had experienced reactive depression following a relationship breakdown many years previously. Since the birth of her child, she suffered chronic depression which she managed with antidepressants (lofepramine) and 'lots of counselling'.

Medications: Susan was taking the following prescribed medications: ramipril and propranolol (hypertension), tolterodine tartrate (bladder), lofepramine (depression), and clonidine (HFNS). She was due to commence anastrozole. She also took a multivitamin, fish oils and glucosamine for arthritis, and calcium.

Additional information: Susan was struggling with her emotions; she was very tearful and described herself as 'emotional' and did not like to talk about cancer.

She had sacrificed hobbies to the demands of her career. Although she had a gym membership, she did not use it.

Relationships: Susan was married. She was very close to her adolescent child. She had experienced three significant bereavements in recent months, including the deaths of her parents and an in-law.

Physical examination: Tongue: Assessed but details not recorded. **Pulses:** Rapid and weak overall.

Diagnoses
CM diagnosis: Spleen qi deficiency, damp, Liver qi stagnation (invading the Spleen), Kidney yin deficiency, Blood deficiency, shen disturbance.

CF diagnosis: My initial thought was water, most notably represented by distinct 'groan' in Susan's voice.

Treatment approach

Susan attended once a week for four acupuncture sessions. The treatments, their rationale, and Susan's progress are discussed below; further details of the techniques used are discussed in Chapter 5, Toolkit.

Needles were not inserted in the arm and hand on the left (affected) side, observing the precautions for breast cancer patients at risk of lymphoedema (see Chapter 9, Cancer Treatment-Related Lymphoedema). When treating breast cancer survivors, I also only moxa chest points on the unaffected side.

Treatment 1

Table 11.2: Susan's first treatment

Abbreviations: Tx treatment; **RS** right side; **bi** bilateral

Tx	Treatment principles	Points	Notes
1	Harmonise qi	Three Gates: Ll-4 *Hegu* (RS) LIV-3 *Taichong* (bi)	Even technique, deqi, needles retained for approximately 20 minutes.

After taking her details, I introduced Susan to acupuncture. For patients who have never experienced acupuncture, I often use Four Gates (or its variant Three Gates for breast cancer survivors) at the first session. I find this procedure:

- reliably elicits distinct needle sensation, giving the patient a good impression of what having acupuncture is like
- gives me valuable information about the patient's energy and how sensitive they are to needling, while using a minimum of needles
- informs how I approach future treatments, by combining the information above with changes in the pulses and in the patient.

This information is augmented by the patient's report of any changes post treatment when they attend for their next session.

It has other advantages. The patient does not have to undress, thus minimising any unease they may feel until there has been time to build rapport and trust. It is potentially deeply relaxing, although acupuncture-naive individuals may be unable to relax very well during their initial session. Susan was one of these; she remained quite tense during the procedure.

During the consultation, I raised the possibility of Susan taking more time off work to allow herself to rest and recuperate – not just from the cancer treatment, but from the stress of her child's illness, as well as her bereavements. Friends, her counsellor, and occupational health in her workplace had also suggested this; however, Susan found this difficult as she felt she had taken enough time away from work already.

Treatment 2

Susan reported that she felt tired and had 'lots of flushes' during the week following her first treatment. These were particularly noticeable in the morning when sweating made it difficult to dress. She attended a breast cancer support group meeting during the week and found it depressing, particularly as an attendee told her that cancer treatment-related fatigue lasts a long time. During our discussion, Susan revealed that although officially part time, she was working 30 hours a week.

My treatment plan was to clear a block to treatment, choosing to focus on Internal Dragons (IDs) (see Chapter 5, Toolkit). Susan had several indications for this, including a history of depression, multiple recent emotional shocks (her cancer diagnosis, her child's severe illness, and three bereavements), as well as the after-effects of two recent surgical interventions.[25]

She also displayed some of the signs of IDs. It was difficult to make eye contact with Susan and taking the case history the previous week had been curiously challenging – it had been very difficult to establish rapport. I also interpreted the recurrent dreams about being locked up as a sign that IDs were indicated.

Furthermore, she had reported very little change after the first treatment (although her diary reflects a decrease in hot flushes, as discussed below). That she perceived very little change could have been the result of several factors; however, considering the other indications and symptoms discussed, I felt this could be part of the block.

Table 11.3: Susan's second treatment

Abbreviations: Tx treatment; **bi** bilateral

Tx	Treatment principles	Points	Notes
2	Clear block to treatment: Internal Dragons (IDs)	Master point 0.25 cun below REN-15 *Jiuwei* ST-25 *Tianshu* (bi) ST-32 *Futu* (bi) ST-41 *Jiexi* (bi)	Insert needles from top to bottom, even technique, deqi, retain for 20 minutes or until changes occur in patient. Remove needles from top to bottom.
	Ground treatment	SI-4 *Wangu* HE-7 *Shenmen*	Needle right arm only.

During the treatment, she was unable to close her eyes and relax. Nonetheless, changes in the pulses were promising, with a marked improvement in rate and depth.

Lifestyle advice at this session included discussing the importance of exercise and rest. I suggested that Susan gradually introduced physical activity into her routine, aiming to do three ten-minute sessions daily. I also encouraged her to rest in the afternoon, suggesting she aim to do this three times during the week. The following day I emailed her a prescription for rest (Box 11.1).

Treatment 3

Susan reported that the HFNS had reduced in frequency and severity after the previous treatment. She had slept through the night all week, which she did not usually do. She had taken exercise twice at the weekend and rested on one day. Her physician had certified her to work reduced hours, or to work from home. She had resumed wearing makeup, which she regarded as a significant change.

Despite these positive changes, Susan was exhibiting signs of poor concentration and high levels of agitation. Travelling to the acupuncture clinic was fraught with difficulties – either with traffic or parking problems. On one occasion during the week, Susan arrived for treatment on the wrong day. I interpreted these difficulties as manifestations of severe Blood deficiency, with the consequent shen disturbance affecting her ability to concentrate. The challenges in her life were increased further by positive test results for high cholesterol and diabetes.

My treatment aims were to calm shen, fortify her spirits, and begin to treat her constitutionally. I also introduced moxa in the form of a 'Toasted Pericardium Sandwich' for its potentially calming effects (see Chapter 5, Toolkit).

Table 11.4: Susan's third treatment

Abbreviations: Tx treatment; **bi** bilateral; **(n)** shows number of direct moxa cones applied

Tx	Treatment principles	Points	Notes
3	Nourish qi and calm shen 'Toasted Pericardium Sandwich'	BL-43 *Gaohuangshu* (7) REN-17 *Shanzhong* (5) BL-14 *Jueyinshu* (bi)	Direct moxa only (number of small moxa cones). Needles retained during moxa on BL-43.
	Test CF – water Yuan source points	BL-64 *Jinggu* (bi) KID-3 *Taixi* (bi)	Tonification, needles removed on deqi.

Treatment 4

Susan reported that she had felt relaxed after the previous treatment. HFNS were much reduced with just a few the previous day. She could now get dressed in the morning without the unwelcome interference of sweating. She reported that she had 'one big one' earlier in the day, which she thought was a response to a very stressful event at work. She would not discuss the details of this event.

She reported that she was feeling tired and emotional. Her sleep pattern was becoming disrupted again, and she was 'struggling to do things'. Her child had a major check-up, and although all was clear, it had been very tiring. When discussing her work pattern, it emerged that although Susan was certified to work reduced hours, she was working almost the equivalent of full time. She left the office early, continued to work at home, and was impatient with suggestions that she work less and rest more.

As HFNS were diminishing consistently, I judged that it was appropriate to begin to tonify qi and Blood. I also wanted to stabilise her emotions after the stressful event that had happened at work, as well as to harmonise Liver qi to address the associated frustration and anger. The response to this treatment was a remarkable pulse change; the pulses seemingly leapt from deep and weak to being strong, vital, and vibrant.

Table 11.5: Susan's fourth treatment

Abbreviations: Tx treatment; **RS** right side; **bi** bilateral; **(n)** shows number of direct moxa cones applied

Tx	Treatment principles	Points	Notes
4	Support spirit Calm shen	KID-24 *Lingxu* (3) (RS) REN-17 *Shanzhong* (5)	Direct moxa only (number of small moxa cones).
	Calm shen Harmonise liver qi Nourish and warm qi	P-7 *Daling* (RS) LIV-3 *Taichong* (bi) SP-6 *Sanyinjiao* (bi) ST-36 *Zusanli* with moxa (7) (bi)	Even technique, needles retained for approximately 20 minutes.

The result

From the pulse response, I anticipated a noticeable positive overall change for Susan. Within a few days, I received a message from her to say that HFNS had increased dramatically after that treatment. Because of this, and the stresses of getting to appointments, she no longer wished to continue treatment.

While disappointing, this was not entirely surprising. The difficulties Susan experienced in making and travelling to appointments had foreshadowed her ability to commit to a longer-term course of treatment.

In addition, I felt I had not been able to penetrate her defences and establish good rapport. This was unfortunate, as there were indications that she was making good progress. Her subjective report of improvement in HFNS is supported by the retrospective analysis of the hot flush diary, which charted HFNS for 14 days starting three days prior to commencing acupuncture. This showed that both the frequency and severity had reduced, especially after the first acupuncture treatment on day 4 (Figure 11.2).

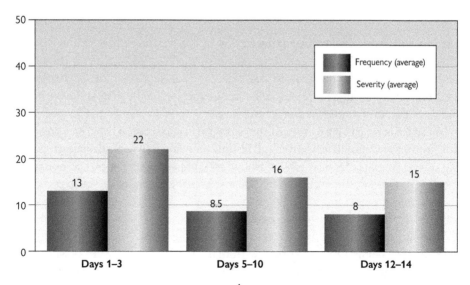

FIGURE 11.2: ANALYSIS OF SUSAN'S HFNS DIARY – ACUPUNCTURE
TREATMENTS WERE ON DAYS 4 AND 11

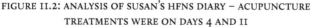

What provoked the upsurge in HFNS? Initially, I was concerned that it was a reaction to the moxibustion. However, Susan had responded well to moxibustion in treatment 3, reporting a noticeable decrease in HFNS afterwards. Perhaps the upsetting incident at work, the details of which Susan chose not to disclose, caused an emotional reaction that triggered HFNS. Susan was exhausted and overburdened, and her seriously depleted energy may have enhanced her vulnerability to such events.

Summary and follow-up

Susan's case study illustrates a situation I frequently find with survivors starting acupuncture treatment immediately after cancer treatment. Busy, often stressful, lives are pushed into overload by cancer and its treatments. Although the resulting symptoms are sufficiently uncomfortable to motivate the survivor to seek acupuncture treatment, the burden of debilitation makes it difficult for them to attend for regular treatment. Progress may seem imperceptible or too slow, and there may be little patience with fluctuations, which are sometimes an inevitable part of the process.

Susan updated me 18 months later when I requested permission for this case study. After the treatment described above, she had received eight sessions of NADA ear acupuncture at the cancer centre. Although relaxing, there was again little improvement in HFNS. She was now walking half an hour every day, and the battle with her weight was ongoing. She was delighted to report that her second annual mammogram was clear.

Year 1: The challenges of recovery

We have looked at the challenges faced by survivors immediately post treatment. It is recognised that the year after the end of primary treatment can be difficult. Although physical consequences can occur at any time after treatment, they are most likely to appear during this period. In a UK survey, 94% of the respondents said they had experienced problems in the first year after treatment.[26]

Physical and emotional consequences

As well as physical changes, emotions may be difficult as people begin the process of adjustment to their changed self and life. Many survivors feel low or depressed, a situation which they find surprising and discouraging. Table 11.6 lists some of the consequences that are common during the first year.

There is also societal pressure in the widespread expectation that once treatment ends, the survivor should feel better and resume previous activities. These expectations may also be generated by the survivor, who may be impatient for a return to normal life, as well as to make up the time lost to cancer treatment. Pressure may also come from others. Family, friends, and colleagues may be eager for the survivor to resume previous activities, often as reassurance that a crisis has passed.

Survivors and those around them often do not anticipate the length of time that problems may persist. I have worked with many survivors who were bewildered or frustrated by this. Acupuncturists can play a vital role in helping survivors to adjust their expectations, and to understand that recovery is a process, rather than an event.

Table 11.6: Some consequences commonly arising during the first year post active treatment (listed alphabetically)

Physical consequences	Emotional consequences
Breathlessness	Anger
Bruising, bleeding	Cancer-related post-traumatic stress[27]
Changed body image	Depression
Changes in function	Fear of recurrence
Early menopause	Inadequacy
Eating difficulties	Insecurity
Fatigue	Isolation
Hot flushes, night sweats (HFNS) (prostate cancer)	Loss of confidence
Insomnia	Negative feelings
Joint stiffness	Stress
Late effects of radiotherapy: dry mouth (head and neck cancers); bowel, urinary disorders (pelvic cancers)	Uncertainty
	Vulnerability
Loss of fertility	**Other consequences**
Lymphoedema	Changes in:
Menopausal symptoms: vaginal dryness, HFNS, libido changes	• employment
	• relationships
Osteoporosis	• role
Pain	• sexuality
Peripheral neuropathy	
Sexual changes: libido changes, erectile dysfunction, vaginal dryness	
Weight changes	

Recovery as a gradual process

Recovery may be a gradual process that takes time. In a consultation exercise, cancer survivors described 'the long process of recovery as important work in the year following the completion of their primary cancer treatment'.[21] This included recovery from physical symptoms, psychological recovery, and adjustment of their expectations.

For many survivors in the transition phase, the thought that recovery may take as much as a year is disappointing. I find that many survivors also measure progress from the date of diagnosis, the moment at which their life changed, rather than from the end of treatment, which is the time from which the body can begin to recover from cancer treatments.

ESSENTIALS

Acupuncturists can play a key role in supporting cancer survivors through the challenges of the first year. As well as addressing physical and emotional symptoms through treatment and lifestyle advice, they can help to adjust expectations associated with the time needed for recovery.

In addition, acupuncturists can reassure survivors about feeling stressed or having negative feelings. There is no strong evidence that stress causes cancer or increases the risk of recurrence.[28] It is also helpful for survivors to know that having negative feelings will not slow recovery or increase the risk of cancer coming back. It is natural for cancer survivors to have times when they feel low or depressed. Survivors can be encouraged to acknowledge difficult feelings, and to feel able to talk about them.

A helpful lifestyle practice – the importance of rest

Recovery from active cancer treatment may be hard work, especially as industrialised societies have lost the concept of convalescence after illness. Cancer survivors are now encouraged to return to normal activities as soon as possible after treatment. Where once doctors advised rest after cancer treatment, the message is now to stay active.[29] This makes sense in terms of the strong evidence for physical activity in cancer recovery (see Chapter 13, Reducing Risk of Recurrence and Subsequent Primary Cancers). Return to work may also be essential from a financial perspective, as well as giving a sense of purpose.

However, rest remains important to the recovery process: 'deliberately resting can be a powerful medicine'[30] and it is vital not to lose that message. Rest is the yin counterpoint to the yang of activity; it is an important way to repair and replenish damage done to qi, Blood, jing, jin ye, and shen by cancer diagnosis and treatment.

As discussed in previous chapters, I regularly prescribe rest in the form of an afternoon nap to my patients (Box 11.1). I repeat this here, as rest is so important to recovery and our society does not give us permission to rest regularly. Had Susan been able to adopt this practice, she may have found gradual relief from her symptoms.

Attitudes to rest

An afternoon nap is regarded by many as a sign of weakness; to be 'caught napping' or told to 'take a nap' are expressions of derision. Nevertheless, many modern business organisations are adopting the concept of the afternoon nap – the 'power nap' – recognising its value for increasing alertness, productivity, and creativity of employees. Research demonstrates that it improves performance in jobs, including long-haul airline pilots, truckers, and factory workers; it also augments perception, facilitates learning, and reduces coronary heart disease.[31]

Theories of rest in East Asian medicine (EAM)

In terms of EAM, a midday rest nourishes the yin as the day's energy transforms from yang to yin. Resting after lunch:

- assists the Spleen's digestive function, helping to overcome the lethargy and tiredness many people experience as a post-lunch dip
- returns Blood to the Liver, especially when lying in the supine position. I recommend lying down between 1pm and 3pm to benefit from the restorative effect on the Liver during its downtime on the 24-hour clock (Figure 11.3).

When patients cannot find time between 1pm and 3pm, a good alternative is between 5pm and 7pm (Kidney time), which will nourish Kidney energy during its peak time.

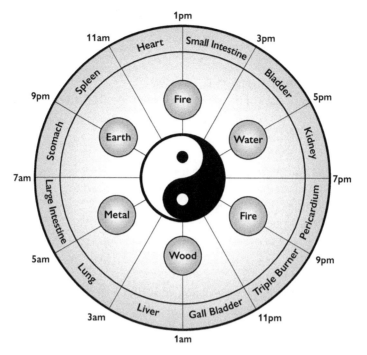

FIGURE 11.3: THE 24-HOUR CLOCK IN CHINESE MEDICINE

How rest impacts symptoms

Many of my patients who adopt this practice report improvements in energy and vitality, along with symptom reduction. This is especially apparent when treating HFNS; however, beneficial effects may extend to many other troublesome symptoms, such as improved memory and concentration.

Patients with sleep disorders express concerns that this practice may disrupt their night sleep; however, I find that mostly this improves the quality and quantity of sleep.

The essence of this practice is to:

- do it as regularly as possible
- restrict rest time to 20 minutes.

Exceeding 20 minutes can cause grogginess and difficulty waking, as well as interfere with night-time sleep. However, when people are seriously depleted, there may be a period during which they need to rest for longer than 20 minutes. This can be encouraged if it does not interfere with night sleep. I find that as people recuperate, their bodies adjust, and they soon automatically time themselves to 20 minutes.

Overcoming resistance to rest

Patients may resist the idea of resting or taking a nap during the day, equating this with laziness. I explain that in adopting this practice, they are taking an *active* role in their recovery. I also encourage them to think about this as 'recharging their batteries' rather than napping.

Box 11.1: Example prescription for rest

Each day (or as many days of the week as possible), ideally between 1pm and 3pm:

- Lie down for 10–20 minutes.
- Close your eyes.
- Imagine you are recharging your batteries.
- Fall asleep – or not – as you choose, or as you need to.
- Avoid reading or watching TV.
- Avoid feeling guilty!
- Do it as often as possible. If you miss a day or two, get back into the swing of it.

Notice how your energy changes when you adhere to this practice and what happens on the days you miss.

Navigating to the five-year milestone
The significance of the five-year milestone

Five years post diagnosis is a significant milestone in cancer survivorship. For most types of cancer, the chances of recurrence are much lower after five years than they are after two years. As more time passes, the likelihood that cancer will recur lessens.

Statistics for cancer survival often are stated as a 'five-year relative survival rate', a way of describing the percentage of people who are expected to survive five years after diagnosis. For example, figures for the UK show that for all cancers diagnosed in 2010–2011, the five-year survival rates are 49% for men and 59% for women.[32] In the US, the five-year relative survival rate for all cancers combined between 2010 and 2016 is 68% among White people and 63% among Black people, an increase from 39% and 27% respectively since the early 1960s.[33]

Survival statistics include survivors who are in remission or undergoing treatment and excludes people who die of other causes. As discussed previously (see Chapter 2, The Consequences of Cancer Treatments), it is difficult to apply the word 'cure' to cancer; cancer cells can remain undetected in the body after treatment, with potential for recurrence or relapse. However, many cancers are considered 'cured' when no cancer is detected five years after diagnosis (bear in mind that recurrence after five years remains a possibility).[34]

Challenges arising during the first five years

Navigating towards the five-year milestone can be challenging. Symptoms arising post treatment and during the first year may continue. Survivors may discover that these have permanent effects, or take longer to diminish than anticipated.[35] Many survivors will still be undergoing long-term adjuvant treatment, and continuing to experience treatment-related side effects.

New consequences may also arise. For example, cumulative incidence of breast cancer-related lymphoedema rises from 13.5% in the first two years post treatment to 41.1% at ten years post cancer treatment.[36] Expectations of others for the survivor to 'move on' may lead to feelings of isolation, as the survivor no longer feels they can discuss their feelings.

There may be changes to the schedule of monitoring and follow-up. For some, annual follow-up appointments may cease at this milestone (although for many cancers in many countries, there is a move to discontinue these at two years). For others, follow-up may continue. Distress may be associated with appointments, scans, and tests, and this may continue for many years.[5] The case study of Rose illustrates the power of check-ups, anniversaries, and new symptoms to trigger fear of recurrence.

CASE STUDY: ROSE AND NAVIGATING FIVE TO TEN YEARS OF CANCER SURVIVORSHIP

Introduction

Rose, who consented to sharing her story, gives us the opportunity to observe one woman's progress around the time of the five-year anniversary and her transition into the second half of her first decade as a survivor.

Rose was deeply affected by a breast cancer diagnosis at the age of 35. Young adults (aged 25–39) have specific experiences that differ from teenage or older people diagnosed with cancer. For example, loss of fertility is a concern. Fear of recurrence is also reported to be particularly pronounced in young adults.[13,19] Her story demonstrates the impact of fear of recurrence and the distress this can cause.

Background

Rose had been having acupuncture for four years, throughout chemotherapy, radiotherapy, and post active treatment. Changes in circumstances necessitated changing acupuncturists, and Rose was referred to me five months before the fifth anniversary of her diagnosis.

Summary of Rose's previous acupuncture treatment

Rose's acupuncturist, who (like myself) practises both Five Elements and TCM styles, provided a summary of treatment. This had varied according to Rose's changing needs over the years:

- During chemotherapy and radiotherapy, treatment focused on clearing heat, strengthening yin and Blood, and clearing blocks to treatment (Internal Dragons).
- Following primary treatment, the focus switched to strengthening, with key treatment principles including clearing stagnation, nourishing yin and Blood, tonifying the Kidney, and supporting the emotions.
- Recently, treatment had shifted to balancing Rose's mood; syndromes included

yin and Blood deficiency, Heart qi deficiency, Liver qi stagnation, and Kidney yin deficiency.
- The CF diagnosis was fire.

Cancer history

Rose's diagnosis and treatment history is detailed in Table 11.7, along with other significant health events. Not included are the regular consultations with her oncologist (initially four-monthly, usually January, May, August) and an annual mammogram (January). As well as having regular acupuncture, Rose saw a nutritionist.

Table 11.7: Rose's cancer and significant health history

Year 1: December 2005 to November 2006	
Dec 2005	Diagnosis T1N1M0 Ductal carcinoma left breast
Dec 2005	Mastectomy and axillary node clearance
Jan 2006	Chemotherapy 4 x FEC (5-fluorouracil, epirubicin, cyclophosphamide), 4 x taxotere
Feb 2006	*Started acupuncture treatment with first acupuncturist*
July 2006	Commenced radiotherapy, 15 fractions
Aug 2006	Radiotherapy ended. Commenced tamoxifen
Years 2–5: December 2006 to November 2010	
June 2008	Hysteroscopy and ovarian cystectomy
July 2010	*Changed acupuncturist*
Dec 2010	Five-year anniversary of diagnosis
Year 6 onward: December 2010 to March 2012	
Feb 2011	Four-monthly consultations with oncologist reduced to twice yearly. Oncologist recommended Rose continue tamoxifen to seven years post diagnosis (to Dec 2012), two years beyond the then recommended five-year duration for tamoxifen.
June 2011	Concern about cancer recurrence; Rose felt her body was 'trying to tell [her] something'. Ultrasound and examination were all clear.
Mar 2012	Rose reported unexplained weight loss since December; this coincided with a friend being diagnosed with breast secondaries. Saw GP, who initially dismissed fears, then realised Rose's anxieties and ordered blood tests. Rose also arranged to see her oncologist. This was at Rose's last treatment with me before she moved away.

Main complaints

Health-conscious Rose made considerable efforts to live as healthily as possible. Acupuncture was part of her strategy for this, and her overall goal when she started seeing me was to 'help maintain a good balance of health'.

Questioning the systems

Sleep: Usually slept well through the night. Recently nights were slightly disturbed by hot flushes (not sweats), and Rose found it difficult to get back to sleep after these incidents. Vivid, often unhappy dreams were becoming more frequent, and Rose often woke up sobbing.

Appetite: Rose described her appetite as 'good', and she enjoyed food. Having adopted a diet recommended by a major cancer centre, she described herself as predominately vegetarian and consumed pulses, fish once or twice weekly, and chicken once a month. She avoided soy and dairy products. All food was organic, and she and her husband grew many of their vegetables. Eating habits were good, and she had regular home-cooked meals. Although she had no difficulties eating and digesting food, she was 'paranoid about weight'. Overweight as a child, Rose became seriously underweight (nearly halving her weight from 14 stone (196lb or 89kg) to 7.5 stone (105lb or 47kg)). Although she had experienced some tamoxifen-associated weight gain, this had stabilised, and Rose's weight was now within the normal BMI range.

Drink: Lots of water, Rose drank bottled water only; one cup of nettle tea per day.

Bowels: Regular daily movement, no issues.

Urination: No significant issues.

Sweating and temperature: Rose's hands and feet were always cold. Tamoxifen-related HFNS had almost disappeared. At the time of this consultation, one month since her last acupuncture treatment, she noticed HFNS were returning, although they were mild.

Pain: No pain in the body; some numbness around left breast.

Gynaecological history: Chemotherapy-induced infertility was 'the hardest thing' for Rose. She had seen a fertility expert, who confirmed she was no longer ovulating. Ovarian cysts had been removed in 2008; it was thought these were a consequence of tamoxifen. Periods had ceased during cancer treatment, although there was an occasional bleed. Rose still experienced a type of hormonal cycle that primarily affected her emotions, leaving her feeling low in mood and introspective.

Head and body: Minor headaches (twice a year); some dizziness associated with HFNS; floaters; no other eye or ear symptoms. Breathing became a problem when Rose was anxious. Her chest tightened, she experienced a slight throbbing sensation, and had difficulty catching her breath.

Personal health history: Perthes disease, a childhood condition in which the blood supply to the femur is insufficient, affected Rose at the age of six and was treated by wearing a brace.

Additional information: Following Rose's diagnosis, she and her husband decided to buy a house that was non-toxic and chemical-free. The challenges of finding such a property combined with those of house-buying in England caused considerable stress.

Relationships: Rose had strong, supportive relationships with her husband and their extended families. There were periodic concerns about the health of both her husband and mother. Rose's father, who had bowel cancer, died on Father's Day the year Rose was diagnosed; the anniversaries of his birthday and death were difficult times for Rose.

Physical examination: Tongue: Wide, with tooth marks on the sides; colour pale overall, orange on the sides; coating thin overall, slightly thickening towards the root; sublingual veins blue and slightly distended. **Pulses:** Deep, weak, thin on both sides, slightly stronger on the right. Choppy front pulse on the left side.

Diagnoses
CM diagnosis: I agreed with Rose's previous acupuncturist, only modifying her diagnosis by adding shen disturbance to the syndromes, as evidenced by the dream-disturbed sleep, anxiety, and emotional lability.

CF diagnosis: I modified the previous diagnosis by focusing on the Pericardium side of fire. I based this on my sense of Rose's energy; although a determined person, Rose had an aura of sadness and vulnerability. Earnest and serious by nature, she was also prone to periods of feeling low and flat. Her choice of 'Rose' as a pseudonym struck me as particularly appropriate, as it encapsulates both the hardiness and delicate fragility of the flower, which was so like Rose's energy.

Treatment approach
Rose attended for 33 treatments over 20 months. Selected treatments, their rationale, and Rose's progress are discussed below; further details of the techniques used are discussed in Chapter 5, Toolkit.

Managing distress and fear of recurrence
Rose's stated priority for acupuncture treatment was to help maintain a good balance of health. As our relationship developed, it became apparent that distress associated with fear of recurrence was a recurring condition. This manifested in a state that Rose referred to as a 'tizwoz', characterised by:

- tightness in the chest
- difficulty breathing
- distressing dreams
- inability to relax
- getting a bit hyper
- becoming emotional.

Triggers included appointments with her oncologist or surgeon, her annual mammogram, anniversaries of diagnosis and cancer treatment dates, and the anniversary of her father's death. Watchful of her body, any changes could initiate fears of cancer recurrence or new cancers.

She was also concerned about ovarian cysts, which had recurred, and were monitored closely by her gynaecologist. Her hormonal cycle increased her sensitivities; although menstruation had ceased, Rose was aware of bodily and emotional changes occurring in a monthly cycle. Added to this was the rollercoaster of house-buying – elation at locating a property matching the required specifications, and the disappointment when it was unsuitable, or when the prospect of a sale fell through. There were also work-related concerns for Rose and for her husband, who also had health concerns.

Treatment planning

In developing Rose's treatment plan, I aimed to accommodate her desire for improving the balance of her overall health and to manage the distress to which she was prone.

BL-43 *Gaohuangshu* was a point that could address many aspects of Rose's health. Among its many actions, those that pertained to Rose were its ability to:

- tonify qi
- strengthen deficiency
- nourish Essence
- invigorate the mind
- tonify and nourish the Lung, Heart, Kidney, Spleen, and Stomach
- calm the spirit
- nourish yin.[37,38]

In the *Thousand Ducat Formulas*, Sun Si-miao wrote 'there is no [disorder] that it cannot treat' and moxibustion on this point 'causes a person's yang qi to be healthy and full'.[38] Maciocia recommends it to tonify the qi of the whole body and lift the spirits when a person has been debilitated after a chronic illness.[37]

As the back transporting point of the *gaohuang* or 'vital region', level with BL-14 *Jueyinshu*, this point is used as an adjunct to treatment on the Pericardium in Five Element acupuncture.[25] As such, it was particularly relevant for supporting Rose's CF. These indications seemed well suited to Rose's presenting symptoms, priorities, and constitution.

Discovering the 'Toasted Pericardium Sandwich'

It was through working with Rose that I developed the concept of the 'Toasted Pericardium Sandwich' (see Chapter 5, Toolkit). I drew on the practice of combining the back transporting and front mu points of an organ to strengthen treatment, matching the back shu point BL-43 *Gaohuangshu* with REN-17 *Shanzhong*, the front mu point of the Pericardium.[38,39]

As recommended in both classical and some modern texts, I prefer to apply moxa only to BL-43 *Gaohuangshu*, and do not needle this point. Classical texts suggest using up to 300 moxa cones on this point;[38] modern texts recommend 7–50.[25,40] Clinically, I use direct moxa and find 15 cones bilaterally works well within the context of a consultation. Typically, I use three or five moxa cones on REN-17 *Shanzhong*.[25]

This combination formed the core of many of Rose's treatments. Its immediate effects were to relieve the tightness in her chest and improve breathing. Rose also found the penetrating warmth helped her to achieve a state of profound relaxation. Longer term and combined with needling on other points on the Pericardium and Ren channels, this calmed the shen to relieve troublesome dreams.

Supplementing the core treatment

I supplemented this according to Rose's condition when attending for treatment, utilising points on the Pericardium and Triple Burner channels to support her CF.

When she experienced a tizwoz, I added points to support her spirit and stabilise her emotions. I also applied gold ear magnets to the ear point *Reverse Shenmen* (see Chapter 5, Toolkit), which Rose could stimulate in the days after acupuncture treatment to prevent or manage the symptoms associated with a tizwoz.

Typical treatments are detailed below. On three occasions, I treated Internal Dragons, as her dreams or emotions were more than usually troubled. Other treatments included addressing acute invasions of wind cold and managing HFNS that resurfaced from time to time.

I judged that the ovarian cysts (three on one side, four on the other) might not respond to the level of acupuncture treatment Rose could commit to and suggested Chinese herbs to disperse these. Rose's preference was to monitor them conventionally.

A sequence of seven of Rose's treatments

I have chosen to detail a sequence of seven of Rose's treatments, which neatly encapsulates events that affected Rose's mood – medical appointments, house-buying, family concerns, and pervasive concerns about her wellbeing. In this sequence, I have only used the 'Toasted Pericardium Sandwich' twice; however, I used it frequently during other phases of treatment.

Notes on treatment

Needles were not inserted in the arm and hand on the left (affected) side, observing the precautions for breast cancer patients at risk of lymphoedema (see Chapter 9, Cancer Treatment-Related Lymphoedema).

- I also only moxa chest points on the unaffected side. However, with Rose I did occasionally needle BL-14 *Jueyinshu* bilaterally and used direct moxa bilaterally on BL-43 *Gaohuangshu*. This was done after discussion and with Rose's agreement.
- In general, I used an even needle technique and direct moxa. When treating the CF, I needle without retention, removing the needles immediately after deqi.
- Details of techniques used are given in Chapter 5, Toolkit.

Table 11.8: Managing low spirits, the house-buying rollercoaster, and a tizwoz

Abbreviations: RS right side; **bi** bilateral; **(n)** shows number of direct moxa cones applied

4 May: Rose arrived feeling down, with low energy and in need of a boost. A potential house purchase had fallen through the previous week on her birthday. Her brand of tamoxifen had also been changed, and she noted that she felt better on her 'usual' brand. She was feeling hot in bed but had no HFNS during the day or night.

Treatment principles	Points	Notes
Calm shen and lift spirits	'Toasted Pericardium Sandwich' BL-43 *Gaohuangshu* (7) REN-17 *Shanzhong* (5)	Direct moxa only (number of small moxa cones).
	BL-14 *Jueyinshu* (bi)	See 'Notes on treatment' above.
Treat CF – Fire (Pericardium)	Yuan source points: P-7 *Daling* TB-4 *Yangchi*	Needled RS only.

24 May: Rose still feeling low and despondent about the house. Described herself as being in a tizwoz and feeling overwhelmed.

Treatment principles	Points	Notes
Support spirit Calm shen	KID-24 *Lingxu* (3) REN-17 *Shanzhong* (5)	Direct moxa only (number of small moxa cones).
Clear block to treatment: Internal Dragons (IDs)	Master point 0.25 cun below REN-15 *Jiuwei* ST-25 *Tianshu* ST-32 *Futu* ST-41 *Jiexi*	
Ground treatment	SI-4 *Wangu* HE-7 *Shenmen*	Needled RS only.
Self-management of stress	Gold ear magnets on earpoint *Reverse Shenmen*	

14 June: Rose said she had been on a rollercoaster over house but now they had found one! Saw her surgeon as felt her body was trying to tell her something; ultrasound and examination confirmed all was well. An occipital headache had lasted five days. Rose asked for a 'pick-me-up'.

Treatment principles	Points	
Harmonise qi	Three Gates: LI-4 *Hegu* (RS) LIV-3 *Taichong* (bi)	
Calm shen	M-HN-3 *Yintang*	

Table 11.9: Managing anniversary and health anxiety, family health, house-buying

Abbreviations: RS right side; **bi** bilateral; **(n)** shows number of direct moxa cones applied

12 July: Rose was fine during the month since her previous treatment. However, she was starting to feel a bit stirred up as a lot was happening. Her scheduled appointment with the oncologist was due next month and she had an appointment to see the gynaecologist about her cysts later in the week. Her husband was unwell, and the house was 'in the air'.

Treatment principles	Points	Notes
Calm shen Support heart protector Treat CF	'Toasted Pericardium Sandwich' BL-43 *Gaohuangshu* (7) REN-17 *Shanzhong* (5) BL-14 *Jueyinshu* (bi)	As per 4 May.
	REN-15 *Jiuwei* P-3 *Quze* (RS) P-6 *Neiguan* (RS)	

Table 11.10: Managing an acute condition and continuing health anxieties (despite good news)

Abbreviations: RS right side; **bi** bilateral; **(n)** shows number of direct moxa cones applied

26 July: Rose presented with a cold, which she thought might be due to stress. They had pulled out of a house deal the previous day.

Treatment principles	Points	Notes
Expel pathogenic factor	BL-12 *Fengmen* BL-13 *Feishu*	Bilateral needling with cupping, cups retained for ten minutes, medium strength.
Release the exterior, expel wind	LU-7 *Lieque* (RS) Ll-4 *Hegu* (RS)	
Clear chest congestion	REN-18 *Yutang* REN-19 *Zigong*	
Calm shen, clear sinuses	M-HN-3 *Yintang*	
Self-management of stress	Gold ear magnets on earpoint *Reverse Shenmen*	

9 Aug: Rose's cold had cleared after the previous treatment. She was left with a little chest congestion. The oncologist had confirmed all was well; he suggested reducing frequency of appointments and alternating them with the surgeon so Rose was seeing a specialist twice a year only. Tamoxifen would be reviewed in 18 months.

Work had picked up, as had her husband's health, and they were due to go on holiday. Despite these up-turns, Rose still felt uneasy about her health. Even though her check-up had been clear, she had had a bad dream about it the previous Saturday.

Treatment principles	Points	Notes
Calm shen	M-HN-3 *Yintang* REN-15 *Jiuwei*	
Warm and nourish qi and Blood, calm spirit	ST-36 *Zusanli* (bi) (7)	Direct moxa plus needling.
Support CF (Metal points of Pericardium and Triple Burner)	P-5 *Jianshi* (RS) TB-1 *Guanchong* (RS)	

Table 11.11: More house-hunting woes and feeling fed up

Abbreviations: RS right side; **bi** bilateral; **(n)** shows number of direct moxa cones applied

23 Aug: Rose reported feeling 'generally okay', but house hunting continued to be disappointing. Her husband was feeling overtired again. Rose was feeling 'fed up' and 'wound up'. She had seen her physician for blood tests, primarily to check Vitamin D levels. She was sleeping well, although was dreaming about houses and experiencing some heat at night.

Treatment principles	Points	Notes
Calm shen and support spirit	REN-17 *Shanzhong* (5) KID-21*Youmen** (3) (bi) KID-22 *Bulang** (3) (bi)	Direct moxa only (number of small moxa cones).
	M-HN-3 *Yintang* REN-15 *Jiuwei*	

6 Sept: Rose felt the previous treatment had lifted her spirits. However, more unsuccessful house hunting meant she was feeling down and was thoroughly 'fed up'.

Treatment principles	Points	Notes
Calm shen	REN-17 *Shanzhong* (5) REN-15 *Jiuwei* M-HN-3 *Yintang* P-6 *Neiguan* (RS)	Needling and moxa as per 23 Aug.
Lift spirits	DU-20 *Baihui*** REN-6 *Qihai*** (9)	

*KID-21 *Youmen* and KID-22 *Bulang* are indicated when a patient is overwhelmed by fearfulness.[25]
**REN-6 *Qihai* (with moxa) and DU-20 *Baihui* are indicated to lift the spirits, and for physical and mental exhaustion and depression.[25,41]

Summary and follow-up

Rose's case provides an insight into how pervasive and burdensome fear of recurrence can be. The frequency of her medical appointments, her sensitivity to anniversaries, and the incidences of cancer in her friends and family combined to create a destabilising effect that was almost continuous for her.

This was very frustrating for Rose. At one of her last meetings with me, she reported that she had been very anxious about a recent appointment with her surgeon, and she felt that she should be 'getting over herself'. To deal with this, she embarked on a specialist course of life-coaching and mind–body therapy offered by a cancer centre.

Although acupuncture did not resolve Rose's deep-seated fears, treatment helped her to cope with the stresses of her health, the challenges of house-buying, and other concerns affecting her daily life.

When I contacted her over two years after her last appointment, Rose declined to read the case study, saying she wished to move on from her cancer experience. She and her husband had found the desired home and were establishing a new business together. Rose kindly gave permission to share her story, for which I am grateful.

Beyond five years of survivorship
Potential changes following the fifth anniversary
From the fifth anniversary of diagnosis, regular check-ups with oncology specialists may cease. This may leave the survivor feeling vulnerable. For Rose, as for many of the cancer survivors I have worked with, the fifth-year anniversary elicited feelings of uncertainty and trepidation rather than being a celebration of a milestone reached.

Long-term consequences may continue, perhaps becoming more severe, and new late effects of treatment may emerge. Survivors may worry about recurrence of their initial cancer, or the possibility of new second cancers.

Ten-year survival
Ten-year survival rates
In general, the news is increasingly positive about cancer survivorship. In the UK, 50% of people diagnosed are now expected to survive for at least a decade, compared with 20% for those diagnosed during 1970–1971.[32] (By comparison, ten-year survival rates for all cancers combined during 2011–2015 in Australia are reported as 63%;[42] in the USA, ten-year survival rates are reported as 84% for breast cancer and 98% for prostate cancers.[34]) The ten-year survival rates of specific cancers are discussed in Chapter 1, Cancer Survivorship and the Role of Acupuncture.

Potential consequences associated with ten-year survival
While ten-year survival is on the increase, it is not problem-free. A UK survey showed that while most survivors (94%) experienced problems in the first year after treatment ended, 71% of those surveyed who were ten or more years post diagnosis had experienced a physical symptom in the previous year that might be linked to cancer and its treatment.[26]

These may be a continuation of consequences that arose in the period during and immediately post treatment, or they may be new long-term consequences that manifest years after treatment ends. Box 11.2 lists some consequences that may persist up to and beyond ten years, with newly arising consequences discussed below.

Box 11.2: Long-term effects of treatment (listed alphabetically)[43]

- Body image problems
- Chronic fatigue*
- Gastrointestinal problems, including faecal incontinence, diarrhoea, bleeding
- Infertility
- Lymphoedema
- Mental health problems, including moderate to severe anxiety or depression, and post-traumatic stress disorder (PTSD)*
- Moderate to severe pain*

- Osteoporosis
- Sexual difficulties**
- Swallowing and speech problems
- Urinary problems, including incontinence

*Reported by survivors up to five years post treatment[43]
**Reported by survivors up to and beyond ten years post treatment[43]

There is also an increased risk of other serious conditions, which may only emerge decades later. Risk of heart disease may be increased by treatments such as the targeted therapy Herceptin® (trastuzumab), chemotherapy using anthracyclines, and radiotherapy to the chest. Second cancers may also be a long-term consequence of cancer treatment. Men who have had prostate cancer are at higher risk of osteoporosis than those who have not had prostate cancer.[44]

Survivors of childhood cancers are a growing population. Treatment of childhood cancers is highly successful, and a high proportion of these people will live into middle and old age. Long-term consequences of childhood cancer include hearing problems, second primary cancers, bone health problems, metabolic syndrome, and fertility or cognitive issues.

Awareness and support for survivors

As discussed in Chapter 1, lack of awareness of these long-term consequences and late effects of treatment is a serious concern. Healthcare professionals working with cancer survivors should be aware of the health issues associated with long-term survivorship in order to help, support, and refer survivors to appropriate care. However, patients discharged from oncology follow-up (typically at the five-year milestone) may subsequently see healthcare professionals who are not cancer specialists. These professionals may not, therefore, be aware of potential late effects of cancer treatment or attribute new symptoms to previous cancer treatments.

Changing needs

As well as symptoms changing over the course of years, survivors' needs may also change. Conditions may become chronic; existing or new comorbidities may complicate the picture, and some symptoms may be intermittent. The case study of Claire illustrates the changing needs of a long-term survivor of breast cancer, as she navigated the milestones over 12 years following her cancer diagnosis and treatment.

CASE STUDY: CLAIRE AND NAVIGATING BEYOND TEN YEARS OF CANCER SURVIVORSHIP
Introduction

Claire is a long-term breast cancer survivor, over two decades post diagnosis at the time of publication of this book. Her decision to continue having acupuncture following management of HFNS, her initial main complaint, provides an opportunity to chart one woman's progress through the milestones up to and beyond a decade since her diagnosis.

Claire consented to and participated in writing this case study. It discusses significant events associated with her long-term survivorship around the ten-year milestone, rather than details of her early or subsequent acupuncture treatment.

Background

I met Claire in March 2003 when she arrived for acupuncture for breast cancer treatment-related HFNS. She was diagnosed at age 36, and I remember my surprise on meeting her – at that time most of my breast cancer patients were older. (Incidence of breast cancer in women under the age of 40 appears to be an increasing trend in many countries.)[45,46]

Tall, stylish, and immaculately groomed, she is an imposing figure. Dynamic, energetic, with a tremendous appetite and enthusiasm for life, Claire is a powerful and vivid personality. Proactive and assertive, her response to life's challenges is to act, to take charge. Applying this approach to her cancer diagnosis, she wrote:

> The only way I felt I could deal with being diagnosed with breast cancer was by taking as much control of the situation as possible. I immediately researched everything about my diagnosis… For me, knowledge was power…it helped me have a positive outlook throughout and I felt I was in control, not the cancer.

Cancer history

Claire's diagnosis of cancer in the right breast and her treatment history are detailed in Table 11.12, along with other significant health events. Not included are the dates of her regular check-ups and mammograms: she saw her consultant twice yearly, in November and May, and had an annual mammogram in May. She also was seeing a counsellor.

Table 11.12: Claire's cancer and significant health history

Year 1: November 2002 to 2003	
Nov 2002	Diagnosis: T1N0 invasive ductal carcinoma (DCIS) of the right breast Wide local excision and axillary node sample of 8 lymph nodes. Tamoxifen started
Dec 2002	Radiotherapy commenced
Jan 2003	Radiotherapy completed Commences Zoladex® injections; administered every 3 months
Mar 2003	*Started acupuncture treatment*
June 2003	Follow-up with consultant. Lump in node confirmed benign
Years 2–5: November 2003 to 2007	
Dec 2004	Zoladex® treatment ended
June 2005	Menstruation resumed
Nov 2007	Tamoxifen due to end. Consultant extended treatment for one year

Years 6–10: December 2007 to October 2012	
Dec 2008	Consultant extended tamoxifen treatment for a further year
July 2008	*Acupuncture treatment to manage anal fissure (Table 11.13)*
May 2009	Concerns about loss of bone density; confirmed negative
Nov 2009	Consultant agreed to extend tamoxifen for a further 3 years, to end 2012
June 2010	Abdominal pain, bloating led to investigations for ovarian cancer. All investigations were normal. These symptoms, and other concerns, convinced Claire to stop tamoxifen
Nov 2010	Lumps discovered in breast; painful. Oncologist confirmed these were cysts
Apr 2011	Recurrence scare!
Apr–Jun 2011	*Acupuncture treatment to manage fear of recurrence (Table 11.14)*
June 2011	Received all clear from oncologist
Nov 2011	Anxiety symptoms preceded routine follow-up with oncologist. Oncologist advised Claire to continue having an annual mammogram
Oct 2012	Ten-year sign off. Claire no longer needed to see the oncologist routinely
Ten years and beyond	
Oct 2013	Discovered lump in left breast; ultrasound and mammogram confirmed it was a cyst

Main complaints

Cancer treatment-related HFNS were Claire's primary complaint. In her pre-treatment HFNS diary, she recorded 9–16 HFNS per day, with severity scores ranging from 12 to 25 (see Chapter 5, Toolkit). The majority were mild, with few severe episodes. Her definitions were:

1. mild = 'increase in temperature, bearable, no sweating'
2. moderate = 'significant increase in temperature to cause a sweat on upper lip; need cooling down'
3. severe = 'sweat breaks out over whole body'.

Incidents occurred mainly during the day, with one or two each night. The flushing sensation felt as if it was rising from her feet, lasted from one to five minutes, and then left her feeling very cold.

Other treatment priorities were to clear the spots and blotches on her upper chest and manage intermittent ankle swelling.

Questioning the systems

Sleep: Usually a very good sleeper but HFNS were waking her once or twice a night. She was able to get back to sleep after going to the toilet. Radiotherapy had made her feel very tired.

Appetite: Enjoyed food 'big time'; had a varied diet and took action to maintain a healthy weight.

Drink: Tended to be thirsty; drank hot and cold water to quench this. Was currently not drinking coffee, alcohol (usually wine) limited to three or four units a week.

Bowels: Tended to constipation; alleviated by drinking ESSIAC® tea, a nutritional supplement of which opening the bowels is a side effect.

Urination: Frequent, copious, pale.

Sweating and temperature: Temperature described as 'erratic'. She had tended to be cold since birth and related how early infant distress was alleviated only by putting her into an incubator. However, prior to her cancer diagnosis she tended to get hot in the summer, and tamoxifen-related HFNS were part of her temperature fluctuations.

Pain: Intermittent low back discomfort managed with osteopathy.

Gynaecological history: Menstruation ceased with cancer treatment. Prior to this, periods had been easy, possibly due to taking the contraceptive pill for ten years, with no premenstrual tension. Had a tendency towards constipation before the period. She and her husband chose to be child-free.

Head and body: No headaches, some dizziness and light-headedness associated with tamoxifen. No eye symptoms. Otosclerosis was causing gradual loss of hearing in the right ear.

Personal health history: Spinal fusion surgery at age 16 for severe childhood scoliosis; there was no associated chronic pain. Prior to this, had scoliosis-related bronchopneumonia. Had never smoked. At the time of presentation, she was taking tamoxifen, having Zoladex® injections every three months, took self-prescribed ESSIAC® tea and a multivitamin.

Other information: Prone to bruising easily. (This was especially noticeable in the period following cancer treatment and has improved remarkably over time.)

Relationships: Claire and her husband had a strong, supportive, and very loving relationship. Deliberately child-free, they enjoyed close relationships with their immediate and extended families and their many friends. They took pleasure in a busy social life, pursuing many interests with great enthusiasm. They shared the same exuberance and *joie de vivre*, treating life as a celebration.

Physical examination: Tongue: Pale with a white coat; swollen, with a centre crack extending from the lung area to the root. Red spots in the Heart and Lung areas, and a red tip. Sublingual veins slightly swollen and blue. **Pulses:** Deep, weak, and thin on left side, especially on the third position. Rhythm regularly intermittent, with every fourth beat very weak or missed. On right side, the pulse on the second position was the strongest of all positions, with some fullness. First position very deep and weak, equivalent to the third position on the left.

Diagnoses

CM diagnosis: Kidney yin and yang deficiency, Spleen qi deficiency leading to Spleen not controlling the Blood, damp.

CF diagnosis: Colour, sound, emotion, odour (CSEO) were challenging to identify. My initial impression centred on wood and fire; when I began to treat the CF, I focused on water. The eventual CF diagnosis is discussed below.

Treatment approach

During the two years of Zoladex® injections, acupuncture treatment focused primarily on managing HFNS, using mainly the HFNS protocol, and sometimes AE Drains, as detailed in Chapter 5, Toolkit. Claire found both effective.

Needles were not inserted in the arm and hand on the right (affected) side, observing the precautions for breast cancer patients at risk of lymphoedema (see Chapter 9, Cancer Treatment-Related Lymphoedema). I also only moxa chest points on the unaffected side.

Finding the CF

Claire's HFNS subsided when Zoladex® injections ended. At this point, I thought it appropriate to change to a Five Element approach to treatment. My rationale was that as it was no longer necessary to manage HFNS, the focus could change to supporting Claire's constitution. As I was struggling to diagnose her CF, I invited her to the Five Element study group I attended, where my colleagues also found diagnosis challenging. The group supervisor suggested treating Claire on earth.

At that session, I needled SP-8 *Diji* and ST-36 *Zusanli* bilaterally; the pulse change was remarkable. At Claire's treatment the following week, I needled the source points of earth: ST-42 *Chongyang* and SP-3 *Taibai*. In addition to significant change in the pulses, the change in Claire's energy was apparent. She was more settled, and less fiery and excitable. When she attended for her next appointment two weeks later, she reported that she felt 'less foggy', that it was as if 'a muzzy cloud has been lifted', and she felt 'awake' and 'very clear'. Her energy was good, she felt less tired, and although she couldn't 'put her finger on it', she felt better – as if 'fog has started to lift'.

I continue to treat Claire using points on the Earth channels in preference to others. This approach has evolved over the years. Claire dislikes needling, to which she responds very strongly. She loves moxa, to which she also has a strong positive response. As a general principle, I treat Claire primarily with moxa and use needles sparingly.

Treating a side effect of Zoladex®

Conventional management of haemorrhoid and anal fissure

Claire's natural tendency towards constipation was exacerbated by Zoladex®, for which constipation is a common side effect. Increased constipation, bleeding on defecation, and continual pain prompted Claire to see her doctor in December 2003. He diagnosed a thrombosed external haemorrhoid and an anal fissure. He prescribed a cream for the fissure and advised Claire to use Fybogel (ispaghula husk) to ease bowel movements.

Because of her dislike of needles, Claire declined the offer to address this aspect of her health with acupuncture until June 2008. The continuous discomfort of a skin tag drove Claire to seek specialist advice. A lateral sphincterotomy was offered. This surgical procedure makes a small cut in the sphincter muscle to reduce tension in the anal canal, allowing the anal fissure to heal and reducing the chance of developing further fissures. Regarded as an effective treatment, it carries a risk of bowel incontinence, and Claire was not enthusiastic about the possible complications.

Acupuncture management of haemorrhoid and anal fissure

Her concerns about surgical side effects outweighed her reluctance to have DU-1 *Changqiang* needled (we had discussed this on several occasions). At the end of July 2008, Claire chose to try acupuncture, and I addressed the haemorrhoids and fissure as outlined below (Table 11.13).

Table 11.13: Treatment principles and points for haemorrhoids and anal fissure

Notes:

All points needled using even technique, deqi, retained for 20 minutes.

Patient positioned on side to allow access to DU-1, and to allow moxa on needle to be in a horizontal rather than vertical position to avoid any possibility of ash falling.

Treatment principles	Points	Notes
Treat haemorrhoids and difficult defecation	DU-1 *Changqiang*	Moxa on needle.
Raise yang and counter prolapse	DU-20 *Baihui*	
Treat haemorrhoids (distal points)	BL-57 *Chengshan* BL-58 *Feiyang*	Needled unilaterally.

This was supplemented with CF treatment on Earth, usually using direct moxa. As well as addressing the CF, this strengthened the Spleen to address two syndromes associated with the condition:

- Spleen qi sinking
- Spleen not controlling Blood.

After the first treatment, Claire reported a dramatic change. Bleeding and pain had both reduced, with the latter occurring only with a bowel movement.

Treatment continued once weekly or fortnightly. After four treatments over eight weeks, Claire said, 'I can't believe the difference':

- Bleeding and pain had substantially reduced.
- She no longer suffered the 'agony' of tears.
- Bowel habits had improved.

- And, best of all, 'I haven't had to have an operation'.

Lifestyle changes

These improvements enabled Claire to identify habits that exacerbated the condition. She increased her consumption of fruit and ensured she drank sufficient water. This improved her bowel movements; however, constipation worsened when she travelled (which was frequently), and when working (as an events manager, she was often on her feet for long hours, eating and drinking irregularly when facilitating an event).

The outcome

We continued with acupuncture treatment as described above. In February 2009, Claire had a follow-up appointment with the consultant, who was amazed at the difference.

His examination found there was no spasm and the scar tissue on the fissure had improved dramatically. He felt surgery would no longer be necessary and advised Claire to 'continue what you are doing'. Nevertheless, he advised an investigation. A sigmoidoscopy a few weeks later showed no polyps and no evidence of a fissure; in short, he declared it 'a perfect colon…whatever you are doing has sorted it out'.

We discontinued this treatment shortly afterwards. Happily, these symptoms have not recurred; Claire self-manages any early signs of problems by addressing diet and fluid intake to avoid any recurrence.

Managing an acute episode of fear of recurrence
Tamoxifen as a safety blanket

Claire took a pragmatic approach to having a cancer diagnosis. She managed her health using a combination of conventional and complementary approaches, along with modifications in her lifestyle. She had confidence in her oncologist, with whom she had a lively relationship. While she experienced some apprehension around the time of her annual check-ups, overall, she was not one to worry unduly.

Tamoxifen played a key role in maintaining Claire's peace of mind. She called it her 'safety blanket'. At a time when tamoxifen was routinely prescribed for five years, Claire persuaded her oncologist to extend her adjuvant treatment for up to ten years (now the recommended prescription). For many women, the end date of tamoxifen cannot come too soon; for Claire, coming off the prescription in June 2010 after seven and a half years provoked a crisis.

The appearance of troubling symptoms

When she attended for acupuncture early in April 2011, Claire mentioned a 'strange sensation in the back of her throat' that was 'hard to explain'. Careful questioning uncovered that she was very worried about her annual mammogram scheduled for mid-May, and this anxiety sprang from discontinuing tamoxifen.

The throat sensation was particularly frightening, as she had experienced this once before – just prior to her cancer diagnosis. Typically, Claire took control of the situation and saw her oncologist the following Monday. She was 'completely relieved' when the physical examination revealed nothing to cause concern; however, he advised that the mammogram be brought forward by two weeks. He also remarked that Claire didn't have anything to worry about as she wasn't experiencing breast pain.

This comment sparked rather than calmed Claire's anxieties, and she explained:

> On leaving the hospital I found I was getting strange pains in my left breast, which I had not experienced before. I couldn't explain what these were and then recalled the earlier comment my consultant had made and my anxiety levels were raised again.

The powerful effects of fear of recurrence

Over the ensuing weeks, she developed multiple symptoms. Normally able to sleep well, she had restless nights. She had difficulty breathing, palpitations, and chest pain. The breast sensations varied from stabbing pains to a dull ache to 'niggling' pains.

These worsened when she noticed veins protruding in her left breast, which were more evident at night. Added to this was the development of a rash between her breasts – another symptom that had preceded her initial cancer diagnosis.

We discussed how these symptoms had followed on from the oncologist's chance remark, and how Claire might be somatising her anxieties around the possibilities of breast cancer recurrence after ceasing tamoxifen. Claire was able to detach somewhat from her distress and observe how fear of recurrence was affecting her. She was fascinated; having never suffered from anxiety before, she was intrigued by the power of her mind over her body.

Managing fear of recurrence

This period spanned ten weeks. As luck would have it, there was a delay in obtaining her mammogram results and again in contacting her oncologist. Mounting anxiety transformed to anger.

During this worrying time, I focused on managing Claire's anxiety and relieving the breast symptoms (Table 11.14). As Claire was normally emotionally stable, the intensity of her reaction and its powerful manifestation suggested Internal Dragons (see Chapter 5, Toolkit), which I addressed several times during this time.

I also regularly applied:

- a heat lamp on the lower jiao, which Claire found immensely comforting and which had a powerful grounding effect
- gold ear magnets to the back of each ear, opposite *Shenmen* (*Reverse Shenmen*) to enable Claire to manage anxiety between treatments.

Table 11.14: Managing fear of recurrence and breast symptoms

Abbreviations: RS right side; **LS** left side; **bi** bilateral; **(n)** shows number of direct moxa cones applied

Date 2011	Treatment principles	Points	Notes
March	Throat symptoms triggered concerns about cancer recurrence		
5 Apr	Calm shen	'Toasted Pericardium Sandwich': BL-43 *Gaohuangshu* (15) REN-17 *Shanzhong* (5)	Direct moxa only.
		M-HN-3 *Yintang*	
	Harmonise Liver qi	LIV-3 *Taichong* (bi)	
10 Apr	Consultation with oncologist; chance remark triggered symptoms		
13 Apr	Calm shen	M-HN-3 *Yintang*	
	Benefit chest, breast, and lateral costal region	SP-4 *Gongsun* (RS) SP-21 *Dabao* (LS) GB-41 *Zulinqi* (LS)	
	Support CF (Earth)	ST-14 *Kufang* (5) (LS) SP-20 *Zhourong* (5) (LS)	Direct moxa only.
19 Apr	Internal Dragons (IDs)	Master point 0.25 cun below REN-15 *Jiuwei* ST-25 *Tianshu* (bi) ST-32 *Futu* (bi) ST-41 *Jiexi* (bi)	
	Ground treatment	SI-4 *Wangu* (LS) HE-7 *Shenmen* (LS)	
28 Apr	Period started (menstruation had restarted in June 2005)		
3 May	Treat pain in left breast	LIV-14 *Qimen* (LS)	
	Repeat IDs and ground treatment	As per 19 Apr	
5 May	Mammogram. Palpitations		
10 May	Calm shen Regulate heart qi Relieve chest and breast pain	'Toasted Pericardium Sandwich': BL-43 *Gaohuangshu* (15) REN-17 *Shanzhong* (5)	Direct moxa only.
		BL-14 *Jueyinshu* (LS) HE-7 *Shenmen* (LS) P-7 *Daling* (LS)	
17 May	Repeat IDs and ground treatment	As per 19 Apr	Claire very agitated.
22 May	Period started 4 days early; unusual for Claire as periods were very regular		
23 May	Repeat IDs and ground treatment	As per 19 Apr	Claire very angry re delays.
	Got all clear		
8 June	Calm shen	M-HN-3 *Yintang*	
	Treat CF/Tonify and warm Stomach and Spleen qi	ST-36 *Zusanli* (7) (bi) SP-3 *Taibai* (3) (bi)	Direct moxa only.
	Support spirit	KID-25 *Shencang* (3) (LS) KID-27 *Shufu* (3) (LS)	

Once Claire received the 'all clear', her symptoms began to disappear. The intensity of this ten-week period was remarkable, particularly as it was so uncharacteristic of Claire's usual approach to life.

Ten years and beyond

As a rule, the more time that passes since diagnosis, the less likelihood there is of recurrence. At her ten-year 'sign-off', Claire's oncologist advised her that her risk of breast cancer was the same as that of the general population.

Claire remained cautious, choosing to continue annual mammograms. This close monitoring was how she chose to maintain peace of mind as she proceeded into the next decade of survivorship. Given the intense reaction detailed above, this was a sensible strategy for managing her anxieties about recurrence.

Summary and follow-up

By agreeing to the publication of her details, Claire has provided a unique insight into how acupuncture can be used in the support of survivorship, up to and beyond the ten-year anniversary of diagnosis.

Initially used to manage immediate side effects of adjuvant treatment (HFNS), acupuncture also addressed longer-term consequences of her treatment (haemorrhoids and anal fissure), and then evolved to support Claire constitutionally. Perhaps the most remarkable aspect of her history is the power of the fear of recurrence, and its capacity to cause uncharacteristic behaviours in one who is as usually pragmatic as Claire.

Coda

At the time of going to press, Claire is poised to mark 30 years since her diagnosis. She remains well, continuing to use acupuncture to manage the menopause transition as well as the stresses of being a carer for her and her husband's ageing parents. She no longer needs the reassurance of an annual mammogram and is screened every three years as per current practice in the UK. I continue to avoid needling in her right arm and hand and use moxa in preference to needles whenever possible.

Survivorship and ageing

Cancer survivorship is a phenomenon of an ageing population. In the USA, nearly two thirds (64%) of the estimated 16.9 million individuals with a cancer history are aged 65 or over.[47]

As survivors age, their health may be affected by other diseases of ageing.[48] For many survivors, the risk of dying from a non-cancer-related condition is greater than death from cancer.[49] Cheryl, a woman treated for breast cancer 30 previously, was shocked when she was diagnosed with type 2 diabetes. She told me that ever since her cancer diagnosis, she had simply assumed that she would die of cancer-related causes.

While studies quoted at the beginning of this chapter report that long-term cancer survivors enjoy quality of life similar to people their age without cancer, preoccupation with cancer-related health worries can last many years, or even a lifetime. Fifty-seven per cent of respondents in a large American survey agreed that cancer would always be part of their lives.[50]

It is important to be aware of the long-term effects that cancer can have on survivors' lives.

CHAPTER SUMMARY

- Cancer survivors may experience consequences of diagnosis and treatment after primary treatment ends. These may be short term or chronic, may change over time, and may cause discomfort and distress.
- The first year following diagnosis and treatment may be especially challenging, as individuals strive to reintegrate their lives. Acupuncturists should be aware that this is a time when depression and anxiety may occur.
- Fear of recurrence is common, may be intermittent or chronic, and may powerfully impact physical and emotional wellbeing. This may occur at any stage of the cancer trajectory.
- Acupuncturists can play a key role in supporting people living with and beyond cancer, and in understanding the immediate and long-term consequences of diagnosis and treatment.

References

1. Doyle N Cancer survivorship: evolutionary concept analysis. J. Adv. Nurs. 2008;62(4):499–509.
2. Ganz PA, Desmond K, Leedham B, *et al.* Quality of life in long-term, disease-free survivors of breast cancer: a follow-up study. J. Natl. Cancer Inst. 2002;94(1):39–49.
3. Hsu T, Ennis M, Hood N, *et al.* Quality of life in long-term breast cancer survivors. J. Clin. Oncol. 2013;31(28):3540–3548.
4. Smith SK, Mayer DK, Zimmerman S, *et al.* Quality of life among long-term survivors of non-Hodgkin lymphoma: a follow-up study. J. Clin. Oncol. 2013;31(2):272–279.
5. Deimling G, Bowman K, Sternes S, *et al.* Cancer-related health worries and psychological distress among older adult, long-term cancer survivors. Psycho-oncology 2006;15:306–320.
6. Carlson LE, Speca M Managing daily and long-term stress. In: Feuerstein M, editor. Handbook of cancer survivorship. New York: Springer; 2007. pp. 339–360.
7. Seiler A, Jenewein J Resilience in cancer patients. Front. Psychiatry 2019;10:208.
8. Ramsey SD, Berry K, Moinpour C, *et al.* Quality of life in long term survivors of colorectal cancer. Am. J. Gastroenterol. 2002;97(5):1228–1234.
9. Cummings A, Grimmett C, Calman L, *et al.* Comorbidities are associated with poorer quality of life and functioning and worse symptoms in the 5 years following colorectal cancer surgery: results from the ColoREctal Well-being (CREW) cohort study. Psychooncology 2018;27(10):2427–2435.
10. Calman L, Turner J, Fenlon D, *et al.* Prevalence and determinants of depression up to 5 years after colorectal cancer surgery: results from the ColoREctal Wellbeing (CREW) study. Colorectal Dis. 2021;23(12):3234–3250.
11. Wu HS, Harden JK Symptom burden and quality of life in survivorship: a review of the literature. Cancer Nurs. 2015;38(1):E29–E54.
12. Elliott J, Fallows A, Staetsky L, *et al.* The health and well-being of cancer survivors in the UK: findings from a population-based study. Br. J. Cancer 2011;105:S11–S20.
13. Simard S, Thewes B, Humphris G, *et al.* Fear of cancer recurrence in adult cancer survivors: a systematic review of quantitative studies. J. Cancer Surviv. 2013;7:300–322.
14. Götze H, Taubenheim S, Dietz A, *et al.* Fear of cancer recurrence across the survivorship trajectory: results from a survey of adult long-term cancer survivors. Psychooncology 2019;28(10):2033–2041.

15. Glaser A, Fraser LK, Corner J, *et al.* Patient-reported outcomes of cancer survivors in England 1–5 years after diagnosis: a cross-sectional survey. BMJ Open 2013;3(e002317).

16. Department of Health Quality of life of cancer survivors in England: report on a pilot survey using Patient Reported Outcome Measures (PROMS). London: National Institute of Health Research; 2012.

17. Koch L, Jansen L, Brenner H, *et al.* Fear of recurrence and disease progression in long-term (≥ 5 years) cancer survivors – a systematic review of quantitative studies. Psycho-oncology 2013;22:1–11.

18. Crist JV, Grunfeld EA Factors reported to influence fear of recurrence in cancer patients: a systematic review. Psychooncology 2013;22(5):978–86.

19. Lidington E, Vlooswijk C, Stallard K, *et al.* 'This is not part of my life plan': a qualitative study on the psychosocial experiences and practical challenges in young adults with cancer age 25 to 39 years at diagnosis. Eur. J. Cancer Care (Engl). 2021;30(5):e13458.

20. Bui KT, Liang R, Kiely BE, *et al.* Scanxiety: a scoping review about scan-associated anxiety. BMJ Open 2021;11(5):e043215.

21. Foster C, Fenlon D Recovery and self-management support following primary cancer treatment Br. J. Cancer 2011;105:S21–S28.

22. de Valois B, Asprey A, Young T 'The monkey on your shoulder': a qualitative study of lymphoedema patients' attitudes to and experiences of acupuncture and moxibustion. Evid. Based Complement. Alternat. Med. 2016;Article ID 4298420.

23. Hewitt M, Greenfield S, Stovall E From cancer patient to cancer survivor: lost in transition. Washington DC: National Academies Press; 2005.

24. Macmillan Cancer Support Two million reasons: the cancer survivorship agenda. London: Macmillan Cancer Support; 2008 September 2008.

25. Hicks A, Hicks J, Mole P Five element constitutional acupuncture. Edinburgh: Churchill Livingstone; 2004.

26. Macmillan Cancer Support It's no life: living with the long term effects of cancer. London: Macmillan Cancer Support; 2009.

27. PDQ˚ Supportive and Palliative Care Editorial Board PDQ Cancer-related post-traumatic stress. Bethesda, MD: National Cancer Institute; 2019. Available from: www.cancer.gov/about-cancer/coping/survivorship/new-normal/ptsd-hp-pdq

28. Cancer Research UK Can stress cause cancer?; 2021. Available from: www.cancerresearchuk.org/about-cancer/causes-of-cancer/cancer-myths/can-stress-cause-cancer#referenceso

29. Macmillan Cancer Support Move more: physical activity the underrated 'wonder drug'. London; 2011. Available from: www.macmillan.org.uk/Documents/Cancerinfo/Physicalactivity/Physicalactivitycampaignreportlores.pdf

30. Deadman P Insufficient rest. In: Live well live long. Hove: The Journal of Chinese Medicine; 2016 p. 47.

31. Ackerman J Sex sleep eat drink dream: a day in the life of your body. New York: Houghton Mifflin Company; 2007.

32. Cancer Research UK Cancer survival statistics for all cancers combined. 2014. Available from: www.cancerresearchuk.org/health-professional/cancer-statistics/survival/all-cancers-combined#heading-Zero

33. American Cancer Society Cancer facts & figures 2021. Atlanta: American Cancer Society; 2021. Available from: www.cancer.org/content/dam/cancer-org/research/cancer-facts-and-statistics/annual-cancer-facts-and-figures/2021/cancer-facts-and-figures-2021.pdf

34. American Society of Clinical Oncology (ASCO) Understanding statistics used to guide prognosis and evaluate treatment. Alexandria, VA; 2020. Available from: www.cancer.net/navigating-cancer-care/cancer-basics/understanding-statistics-used-guide-prognosis-and-evaluate-treatment

35. Corner J, Wagland R, Glaser A, *et al.* Qualitative analysis of patients' feedback from a PROMs survey of cancer patients in England. BMJ Open 2013;3:e002316.

36. Ribeiro Pereira ACP, Koifman RJ, Bergmann A Incidence and risk factors of lymphedema after breast cancer treatment: 10 years of follow-up. Breast 2017;36:67–73.

37. Maciocia G The foundations of Chinese medicine. London: Churchill Livingstone; 1989.

38. Deadman P, Al-Khafaji M, Baker K A manual of acupuncture. Hove: The Journal of Chinese Medicine; 2007.

39. Maciocia G The channels of acupuncture: clinical use of the secondary channels and eight extraordinary vessels. Edinburgh: Churchill Livingstone; 2006.

40. Xiaorong C, Jing H, Shouxiang Y Illustrated Chinese moxibustion: techniques and methods. London: Singing Dragon; 2012.

41. Maciocia G The psyche in Chinese medicine. London: Churchill Livingstone; 2009.

42. National Cancer Control Indicators (NCCI) 10-year relative survival. Australia: Cancer Australia; 2020. Available from: https://ncci.canceraustralia.gov.au/outcomes/relative-survival-rate/10-year-relative-survival

43. Macmillan Cancer Support Cured – but at what cost: long-term consequences of cancer and its treatment. Macmillan Cancer Support; 2013. Available from: www.macmillan.org.uk/documents/aboutus/newsroom/consequences_of_treatment_june2013.pdf

44. Hussain A, Tripathi A, Pieczonka C, *et al.* Bone health effects of androgen-deprivation therapy and androgen receptor inhibitors in patients with nonmetastatic castration-resistant prostate cancer. Prostate Cancer Prostatic Dis. 2021;24:290–300.

45. Leclère B, Molinié F, Trétarre B, *et al.* Trends in incidence of breast cancer among women under 40 in seven European countries: a GRELL cooperative study. Cancer Epidemiol. 2013;37(5):544–549.

46. Huang J, Chan PS, Lok V, *et al.* Global incidence and mortality of breast cancer: a trend analysis. Aging (Albany NY) 2021;13(4):5748–5803.

47. American Cancer Society Cancer Treatment & Survivorship Facts & Figures 2019–2021. Atlanta: American Cancer Society; 2019.

48. Leach CR, Bellizzi KM, Hurria A, *et al.* Is it my cancer or am I just getting older? Impact of cancer on age-related health conditions of older cancer survivors. Cancer 2016;122(12):1946–1953.

49. Zaorsky NG, Churilla TM, Egleston BL, *et al.* Causes of death among cancer patients. Ann. Oncol. 2017;28(2):400–407.

50. Wolff S The burden of cancer survivorship: a pandemic of treatment success. In: Feuerstein M, editor. Handbook of cancer survivorship. New York: Springer; 2007. pp. 7–18.

Chapter 12

Supporting Resilience and the Immune System

The importance of living well after cancer treatment, and the role acupuncture can play in this, are summarised in these quotations:

> To live as well as possible in every area of our lives we need more than medicine. (Dr Catherine Zollman, Medical Director, Penny Brohn UK)[1]

> My quality of life has improved... I now feel I can lead a normal life again. (Dolores, a breast cancer survivor on her course of acupuncture treatment)

Background

Cancer and its treatments take their toll on the body's immune function. During or following cancer treatments, many survivors are keen to support their immunity. They may wish to reduce risk of recurrence, deal with the long-term and late effects of treatment, and minimise their chances of developing other illnesses. Acupuncture, moxibustion, and lifestyle habits can be beneficial in supporting the immune system, helping it to recover and function at optimum levels. This in turn facilitates the development of resilience and the ability to cope with life's challenges.

Resilience

TERMINOLOGY

Resilience is the 'process of adapting well in the face of adversity, trauma, tragedy, threats, or significant sources of stress – such as family and relationship problems, serious health problems, or workplace and financial stressors. It is the ability to "bounce back" from difficult circumstances and may involve profound personal growth.'[2]

Resilience is enabled through many factors, including personal control, positive affect (having positive emotions), optimism, and social support. Anyone can develop resilience by learning or adopting behaviours that enable one to cope with significant life challenges. An individual's resilience may vary through the course of life; cancer diagnosis

380

and treatment are major stressors that can both test and develop an individual's resilience. So too is survivorship.

The relationship between resilience and the immune system

In an extensive review, Dantzer et al.[3] discuss the bi-directional relationship between resilience and immunity. While there is considerable evidence about the impact of psychological factors on resilience, Dantzer's team are interested in the effect of the immune system on resilience. Arguing that 'immune mediators can influence factors that contribute to resilience and stress outcomes', they cite evidence that chronic inflammation and infectious diseases often trigger 'sickness behaviour'. This comprises non-specific psychological and behavioural changes including fatigue, malaise, the inability to feel pleasure (anhedonia), disturbed sleep, poor concentration, and social withdrawal. In short, poor immunity may impact the factors needed to develop resilience.

The case studies of Dolores and Molly (below) tell the stories of two cancer survivors struggling to cope with life after having successfully negotiated cancer diagnosis and treatment. Repeated chronic infections impact their resilience and ability to deal with the stressors of life, such as Dolores's multiple bereavements. These cases demonstrate how acupuncture can relieve the burden of infections and facilitate the 'bounce back' effect. This important role that acupuncture can play is recognised by cancer centres such as Penny Brohn in the UK, which incorporate acupuncture in their wellness programmes for people living with cancer.[4]

The immune system and cancer
Function of the immune system

A healthy immune system functions to create the immune response – a chain of reactions designed to rid the body of foreign material, including external microorganisms that invade the body and abnormal cells that develop within the body. A complex network comprising white blood cells (leukocytes), and the organs and tissues of the lymph system (including the thymus, spleen, tonsils, lymph nodes, lymph vessels, and bone marrow), it provides:

- **Non-specific immunity** – a general defence against anything recognised as 'not self', comprising neutrophils, monocytes, macrophages, and natural killer (NK) cells.
- **Specific immunity** – whereby lymphocytes (T cells and B cells) recognise and target specific threatening agents.

Cancer and the immune system

A weakened immune system may contribute to the formation of some cancers when the body's natural defences are unable to deal with potentially harmful microorganisms or to identify and eliminate abnormal cells. Cancer itself can weaken the immune system, especially if it spreads to the bone marrow and interferes with the production of blood cells that help fight infection. This is most associated with leukaemia and lymphoma and may happen with other cancers as well.

Cancer treatments and the immune system

Cancer treatments may also weaken the immune system. Surgery elicits a 'surgical stress response', characterised by profound changes in the neuroendocrine, metabolic, and immune systems. Interventions associated with surgery, including anaesthesia, blood transfusion, as well as post-operative pain and hyperglycaemia, also disrupt immune performance.[5] It may take several months for the immune system to recover from surgical stress. (This applies to surgery for any reason and is not restricted to cancer treatment.) Surgery involving removal of lymph nodes, which filter out harmful substances while triggering an immune response, may further impact immune performance.

Chemotherapy affects the immune system primarily during the chemotherapy cycle, when damage to the neutrophils (white blood cells) is most severe. This begins in the week following treatment, reaches its nadir (the point at which white blood cell production is lowest) at 7–14 days, and then begins to recover in time for the next treatment (usually the third week). It is generally expected that the immune system will recover in 21–28 days after all chemotherapy treatment is completed.[6] However, recovery may take a more prolonged period and many survivors continue to experience signs of suppressed immunity, including increased susceptibility to colds, flu, and other infections, for some time.

While the effect of radiotherapy on the immune system is regarded as generally mild, radiotherapy to areas of lymph nodes may contribute to infection in the associated limb(s) or trunk, leading to lymphoedema. Production of blood cells in the bone marrow may be affected by radiation to the bone, particularly in relation to the pelvis, or the head and neck (e.g. osteoradionecrosis).

Each of these treatment modalities impacts the immune system. As cancer survivors may have experienced multiple modes of cancer treatment, the cumulative effects on the immune system can be extensive.

Biomedical advice for supporting the immune system

Cancer organisations[7,8] provide advice to people with cancer who wish to support their immune system, giving the recommendations for healthy living (Box 12.1). These recommendations are appropriate for any person and may improve outcomes for many other chronic conditions (e.g. cardiovascular disease).

Box 12.1: Taking care of the immune system

- Sleep: aim to obtain at least seven hours of good quality sleep. Evidence shows there is a relationship between poor sleep and reduced immune function.[9,10]
- Nutrition: eat a healthy, well-balanced diet. Rely on fresh, whole foods rather than vitamins and supplements to obtain optimum nutrition.

- Physical activity: moderate regular physical activity has positive benefits on the immune system (see Chapter 13, Reducing Risk of Recurrence and Subsequent Primary Cancers).
- Stress reduction: chronic, high levels of stress hormones (such as adrenaline and cortisol) can suppress the immune system, thereby reducing the body's capacity to defend or repair itself.[11] Finding ways to manage long-term stress can be helpful during and after cancer treatment. Many techniques may be helpful; some examples include meditation, mindfulness, tai qi and qigong, yoga, acupuncture, massage, reflexology, support groups.
- Avoid smoking and alcohol.

East Asian medicine approaches to supporting the immune system
Chinese medicine approaches to supporting the immune system
In Chinese medicine (CM), defensive (Wei) qi is the first line of defence against external pathogenic factors. Defensive qi is controlled by the Lung; however, it is rooted in the Kidney (originating from essence and original qi, and transformed by Kidney yang), and is nourished by food qi produced in the Spleen and Stomach. Thus, even this first line of defence relies for its strength on the health of the Kidney, Stomach, Spleen, and Lung.

The health of all the organs, the vital substances, and yin and yang all contribute to a strong immune system. No one pattern equates with the immune system; and conversely, an imbalance in any of these aspects may lead to diminished immunity. Thus, the immune system is supported through the normal mechanisms of CM diagnosis of the individual and the associated treatment. The case studies below illustrate two different approaches to supporting the immune system using CM approaches.

The evidence for using acupuncture to support the immune system
Chinese research on animals and humans reports significant improvements in many mechanisms of immune function after acupuncture.[12] Human studies tend to focus on chemotherapy-related myelosuppression, which causes a decrease in blood cell production, including the leukocytes responsible for immunity. Most published studies have been conducted in China, are available in the Chinese language only, and use a variety of modalities including acupuncture, electro-acupuncture, and warm needling. A meta-analysis of Chinese studies noted that there appeared to be a clinically significant level of improvement in white blood cell counts in chemotherapy patients treated with acupuncture; however, due to the poor quality of the studies, the authors caution that these results 'should be treated in an exploratory nature only'.[13]

ST-36 Zusanli, the immune-enhancing acupoint
In their review of acupuncture for chemotherapy-related myelosuppression, Wong and Sagar note that ST-36 Zusanli (see Figure 5.16) was used in all the studies they reviewed.[14] Johnston et al. also note its frequent use to enhance immune function, calling it the 'immune-enhancing acupoint'.[15] They comment that while ST-36 Zusanli alone appears

to produce a measurable effect on immune function in animal studies, its use in humans 'in conjunction with other well-chosen points would lead to even more effective immune enhancement'.[15]

The evidence for using moxibustion to support the immune system

Chinese studies on animals report marked improvements in immune cell function of tumour-bearing mice, using single points such as DU-14 *Dazhui*, REN-4 *Guanyuan*, or REN-8 *Shenque*.[12]

A systematic review of moxibustion for chemotherapy-induced leukopenia in humans, which identified six Chinese randomised controlled trials, concluded that 'moxibustion was more effective than various types of control interventions in increasing white blood cell counts'.[16] The number of sessions, duration of treatment, and moxibustion style varied across the studies, which used a variety of indirect moxibustion techniques (e.g. moxa on herbs or ginger, or a thermal moxa stick). Points used included ST-36 *Zusanli*, REN-8 *Shenque*, and DU-14 *Dazhui*. The studies reported increased leukocytes (white blood cells and platelets) and reduced side effects of chemotherapy.

Using acupuncture and moxibustion to support the immune system
Reflections on my clinical experience

Over the years, many survivors have come for acupuncture to 'boost' their immune systems. I have always tailored treatment to their individual presentation; in my opinion, there is no standard treatment that fits all circumstances.

A healthy immune system relies on the balance and harmony of all the body's systems. To meet the needs of an individual, all their presenting symptoms and circumstances should be considered. Addressing physical and emotional symptoms, as well as lifestyle practices, forms part of addressing the toll that cancer and its treatment takes, as shown in the case of Dolores below.

Five Element approaches to supporting the immune system

Five Element acupuncture is well suited to treatment of chronic conditions and is an elegant way to strengthen the immune system. Using minimal intervention, it aims to return the Five Elements to a balanced state by restoring the underlying imbalance, the constitutional factor (CF), to a state of health. This enables individuals to enjoy better physical and psychological health, as well as reducing their predisposition to suffer from future health problems.[17] I often treat patients solely using Five Elements acupuncture, or use it in conjunction with other approaches, as demonstrated in the case studies throughout this book.

Moxibustion approaches to supporting the immune system

Moxibustion for health cultivation has been used throughout East Asia historically and in modern times. It is used to treat disease, to restore health to patients weakened by illness, and to preserve health and prevent disease. With its abilities to 'regulate qi and blood, warm and open the channels and collaterals, warm and nourish the organs, and prolong life', moxibustion can play a key role in rehabilitating survivors weakened by cancer and its treatments, as well as improving their health long term.[18]

Chapter 5, Toolkit, discusses moxibustion. Table 12.1 lists some moxibustion techniques I commonly use to enhance the immunity of cancer survivors (see also Table 6.4).

Table 12.1: Some points to use with moxibustion to support the immune system of cancer survivors

Points	Indications[19]	Method
ST-36 *Zusanli*	General tonic; to nourish Blood; tonify qi and yang; tonify qi of the entire body, and support the upright qi.	Stick, warm needle, or direct (7–20 cones). Also, for self-moxa by the patient.
BL-43 *Gaohuangshu*	General tonic; to tonify and nourish the Lung, Heart, Kidney, Spleen, and Stomach; nourish yin; treat all types of deficiency taxation. I often combine this with direct or indirect moxa on REN-17 *Shanzhong*, especially for anxious patients – see the 'Toasted Pericardium Sandwich' in Chapter 5, Toolkit.	Direct (7–50 cones, usually 15 on each point). I use this bilaterally or unilaterally, depending on the lymphoedema status of the individual. For REN-17, direct moxa (3–5 cones).
REN-4 *Guanyuan*	General tonic, especially for those in later life; to nourish Blood; fortify original qi; tonify and nourish the Kidney; warm and strengthen the Spleen; benefit the Bladder; restore the yang.	Stick, warm needle, or direct (7–20 cones).
REN-8 *Shenque*	Exhaustion; to warm and rescue yang.	Moxa box, moxa on salt or ginger; stick.

Self-management with moxa

I often teach patients to self-moxa ST-36 *Zusanli* (Figure 12.1). Many survivors find this gives them a sense of control, and they feel they are actively contributing to improving their health. It is a procedure that is easy to teach and for patients to self-administer in their own homes. See Chapter 5, Toolkit, for instructions on how to teach patients to do this.

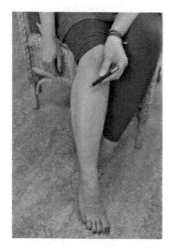

FIGURE 12.1: SELF-MOXA ON ST-36 *ZUSANLI*

Seasonal treatment for deficiency of defensive qi

For repeated, debilitating respiratory infections associated with deficiency of defensive qi, I follow Maciocia's seasonal treatment (Table 12.2).[20] Maciocia recommends doing this three times a week for a month, ideally from mid-August to mid-September. This corresponds to autumn (on the Chinese Farmer's calendar) with its association with the metal element and the Lung. Over time, this can help reduce susceptibility in those who need repeated antibiotic treatment for bronchial and other respiratory infections.

To administer this treatment:

- I ask the patient to bring a companion to the initial appointment. Using surgical pen, I mark up the points and show the companion how to use stick moxa.
- For patients attending for acupuncture on a weekly basis, I administer this treatment using direct moxa, and have the companion carry out the treatment twice more during the week using indirect stick moxa.
- For patients who do not have a helpful companion, I recommend self-moxa on ST-36 *Zusanli* in addition to attending for weekly treatment on the points in Table 12.2.

Table 12.2: Seasonal treatment to tonify defensive qi[20]

Points	Method	Frequency and timing
BL-12 *Fengmen* BL-13 *Feishu* DU-12 *Shenzhu* ST-36 *Zusanli*	Indirect stick moxa, 3 minutes each point OR, direct moxa, usually 7 cones per point OR, a combination of both methods (as discussed above).	Carry out this procedure 3 times per week, for one month. Mid-August through mid-September is the optimum time for adminstering.

Other moxa techniques

Many points and moxibustion techniques can be used to enhance the immune system. In *Illustrated Chinese Moxibustion: Techniques and Methods,* Xiarong *et al.* devote a chapter to the modern clinical use of moxibustion for health cultivation, recommending the following points as being effective when used on their own with moxa (Table 12.3).[18]

Table 12.3: Acupoints for health cultivation moxatherapy

Ll-4 *Hegu* Ll-11 *Quchi* SP-6 *Sanyinjiao* BL-12 *Fengmen*	BL-23 *Shenshu* KID-1 *Yongquan* REN-6 *Qihai* REN-12 *Zhongwan*	DU-4 *Mingmen* DU-12 *Shenzhu* DU-14 *Dazhui*

In a comprehensive discussion of moxa techniques and procedures, Abbate provides several moxa points and prescriptions to enhance immunity, as listed in Table 12.4.[21]

Table 12.4: Moxa prescriptions to enhance immunity

Points	Energetics	Notes
Ll-4 *Hegu* ST-36 *Zusanli* BL-12 *Fengmen* BL-23 *Shenshu* BL-43 *Gaohuangshu* TB-5 *Waiguan* REN-4 *Guanyuan* REN-17 *Shanzhong* DU-4 *Mingmen* DU-14 *Dazhui*	A repertoire of tonic points to strengthen immunity for immunodeficient patients and to increase white blood cell production.	Use a non-scarring method. Use small cones, few moxas, and monitor for heat aggravation as immune deficient patients are also often yin deficient. • For BL-12 *Fengmen* and DU-14 *Dazhui*, moxa until the skin reddens and the neck feels warm. • For REN-17 *Shanzhong* use mild moxa (indirect stick or 3 moxa cones) due to its proximity to the heart.
ST-36 *Zusanli* REN-4 *Guanyuan* REN-6 *Qihai* DU-4 *Mingmen*	Points to increase longevity.	Moxa each point every other day for 10 minutes.
KlD-1 *Yongquan*	Tonify the Kidney.	Use tiger warmer, with pressure.
Ll-11 *Quchi* KlD-6 *Zhaohai* TB-16 *Tianyou* DU-14 *Dazhui*	Known as 'tonsillar treatment' – strengthens immunity by activating lymphatic tissues.	

Cautions and contraindications

There is a wide choice of approaches for using moxibustion to enhance immunity. Treatments using moxibustion should be tailored to the diagnosis and the treatment principles selected for the individual patient.

Observe the usual cautions and contraindications. Exercise caution with patients who may be at increased risk of burns due to inability to feel or communicate about temperature sensation, including those with:

- decreased neurological functioning due to nerve damage (the result of some chemotherapy regimens)
- diabetes
- reduced mental status
- extreme age.

Painkillers and steroids may also affect pain perception, so exercise caution with patients taking these.[21] Head and neck cancer patients who have a breathing stoma may be sensitive to moxa, including smokeless moxa.[22]

I am also guided by patient response. I find many cancer survivors really love moxa, enjoying the warmth, aroma, and comfort it provides. When patients actively dislike moxa, or are sceptical about it, I do not use it.

Lifestyle advice

The lifestyle advice I offer follows that listed in Box 12.1, modified according to the individual's needs. For example, this might include recommending introducing foods that nourish the Blood for survivors who are Blood deficient. I encourage those prone to colds and flu to protect themselves from invasions of wind by wearing appropriate clothing and avoiding drafts.

Case studies

Several case studies in this book illustrate how acupuncture can support the immune system and facilitate increased resilience, including Ann in Chapter 14, Getting My Life Back. The studies of Dolores and Molly, presented below, illustrate two different approaches to achieving these goals.

CASE STUDY: DOLORES AND TREATING METAL AND EARTH TO SUPPORT THE IMMUNE SYSTEM

Introduction

Dolores was a reserved, soft-spoken woman who worked full time as a health professional. She attended initially for 13 acupuncture treatments during 2009 as part of the research study into using acupuncture to improve wellbeing and quality of life of people with lymphoedema (see Chapter 9, Cancer Treatment-Related Lymphoedema). She later attended briefly for private treatment in 2010 and again in 2011.

This case study presents her 2009 treatment, during which she reported benefits relating to her lymphoedema and general wellbeing. It focuses on the role acupuncture played in supporting Dolores's immune function as well as contributing to building her resilience. This case demonstrates the complex interrelationship between emotions, cancer-related fatigue, and immune function. I am grateful to Dolores for her permission and her informative written comments about her acupuncture treatment.

Background and main complaints

Dolores, aged 57, was diagnosed six years previously (2003) with ductal carcinoma in situ (DCIS) of the left breast. Surgery, comprising a wide local excision and sentinel node biopsy, was followed by radiotherapy and adjuvant hormonal treatment with tamoxifen. Five years later (in 2008), cellulitis in the left breast triggered lymphoedema in her hand. The lymphoedema was mild, and Dolores was concordant with prescribed exercises to manage this.

More troublesome for Dolores were repeated chest infections experienced over the previous two years. Salbutamol and Becotide had been prescribed, although Dolores was not asthmatic. When she came for acupuncture in March 2009, she had suffered a chronic cold and sinusitis since the previous Christmas and was on sick leave from work for a month.

Questioning the systems

At her initial consultation, Dolores spoke of experiencing recurrent respiratory infections since her mother's death the previous year. Antibiotics, inhalers, and time off work were proving ineffective against the current infection, characterised by severe and painful sinusitis, which had continued for over three months. Breathing was difficult, and she had lost her senses of smell and taste. There was no discharge of mucous.

Sleep: Sinusitis disturbed her usually good sleep pattern; consequently, she felt tired in the morning. She sometimes experienced dream-disturbed sleep.

Appetite: Dolores loved food and cooking, aiming to buy quality foods and avoid cakes, biscuits, and sweets. She sometimes skipped breakfast. Comfort eating during cancer treatment and after her mother's death had resulted in weight gain; she had recently lost 3kg (6.6lb) and still had some way to go to reach her desired weight.

Drink: Although she did not experience thirst, she drank ten cups of tea a day plus a litre of water when at the gym.

Bowels: Regular, with a daily movement.

Urination: Frequent, copious, often urgent, with pale urine; she got up once or twice during the night to go to the toilet.

Sweating and temperature: No longer troubled by tamoxifen-related hot flushes (she had completed tamoxifen treatment the previous summer).

Gynaecological history: Hysterectomy six years previously (age 51). Prior menstrual history characterised by regular periods that were 'flooding' with clots and preceded by 'disabling PMT'.

Relationships: An only child with a difficult family history, Dolores had a stable marriage and close relationships with her only child and grandchild. Her parents had died recently within two years of each other.

Other information: Dolores aimed to have a healthy lifestyle. She had done the pre-scribed exercises for her arm diligently following breast cancer surgery. While it was important for her to go to the gym regularly, chronic exhaustion now made this an effort.

Dolores described herself as determined and made considerable effort to take care of herself. However, she spoke of getting 'depressed in a certain way' and although she felt she could 'cope with life' she quite often 'burst into tears'.

Physical examination: Tongue: Short, red, and swollen towards the front with a long central crack extended from the tip to the rear; sublingual veins distended. **Pulses:** Deep and weak overall, especially on the third positions on both sides.

Diagnoses

CM diagnosis: Lung qi deficiency, Stomach and Spleen qi deficiency, Kidney yin and yang deficiency.

CF diagnosis: Although I was unsure whether Dolores was a metal CF, metal was the element in distress, and I chose to focus on this initially.

Treatment approach

Dolores's priorities for acupuncture treatment were to:

- treat the sinusitis
- address the grief for her mother.

Going to the gym was the activity she wished to improve. In the research study, it was usual to administer an Aggressive Energy (AE) Drain at the first treatment, followed by Internal Dragons (IDs) at the second session (see Chapter 9, Cancer Treatment-Related Lymphoedema). However, Dolores's physical distress was so great that I prioritised relieving the sinusitis.

I drew on the dual function of points, using points on the Lung and Large Intestine channels to clear the physical symptoms, and relied on their connection to the emotional aspect of metal, grief, to simultaneously address the emotions. Points on these metal channels were appropriate for addressing Dolores's grief, especially as it appeared to be so closely associated with her physical symptoms.

Treatment notes

- As with all participants in this study, needling was avoided in the arm and torso of the side of the body affected by lymphoedema (see Chapter 9, Cancer Treatment-Related Lymphoedema).
- All points were needled with even technique to obtain sensation (deqi). Needles retained for 20 minutes with no further stimulation.
- Many of the techniques used are described in Chapter 5, Toolkit.

Progress through initial treatments

Table 12.5: Dolores's initial treatments 1–3

Abbreviations: Tx treatment; **RS** right side; **bi** bilateral

Tx	Treatment principles	Points
1	Treat sinusitis: clear Large Intestine (LI) channel	LI-4 *Hegu* (RS) LI-20 *Yingxiang* (bi)
	Use local points for sinuses	DU-23 *Shangxing* M-HN-3 *Yintang* M-HN-14 *Bitong* (bi)
	Resolve phlegm	ST-40 *Fenglong* (bi)

2	As per Tx 1 plus a distal point for nasal congestion	BL-67 *Zhiyin* (bi)
3	Clear entry/exit (E/E) block between Small Intestine and Bladder	SI-19 *Tinggong* (bi) BL-2 *Zanzhu* (bi)
	Clear Ll channel	Ll-4 *Hegu* (RS) Ll-20 *Yingxiang* (RS)
	Resolve phlegm	LU-5 *Chize* (RS) ST-40 *Fenglong* (bi) SP-6 *Sanyinjiao* (bi)

Tx 1: LI-20 *Yingxiang* and M-HN-14 *Bitong* are not points I usually use in the first treatment of an acupuncture-naive person, as they can be uncomfortable and potentially off-putting. However, Dolores tolerated needling in these sensitive areas. During this session, I also suggested improvements to her lifestyle, which was already quite good, recommending that she try to:

- eat a warm breakfast regularly
- rest every afternoon (see prescription for rest in Chapter 5, Toolkit)
- do gentle exercise only, until her health improved.

Tx 2: Dolores reported feeling a 'bit bizarre' after the first treatment and experienced a slight headache that evening. She was tired for two days following treatment and had rested (despite feeling guilty about resting). Her sleep began to improve, and by this second treatment she was sleeping through the night. She said she felt much better physically and psychologically, and her husband and daughter noticed a change.

Tx 3: Dolores reported that her sinuses felt clearer, she was starting to discharge (yellow) mucous, and she had more energy. She was eating porridge for breakfast every morning.

Treating an entry/exit block

Rachel Peckham, my colleague who administered this treatment, identified an entry/exit (E/E) block. This is a Five Element block to treatment that occurs when the qi flow between channels is partially or completely blocked.

It is detected by pulse diagnosis, indicated by a relatively full pulse on one organ or channel followed by a very deficient pulse on the next. An entry/exit block may also be indicated by signs and symptoms around the area of the blockage.[17] These indications applied to Dolores, and Rachel cleared the block between the Small Intestine and Bladder channels, using the exit point of the Small Intestine channel, SI-19 *Tinggong*. She substituted BL-2 *Zhanzhu* for the entry point of the Bladder channel, BL-1 *Jingming*, to avoid needling close to the eye.

Moving from the physical to the emotional

Table 12.6: Dolores's further treatments 4–7

Abbreviations: Tx treatment; **RS** right side; **bi** bilateral; **(n)** shows number of direct moxa cones applied

Tx	Treatment principles	Points	Notes
4	Clear block to treatment: Internal Dragons (IDs)[2]	Master point 0.25 cun below REN-15 *Jiuwei* ST-25 *Tianshu* ST-32 *Futu* ST-41 *Jiexi*	All points bilateral except Master point. For method, see Chapter 5, Toolkit.
	Address sinusitis	M-HN-3 *Yintang*	
	Tonify Stomach qi	ST-36 *Zusanli* (bi)	
5	Clear heat in the Lung	LU-5 *Chize* (RS)	Method as in Table 12.5.
	Tonify Stomach qi	ST-36 *Zusanli* (bi)	
	Harmonise, balance emotions	ST-25 *Tianshu* (bi) SP-15 *Daheng* (bi)	
	Address grief	LU-1 *Zhongfu* (RS)	
6	Clear sinuses	LI-4 *Hegu* (RS) LI-20 *Yingxiang* (bi) DU-23 *Shangxing* M-HN-3 *Yintang*	
	Resolve phlegm	ST-40 *Fenglong* (bi)	
	Tonify Stomach qi	ST-36 *Zusanli* (bi) REN-12 *Zhongwan*	
	Tonify Lung qi, support spirit	BL-12 *Fengmen* (bi) LU-1 *Zhongfu* (RS)	
7	As per Tx 6 plus tonify and nourish qi and calm the spirit	Points as per Tx 6 plus direct moxa (7) on BL-43 *Gaohuangshu* (RS)	

Progress through treatments 4–7

Tx 4: Dolores reported that in spite of some congestion, her sinuses were much improved, and she felt much better in herself. She was feeling low about the upcoming anniversary of her mother's death.

At this treatment, I administered Internal Dragons (IDs). Although her physical symptoms were improving, the proximity of their onset to her mother's death suggested they might be connected to the shock of loss and the intensity of the emotions at this time. These may have been overwhelming, and in such circumstances, IDs are indicated.[17] Her pulses, which were very subdued after this, became more even, harmonious, and vital after I needled ST-36 *Zusanli* to ground the treatment.

Tx 5: Dolores reported feeling tired for two days after the IDs and had rested. Her physical symptoms continued to improve, and she made further lifestyle changes – she reduced comfort eating, and was doing regular gentle exercise. Emotionally, she 'had moments' but now her emotions seemed 'more like grieving than depression'.

Dolores's sinusitis was improving, and her emotional state was changing. However, she was still feeling tired. At this stage I introduced more points on the Stomach channel, aiming to:

- strengthen Lung qi by 'cultivating the Earth to generate Metal'[19]
- resolve phlegm by strengthening the Stomach and Spleen using Stomach points and REN-12 *Zhongwan* according to the saying of Chinese medicine that 'the Spleen is the origin of phlegm and the Lung is the container of phlegm'[19]
- improve energy by tonifying Stomach qi
- enhance immunity (relying particularly on ST-36 *Zusanli*; in later treatments, I used moxa on this, aiming to preserve and maintain health)
- calm the spirit and harmonise the emotions (with points such as ST-36 *Zusanli*, SP-15 *Daheng*, and ST-25 *Tianshu*).

I used metal points to continue to relieve the residual sinusitis and support the grieving process, choosing:

- LU-5 *Chize* to address any heat in the Lung, indicated by the yellow discharge
- LU-1 *Zhongfu*, which in Five Element acupuncture is indicated for people who are grief stricken, enabling them 'to reconnect with inspiration from Heaven and experience greater meaning in life'.[17] As the meeting point of the Lung and Spleen channels, it is a place where the nourishment of the Earth element and the inspiration of metal unite,[23] and in combination with ST-36 *Zusanli*, 'fills Earth to generate Metal'.[24]

Tx 6: Dolores reported improvements in her energy and emotions. She had managed well during a trip away to mark the anniversary of her mother's death. However, upsetting news had arrived, as a close family member was undergoing tests for suspected bowel cancer. I continued to support the Stomach, Spleen, and Lung qi and address the emotions. I used points on the front and back, the front mu point LU-1 *Zhongfu* and the back shu point of the Lung BL-12 *Fengmen* to balance the treatment, as indicated for chronic cases.[24]

Tx 7: This was a review point for the study. Dolores was feeling much better: her left nostril had cleared completely; breathing was easier, making her less reliant on inhalers, and she had started a phased return to work. Dolores found acupuncture beneficial and opted to continue with a further six treatments, as offered in the research study.

Progress through treatments 8–13

Tx 8–13: During the subsequent six weeks of treatment, Dolores increased her working hours to full time. She found this tiring, and her sinusitis would ebb and flow with her energy levels. I continued to treat her using the principles outlined above. I also added in moxa on BL-43 *Gaohuangshu*, using up to 15 cones per session on the right side only. This was to tonify and nourish the Lung, Heart, Kidney, Spleen, and Stomach, and to calm the spirit, foster original qi, and resolve phlegm.[19]

At her 13th treatment and final treatment of the study, Dolores spoke of the difference acupuncture had made. She felt she had 'turned a corner'. She was working full time without feeling exhausted, going to the gym, and waking at 6–7am feeling refreshed and energised. Although she still had some mucous and congestion, she was not snoring at night and was less dependent on inhalers. Lymphoedema had reduced to be negligible.

Prior to starting acupuncture, she had considered retiring as work was too draining. She now felt 'alive', 'vital', and more as she should for her age. Her interest in her appearance and dress revived, and she was taking action to lose weight. Most of all, she was delighted to recover her 'old self'. I too was delighted to see such a changed person. My notes record:

> [Dolores] is looking fantastic. She has colour, the bags and circles under her eyes have gone, she looks vital and alive, glowing. [She] is quite a different person to when she started treatment.

Short- and long-term feedback
At the end of 13 treatments, Dolores wrote:

> When I entered the trial, I was at a very low ebb in my life. My mother had died in the previous year and I experienced exacerbation of my lymphoedema (i.e. my hand had started to swell). I also had had recurrent infections since my mother's death. I had at this time severe sinusitis being treated with antibiotics and various therapies but nothing seemed to resolve my symptoms.
>
> Since starting the treatment my sense of smell has returned; previously I could not even smell Olbas oil. When at work I could not even answer the phone due to the severity of sinusitis and related ear infection. I often had days off sick. I have now returned to work and can complete a day's shift without feeling exhausted. My sleeping has improved dramatically. I don't snore now.
>
> Due to my physical problems being greatly resolved, I now have a feeling of wellbeing. The lymphoedema in my arm has reduced. When I started, the swelling was classified as 8; it is now 0.7.
>
> My quality of life has improved... I now feel I can lead a normal life again.

Eighteen weeks later, in September 2009, she wrote:

> When I started the treatment...I also had medical problems which despite going to the doctor numerous times had not resolved. The treatment gradually resolved my physical problems, thus allowing me to gradually return to work and participate in normal everyday living ...I have returned to work and not had to have a day off sick... I also go to the gym...eat more sensibly, and have lost some weight. I feel more positive about myself.

Treatment longer term

Dolores returned for private treatment the following spring, having experienced several bereavements early in the year. Her husband had also been in a serious accident. She sought treatment to manage stress and 'get back on track'. Despite the stressful events, Dolores said she had been well, her energy was good, she was exercising, losing weight, and coping with work. The sinusitis had not returned, and she had not had a cold that year.

Dolores had four treatments in 2010 and returned in the spring of 2011, when once again bereavements during winter triggered symptoms. (In total, Dolores experienced five significant bereavements during 2010–2011, one of which was extremely traumatic.) In 2011, the sinusitis returned, but not as severely as when she first came for acupuncture in 2009. She had felt well in herself, was continuing to look after herself well, and had lost another stone in weight. I saw her again for four treatments.

Summary

Dolores's case illustrates how acupuncture can improve resilience, as illustrated in the model below (Figure 12.2). Through relieving symptoms, improving immune function, and simultaneously addressing physical and emotional symptoms, Dolores's energy improved, and she was able return to normal functioning, actively enjoying life and work again. It enabled her to improve her self-care, which included returning for brief courses of acupuncture treatment when life events mounted up, causing symptoms to return.

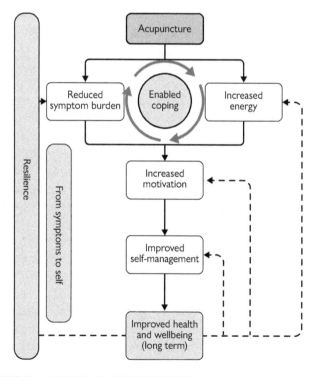

FIGURE 12.2: A MODEL OF ACUPUNCTURE FOR IMPROVING LONG-TERM
HEALTH AND WELLBEING AND DEVELOPING RESILIENCE

CASE STUDY: MOLLY AND USING THE EXTRAORDINARY VESSELS TO SUPPORT THE IMMUNE SYSTEM

Introduction

Molly's case study presents a different approach. Like Dolores, Molly experienced lymph-oedema following cancer treatment. She was referred to the lymphoedema study, where she was treated by my colleague Rachel Peckham during the spring of 2009. Molly was delighted to report improvements in her energy and sleep, a feeling of calm, and fewer incidents of facial swelling, which helped her to feel more in control of her lymphoedema. Molly contacted me for follow-up treatment in autumn 2012, as the location of my private clinic was convenient for her to access.

I am grateful to Molly for her permission and involvement in sharing these details of her private treatment.

Background and main complaints

Molly, aged 67, was diagnosed with medullary thyroid cancer with spread to the lymph nodes and salivary glands in March 2004. Surgery to remove the thyroid, salivary glands and associated lymph nodes was followed by a six-week course of external beam radio-therapy. Molly was prescribed daily thyroxine for life to prevent recurrence and manage hypothyroidism. Follow-up appointments with her oncologist were scheduled for every three months.

In the four months prior to her seeing me, she had two ear infections. These triggered episodes of cellulitis and lymphoedema, which were treated with antibiotics. These episodes, which had become infrequent after her treatments with Rachel, were returning. Molly wished to avoid taking antibiotics long term, and she felt that acupuncture could improve her immunity.

Questioning the systems

Although Molly is usually economical with details, she described the facial swelling as 'horrendous', 'like a huge football', making her look 'like a puppet from Spitting Image'. Episodes were triggered by an ear infection characterised by discharge from the ears. Treatment with antibiotics and steroids controlled this; however, Molly admitted that she often left it too long before seeing the doctor. The aftermath of these episodes left her with residual swelling under the eyes, in front of the ears, and on the neck. Itchiness affected her ears as well as the skin on her face, which became dry with red splotches around the mouth. A cold would often follow, leaving her feeling under par.

Sleep: Her sleep was 'alright'; able to get to sleep easily, she would wake up in the night when worried.

Appetite: A vegetarian, her appetite was good. The consequences of her treatment made swallowing difficult, restricting her to eating soft foods, and she was anxious about eating in public (these consequences also caused her to snore loudly when sleeping).

Drink: She drank sufficient fluids.

Bowels: Regular.

Urination: No problems reported.

Sweating and temperature: Tendency to feel hot.

Relationships: Married, with three adult children.

Other information: She did not experience headaches, dizziness, or vision problems. Molly described herself as an anxious person – she 'came from an anxious family'. She was physically active, enjoying swimming, cycling, and walking, and loved nature.

Physical examination: Tongue: Short, red, had no coat, and no cracks. **Pulses:** Full, big, and rapid on all positions.

Diagnoses
CM diagnosis: Damp heat in the Gall Bladder (ear discharge), heat in the Lung and Stomach, shen disturbed.

CF diagnosis: I had no Five Element diagnosis at this stage.

Treatment approach
Molly's priorities for acupuncture treatment were to 'not to have ear infections so often', and if she had them, 'to recover more quickly'.

My priority was to address the itching sensation of the ears and clear heat from the skin. I also wanted to address other symptoms, including anxiety and facial swelling.

Table 12.7: Molly's first three acupuncture treatments

Abbreviations: Tx treatment; **RS** right side; **LS** left side; **bi** bilateral; **(n)** shows number of direct moxa cones applied

Tx	Treatment principles	Points	Notes
1	Benefit the ears; clear heat	TB-5 *Waiguan* (bi)	
	Clear heat from face	LI-4 *Hegu* (bi)	
	Relieve facial swelling, clear heat, calm the spirit	ST-45 *Lidui* (bi)	
2	Open Yang Linking Vessel	TB-5 *Waiguan* (RS) GB-41 *Zulinqi* (LS)	See Chapter 5, Toolkit, for details.
	Benefit the ears	TB-3 *Zhongzhu* (RS)	
	Clear heat from face, skin	LI-4 *Hegu* (LS) LI-11 *Quchi*	
	Relieve facial swelling, clear heat, calm the spirit	ST-45 *Lidui* (RS)	

cont.

Tx	Treatment principles	Points	Notes
3	Open Yang Linking Vessel	TB-5 *Waiguan* (RS) GB-41 *Zulinqi* (LS)	
	Benefit the ears	TB-3 *Zhongzhu* (RS)	
	Clear heat from face, skin	Ll-4 *Hegu* (LS) Ll-11 *Quchi*	
	Relieve facial swelling, clear heat, calm the spirit	ST-45 *Lidui* (RS)	
	Nourish qi and calm shen	'Toasted Pericardium Sandwich': BL-43 *Gaohuangshu* (bi, 15 moxa cones each point) REN-17 *Shanzhong* (5)	Direct moxa only; no needling.

Tx 1: To address her symptoms, I chose:

- TB-5 *Waiguan* to benefit the head and ears and clear heat; indicated for itching, pain, and swelling of the ear[19]
- LI-4 *Hegu* to regulate the face and ears; as the 'single most important point to treat disorders of the face and sense organs',[19] it is said in Chinese medicine that 'the face and mouth are reached by LI-4'[24]
- ST-45 *Lidui* to clear heat from the Stomach channel and calm the spirit; indicated for facial swelling and insomnia.[19,24]

Tx 2: Molly reported feeling well after the first treatment. The itchiness in her ears had diminished; the skin on her face was still dry. I introduced using the Yang Linking Vessel (*Yang Wei Mai*) (see Chapter 5, Toolkit) for its beneficial effects on ear problems (such as ear discharge from damp heat in the Gall Bladder).[25] In prior work with survivors of head and neck cancers, I found this extraordinary vessel useful to address the consequences of treatment affecting the mouth, tongue, and teeth, and felt this might also benefit Molly's ability to eat. I also introduced:

- TB-3 *Zhongzhu* to benefit the ears and address itching of the face[19,24]
- LI-11 *Quchi* to clear heat, cool Blood, and alleviate itching.[19,24]

Tx 3: Molly said the itching in her ears disappeared after the treatment one week previously. Her energy was good, and she felt relaxed after treatment. Sleep had not improved, and it was at this appointment she spoke about coming from an anxious family. Her skin was still dry; she felt neither hot nor cold.

Building on the previous treatments, I began to nourish qi, using direct moxibustion on BL-43 *Gaohuangshu* and REN-17 *Shanzhong*. While it seems contradictory to treat a 'hot' person with moxibustion, these points are contraindicated to needling in many classical texts, and it is my usual practice to use moxa only on these. I wanted to invoke the potential of:

- BL-43 *Gaohuangshu* to tonify and nourish the Lung, Heart, Kidney, Spleen, and Stomach[19]
- REN-17 *Shanzhong* to tonify Lung qi,[24] with the aim of fortifying Molly's immune system.

I also used this combination, which I call the 'Toasted Pericardium Sandwich', to calm the shen, relieve anxiety, and improve sleep (see Chapter 5, Toolkit). Many patients find this to be a profoundly relaxing treatment.

Tx 4: The following week, Molly reported that she was feeling 'really well'. She had lots of energy, and her adult children noticed a difference in her. The skin dryness had disappeared. Although she enjoyed the moxa treatment, there was no difference in her sleep.

Developing a long-term maintenance programme
Over the next few treatments, I modified the treatment protocol by:

- adding extra point M-HN-3 *Yintang* to calm the shen
- substituting ST-44 *Neiting* for ST-45 *Lidui*. ST-44 *Neiting* has a similar ability to clear heat and calm the shen, and Molly found it slightly more comfortable than ST-45 *Lidui*.

Except when Molly presented with an acute condition, I used this protocol (detailed in Table 12.8) to manage the ear problems, bouts of swelling, and support her immune system. In hot weather, I did not use the moxa, and needled LI-11 *Quchi* if Molly was feeling exceptionally warm.

Table 12.8: 'Molly's protocol'

Abbreviations: RS right side; **LS** left side; **bi** bilateral; **(n)** shows number of direct moxa cones applied

Treatment principles	Points	Notes
Open Yang Linking Vessel	TB-5 *Waiguan* (RS) GB-41 *Zulinqi* (LS)	
Benefit the ears	TB-3 *Zhongzhu* (RS)	
Clear heat from face, skin	LI-4 *Hegu* (LS) LI-11 *Quchi* (LS) as needed	
Relieve facial swelling, clear heat, calm the spirit	ST-44 *Neiting* (RS)	
Calm shen	M-HN-3 *Yintang*	
Nourish qi	BL-43 *Gaohuangshu* (bi, 15 moxa cones each point) Ren-17 *Shanzhong* (5)	Direct moxa only; no needling.

Progress through treatment

Managing through setbacks

Tx 7: Initially, Molly had weekly treatment, and reported mostly continual improvements. At her seventh treatment, she reported that an ear infection had flared the previous week. She had immediately seen her consultant, who prescribed a five-day course of antibiotics and steroids. Molly was not disappointed with this – recovery from an episode usually took four to six weeks, and she had bounced back after five days. Her consultant was also impressed by this improved resilience.

Lifestyle advice

This was in December, with cold winter weather descending. Molly's tendency to feel warm meant she was casual about wrapping up well. I discussed the importance in Chinese thought of protecting the body from cold and drafts, regarded as a trigger for invasions of wind (the CM equivalent of the common cold). Given the vulnerability of her ears, I also suggested she adopt the habit of wearing a hat or earmuffs to protect them.

Supporting recovery

Tx 8: Molly presented with the usual aftermath of these episodes – residual swelling under the eyes, in front of the ears, and around the neck. Her skin was dry and itchy, and she felt hot all the time. I adjusted her treatment, excluding moxibustion and introducing extra point M-LE-34 *Baichongwo* to alleviate itching.

Tx 9: At her next treatment three weeks later, itching was still troublesome, and she had red patches round her neck.

While she had tested negative for diabetes before Christmas, blood tests revealed a low white cell count, and her doctor said she had a 'very low immune system'. To address her desire to improve further her immunity, I taught Molly to self-moxa ST-36 *Zusanli*, recommending that she carry out this procedure daily, if possible (see Chapter 5, Toolkit).

Moving toward self-management

At this appointment, Molly also expressed a desire to have treatment less frequently. We agreed to phase treatments, beginning with fortnightly sessions, and gradually extending the time between treatments. Molly reported that she was self-administering moxa three to four times a week.

Tx 13: In early March, Moly contracted a chest infection, and was coughing up green phlegm. My treatment principles aimed to:

- expel the invasion of wind heat in the Lung using BL-12 *Fengmen*, Bl-13 *Feishu*, and LI-4 *Hegu*
- resolve phlegm heat using LU-5 *Chize* and ST-40 *Fenglong*
- unbind the chest and descend qi using REN-18 *Yutang*
- calm shen and deal with any nasal discharge using extra point M-HN-3 *Yintang*.

Tx 14: Molly attended three weeks later, reporting she had shaken off the chest infection, and realised her aim of not having to use antibiotics. However, she now had a urinary infection, characterised by frequent, yellow urine, discomfort in the bladder, and itching. To treat this, I:

- opened the Girdle Vessel (Dai Mai) to resolve damp in the lower burner, needling the opening point GB-41 *Zulinqi* on the right and the coupled point TB-5 *Waiguan* on the left[25]
- cleared heat in the Bladder using BL-63 *Jinmen* and BL-66 *Zutonggu*
- regulated the Bladder function using BL-28 *Pangguangshu*, REN-2 *Qugu*, and REN-3 *Zhongji*
- resolved damp using SP-9 *Yinlingquan* and SP-6 *Sanyinjiao*.

This resolved the infection.

More challenges

Molly was having acupuncture every four to five weeks and self-administering moxa three times a week. It was now the summer of 2013, and a challenging time for Molly. A lump under her left collarbone fortunately proved benign. There were family problems and changes affecting Molly's employment. In August, she had a troublesome eye infection, with redness, swelling, continuous watering, and discomfort. A specialist eye hospital prescribed ointment and a lubricating gel.

Tx 18: She attended for acupuncture ten days later, and I treated this by:

- opening the Yang Linking Vessel (conveniently useful for both eye and ear problems)
- using local points ST-2 *Sibai* and extra points M-NH-1 *Sishencong* and M-HN-3 *Yintang*, all indicated for eye disorders.

Tx 19: At her treatment four weeks later, Molly said this had cleared the problem for a week, and then it returned. She was now taking antibiotics. I repeated the treatment to alleviate her continuing discomfort. When she returned in November, Molly reported that the eye infection had cleared, and we returned to using the protocol set out in Table 12.8.

Realising her goal

During the ensuing 13 months, Molly had acupuncture every six weeks. She had no further serious infections, and no episodes of cellulitis or lymphoedema. She had avoided antibiotics during those 13 months, had managed to fight off several colds, and generally felt well. Her oncologist reduced her follow-up appointments to every four months. She discontinued self-administering moxa, and I never succeeded in persuading her to cover her head, ears, and neck in cold weather.

Short- and long-term feedback

In reviewing this case study with Molly, she said:

> Acupuncture has been very beneficial and helpful. If finances had allowed, I would have had more frequent treatment. I consider myself very fortunate to have had this. I have to say, I've valued having treatment from someone who is able to identify with my cancer treatment – a specialist who understands my special needs. I've also valued – at the back of my mind – that I could communicate with my acupuncturist if I needed to. Beverley was available if needed, and was encouraging.

Afterward

As luck would have it, while writing this case study, Molly contracted an ear infection. She had been free of these for 14 months. She saw her specialist immediately and took antibiotics. Although disappointing, this provided the opportunity to discuss the importance of daily self-moxa of ST-36 *Zusanli*. Molly had given it up; she said she had become complacent.

Summary

Molly's case illustrates the potential challenges of managing immune-related conditions. Her symptoms and their treatment are markedly different from Dolores's, and this supports the need for an individualised approach. Molly might have benefitted from more frequent treatment, especially when having acute episodes. Continuing self-administered moxa and covering up in cold weather may also have improved outcomes. Nevertheless, it appears that her immune system was strengthened sufficiently to meet her goals for treatment – to have fewer ear infections and facilitate better recovery from any she does have.

CHAPTER SUMMARY

- Many cancer survivors wish to improve their immunity, and treatment with acupuncture and moxibustion offer a means of doing this.
- Restoring and building good health is at the heart of acupuncture treatment, which can go beyond treating specific symptoms to treat the whole person.
- We can draw on the points and protocols offered by CM theory or use Five Element approaches to fortify the constitution.
- A further benefit is that improving immunity may increase resilience, helping survivors to 'bounce back' and have the capacity to 'lead a normal life again'.

References

1. Genesis Care Live well with cancer. Waterlooville, UK: Genesis Care; 2019. Available from: https://image-assets.genesiscare.com/wp-content/uploads/2020/05/13032918/Penny-Brohn-Patient-Brochure_LOCKED.pdf

2. American Psychological Association Building your resilience. Washington DC: APA; 2020. Available from: www.apa.org/topics/resilience/building-your-resilience
3. Dantzer R, Cohen S, Russo SJ, *et al*. Resilience and immunity. Brain. Behav. Immun. 2018;74:28–42.
4. Zollman C, Walther A, Seers HE, *et al*. Integrative whole-person oncology care in the UK. JNCI Monographs 2017;2017(52).
5. Scholl R, Bekker A, Babu R Neuroendocrine and immune responses to surgery. The Internet Journal of Anesthiology 2012;30(3).
6. Breastcancer.org How chemotherapy affects the immune system. Ardmore, PA: Breastcancer.org; 2022. Available from: www.breastcancer.org/managing-life/immune-system/cancer-treatments/chemotherapy
7. Chemaly R How to boost your immune system. University of Texas: MD Anderson Cancer Center; 2020. Available from: www.mdanderson.org/publications/focused-on-health/how-to-boost-your-immune-system-.h13-1593780.html
8. Breastcancer.org Taking care of your immune system. Ardmore, PA: Breastcancer.org; 2022. Available from: www.breastcancer.org/managing-life/immune-system/self-care
9. Besedovsky L, Lange T, Born J Sleep and immune function. Pflugers Arch. 2012;463(1):121–137.
10. Aldabal L, Bahamman AS Metabolic, endocrine and immune consequences of sleep. Open Respir. Med. J. 2011;5:31–42.
11. Segerstrom SC, Miller GE Psychological stress and the human immune system. Psychol. Bull. 2004;130(4):601–630.
12. Zhang R, Lao L Acupuncture and moxibustion in animal models of cancer. In: Cho W, editor. Acupuncture and moxibustion as an evidence-based therapy for cancer. Dordrecht: Springer; 2012. pp. 291–311.
13. Lu W, Hu D, Dean-Clower E, *et al*. Acupuncture for chemotherapy-induced leukopenia: exploratory meta-analysis of randomized controlled trials. Journal of the Society for Integrative Oncology 2007;5(1):1–10.
14. Wong R, Sagar SM Acupuncture and moxibustion for cancer-related symptoms. In: Cho W, editor. Acupuncture and moxibustion as an evidence-based therapy for cancer. Dordrecht: Springer; 2012. pp. 83–120.
15. Johnston M, Sanchez E, Vujanovic NL, *et al*. Acupuncture may stimulate anticancer immunity via activation of natural killer cells. Evid. Based Complement. Alternat. Med. 2011;2011:481625.
16. Choi TY, Lee MS, Ernst E Moxibustion for the treatment of chemotherapy-induced leukopenia: a systematic review of randomized clinical trials. Support. Care Cancer 2015;23(6):1819–1826.
17. Hicks A, Hicks J, Mole P Five element constitutional acupuncture. Edinburgh: Churchill Livingstone; 2004.
18. Xiaorong C, Jing H, Shouxiang Y Illustrated Chinese moxibustion: techniques and methods. London: Singing Dragon; 2012.
19. Deadman P, Al-Khafaji M, Baker K A manual of acupuncture. Hove: The Journal of Chinese Medicine; 2007.
20. Maciocia G The practice of Chinese Medicine. London: Churchill Livingstone; 1994.
21. Abbate S An overview of the therapeutic application of moxibustion. J. Chinese Med. 2002;69(June):5–12.
22. de Valois B, Peckham R Treating the person and not the disease: acupuncture in the management of cancer treatment-related lymphoedema. Eur. J. Orient. Med. 2011;6(6):37–49.
23. Hatton CL Acupuncture point compendium. Leamington: College of Traditional Acupuncture; 2004. Available from: www.dropbox.com/s/eso5a5mm2vpgod7/Acupuncture%20Point%20Compendium%202014.pdf?dl=0
24. Maciocia G The foundations of Chinese medicine. London: Churchill Livingstone; 1989.
25. Maciocia G The channels of acupuncture: clinical use of the secondary channels and eight extraordinary vessels. Edinburgh: Churchill Livingstone; 2006.

Chapter 13

Reducing Risk of Recurrence and Subsequent Primary Cancers

Introduction

The potential threat of cancer recurrence or developing subsequent primary cancers is summarised in these quotations:

> As the population of cancer survivors has increased and continues to age, the occurrence of second cancers has risen dramatically – from 9% of all cancer diagnoses in 1975–1979 to 19% in 2005–2009. (Morton *et al.*)[1]

> Cancer loves me more than I love it. (Rosa, a colorectal cancer survivor)[2]

Many people fear a return of their disease after treatment. As more people live longer after cancer treatment, a new threat arises, which is the potential to develop new primary cancers.

Diagnosis of new tumours, different from the first primary tumour, is now a substantial healthcare concern. The number of diagnoses in the USA for first primary malignancies rose from 317,000 in 1975–1979 to 548,000 in 2005–2009, an increase of 70%. During that time, the number of diagnoses of subsequent primary cancers increased by over 300%, from 30,000 to 125,000.[1]

It appears necessary to add a new potential event to the diagram of the cancer pathway – 'Subsequent primary diagnosis of another type of cancer', and I have taken the liberty to draw this in Figure 13.1.

This chapter explores the topic highlighted in Figure 13.1. It also offers information on the signs and symptoms of cancer, as all healthcare professionals should be able to identify the early indicators of cancer and refer patients on for investigation, remembering that early diagnosis and treatment lead to better outcomes. Also discussed is how to help all patients (cancer and non-cancer) reduce risk of developing primary or subsequent primary cancers.

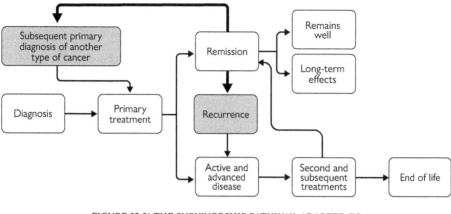

FIGURE 13.1: THE SURVIVORSHIP PATHWAY, ADAPTED TO
INCLUDE SUBSEQUENT PRIMARY CANCER

Recurrence, metastases, and subsequent primary cancers[3,4]
Recurrence
Recurrence, or recurrent cancer, is the term used when cancer returns after anti-cancer treatment. Cancer can recur anywhere in the body and may be:

- **Local** – in the same part of the body as the primary cancer.
- **Regional** – near where the primary cancer was located.
- **Distant** – in another part of the body; also called metastatic cancer.

Recurrent cancers are named after the location of the primary cancer, even when they occur in another part of the body. For example, if prostate cancer recurs distally in the liver, it is prostate cancer, not liver cancer, and referred to as 'metastatic prostate cancer'.
    The prognosis of recurrent cancer depends on many factors, including the type of primary tumour, the treatment, and the stage of recurrence.

Metastases
Metastatic cancer, also called metastatic disease, secondary cancer, metastases, or distant recurrence, is cancer that has spread from the primary site to another part of the body. Common sites of metastatic spread from solid tumours include the bones, lungs, liver, and brain, with each type of cancer having its own characteristic route of spread.
    In general, people with metastatic disease die of their primary cancer, although some may live for many years and are considered to be 'incurable but treatable'.[3]

Subsequent primary cancer(s)
This is the development of a new cancer that is unrelated to any previous cancer diagnosis. Sometimes called a 'second' cancer, more accurate terms are 'subsequent primary cancer' or 'new primary cancer'. 'Multiple primary cancers' is also used, as survivors may be diagnosed with more than one 'second' cancer in their lifetime. New primary cancers may be:

- unrelated to the initial diagnosis
- a late effect of the initial cancer or its treatment.

Subsequent primary cancers are becoming more common as more people are living longer after their first cancer diagnosis.

Understanding recurrent and subsequent primary cancers
Recurrent cancers
Cancer recurs for many reasons, including:

- The original treatment did not eradicate all cancer cells, which have formed a new tumour.
- Some cancer cells spread elsewhere in the body (metastasised) and formed tumours in new locations (metastases).

Rates of recurrence will vary depending on the type of primary tumour, stage of the disease, previous treatments, and the time from initial treatment. While recurrence usually happens within the first three years after primary treatment, any cancer may recur at any time from weeks to decades after treatment.

Subsequent primary cancers
Between 2009 and 2013, 18% of all cancers diagnosed in the USA were subsequent primary cancers, meaning nearly one in five people diagnosed with cancer previously had a different type of cancer.[5] Studies from Japan[6] and pan-Europe[7] report that rates of 8.1% and 6.3% of the studied populations developed a second primary cancer. There are some risk factors for developing these cancers:

- **Type of first cancer (first primary site):** incidence of subsequent primary cancers ranges from 2% in survivors of malignant lymphoma to 30% in small lung cancer and 34% in bladder cancer survivors.[8]
- **Age at first diagnosis:** differences by age at first diagnosis have been reported, with prevalence of 11% among those aged 20–64 years, rising to 25.2% among those aged 65 years and older.
- **Tobacco and alcohol:** survivors with tobacco-related cancers have a high risk of developing subsequent tobacco-related cancers, while alcohol consumption is also associated with high risk of developing cancers (Table 13.1).

Radiotherapy and chemotherapy may also be associated with an increased risk of subsequent cancer, especially in those who were treated for a first primary cancer as a child, teen, or young adult. It is important to note that the benefits of treating the first primary cancer generally outweigh the risk of developing subsequent primary cancers.[5]

Table 13.1: Cancers associated with tobacco and alcohol usage[5]

Note:

Combined use of alcohol and tobacco is estimated to account for 75–85% of cancers of the oral cavity, pharynx, larynx, and oesophagus in the USA.

Tobacco-related cancers	Alcohol-related cancers
• Kidney and renal pelvis	• Colon
• Lung and bronchus	• Female breast
• Oesophagus (men only)	• Larynx
• Oral cavity and pharynx	• Liver
• Urinary bladder	• Oesophagus
	• Oral cavity and pharynx

Signs and symptoms of cancer

As survivors of a first primary cancer may have a recurrence or develop a subsequent primary cancer, it is important that healthcare professionals, including acupuncturists, are aware of possible signs and symptoms (Table 13.2) in these patients.[3] As acupuncturists, we can also use these to monitor patients who have never had a cancer diagnosis.

Patients can be reassured that the appearance of these phenomena are not necessarily cancer and may be signs of other things. However, patients should be encouraged to have investigated:

- any of these signs or symptoms
- changes in the body that are not normal for them
- symptoms or body changes that persist or worsen.

It is essential to remember that early diagnosis and treatment lead to better outcomes.

Table 13.2: Signs and symptoms of cancer[9,10]

Symptoms affecting	
General	• Bleeding, blood or bruising that is unusual. • Fatigue or extreme tiredness that does not improve with rest. • Lump or swelling anywhere in the body that is persistent. • Night sweats that are heavy and drenching. • Pain or ache that is unexplained (i.e. not due to injury, exertion, ageing, comorbidity). • Weight loss or gain of 10lb (4.5kg) or more that are unexplained.
Respiratory system	• Breathlessness that is unusual or unrelated to activity. • Cough that is persistent. • Coughing up blood. • Voice that is persistently croaky or hoarse.

cont.

Symptoms affecting	
Digestive system	• Appetite loss that is persistent. • Bloating, especially if experienced most days. • Blood in stools. • Bowel changes, including constipation, looser stools, more frequent movements. • Heartburn or indigestion that is frequent and may be painful. • Mouth or tongue ulcer that persists beyond 3 weeks. • Swallowing that is difficult and unrelated to other medical conditions (dysphagia). • Vomiting blood.
Urinary system	• Blood in urine. • Urinary problems, including difficulty or pain on urinating, or needing to go urgently or more frequently.
Skin	• Changes in a patch of skin or nail. • Jaundice. • Moles that are new, or changing, especially those that become crusty, itchy, painful, or that bleed or ooze. • Sores, spots, warts that do not heal.
Breast (for all genders)	• Breast lump. • Breast changes, including change in size, shape, or feel, skin changes, redness, pain in breast. • Nipple changes, including leaking fluid (which may be blood-stained) in women who are not pregnant or breastfeeding.
Gynaecological	• Vaginal bleeding that is unexplained, including after intercourse, between periods, or post menopause.
Other	• Headaches and vision or hearing problems.

Understanding risk factors for primary, recurrent, and subsequent primary cancers

There is no guaranteed way to prevent cancer. However, individuals can take action to reduce risk. Some risk factors, such as ageing, are beyond our control; others can be changed and may decrease risk. Acupuncturists can play an important role in supporting individuals to make these changes.

Understanding risk factors

Risk is the chance that an event will occur. In relation to cancer, risk is the term used to describe the chance that an individual will develop cancer, or that cancer will recur. A cancer risk factor is anything that increases an individual's chance of developing cancer. However:

- most risk factors do not directly cause cancer – numerous mistakes in the DNA must accumulate before a cancer develops[5]
- some people with multiple risk factors never develop cancer

---

408

- some people with no known risk factors develop cancer.[11]

General risk factors for developing cancer

Understanding risk factors can help an individual to make choices to reduce risk of a cancer diagnosis or recurrence. While these may vary for different types of cancer, there are key general risk factors:

- Older age.
- Personal or family history of cancer.
- Use of tobacco and/or alcohol.
- Some viral infections such as human papillomavirus (HPV).
- Specific chemicals.
- Exposure to radiation, including ultraviolet radiation from the sun and tanning equipment.[11]

Risk factors for developing subsequent primary cancers

Factors associated with increased risk of developing subsequent primary cancer(s) fall into three broad categories:

- Hereditary cancer syndromes.
- Common exposures, such as tobacco and alcohol usage, hormonal factors, and immune deficiency and infection.
- Effects of treatment of a previous primary cancer.[5]

Hereditary cancer syndromes

Hereditary cancer syndromes are associated with about 1–2% of all cancers. This means individuals have a mutation in every cell that may have been inherited from a parent or arisen early in development. Although individuals with hereditary cancer syndromes have a high lifetime probability of developing certain cancers, development of a malignant tumour depends on acquiring additional mutations of the DNA and is not down to genetic factors alone.[5]

There are some hereditary syndromes associated with increased risk of developing multiple primary cancers:

- Inherited mutations in cancer susceptibility genes BRCA1 and BRCA2: associated with early onset breast and ovarian cancers, and increased risk of subsequent primaries in the breast, ovary, and other sites.
- Familial adenomatous polyposis (FAP) and hereditary non-polyposis colorectal cancer (HNPCC): two genetic syndromes associated with high risk of colorectal cancer at a young age and at multiple sites within the colon and rectum.

Common exposures

Tobacco and alcohol use are risk factors for developing first primary cancers and provide increased risk of developing subsequent primary cancers.

Hormonal factors associated with the development of first primary cancers are also linked to increases in relative risks for breast, ovarian, and uterine corpus cancers. These are thought to be linked to the risk factors associated with menstruation and pregnancy, use of hormonal medications, and genetic susceptibility.[5]

Multiple primary tumours are associated with immunodeficiency syndromes, for example:

- Kidney transplant patients receiving immunosuppressive therapies are at increased risk of non-Hodgkin lymphoma, Kaposi sarcoma, and squamous cell cancer on sun-exposed areas of skin.
- HIV (human immunodeficiency virus) patients are at increased risk of non-Hodgkin lymphoma, Kaposi sarcoma, and cervical and anal cancer.

Human papillomavirus (HPV) infections are the main cause of cancer of the uterine cervix and are implicated in other cancers including those of the vulva, vagina, perineum, anus, and penis.

Effects of treatment of a previous primary cancer

Radiotherapy and chemotherapy can increase risk of subsequent cancer, with risk lasting years or decades after treatment of a first primary cancer. Some examples include:[1,5]

- Radiotherapy-related second cancers: leukaemia (acute, chronic myelogenous); cancers of the breast, brain, gastrointestinal tract, lung, bladder, or thyroid; non-melanoma skin cancers; cancers of the bone and connective tissue in individuals receiving high-dose radiation.
- Chemotherapy agents: acute myeloid leukaemia is associated with alkylating agents, topoisomerase II inhibitors, and anthracyclines.
- Both radiotherapy and chemotherapy can cause treatment-related leukaemia.

Improved radiotherapy techniques and development of less toxic chemotherapy agents aim to produce treatments that are more effective in targeting the cancer cells while reducing short- and long-term toxicities, including risk of second cancers.

It is important to re-state that the benefits of treating a first primary cancer are considered to outweigh the risks of developing subsequent primary cancers.[5]

Reducing risk of primary, recurrent, and subsequent primary cancers
Preventable cancers

Globally, 30–50% of cancers are said to be 'preventable',[12] with around four in ten cancer cases regarded as preventable in the UK[13] and USA.[14,15] To be preventable, there must be a causal relationship to a potentially modifiable risk factor. Worldwide, smoking is the single greatest avoidable risk factor for cancer mortality, responsible for eight million deaths annually.[12] Smoking cessation in the UK and USA would potentially avoid the 15% and 19% (respectively) of total cancer diagnoses caused by smoking.[13,15]

A study linking cancer risk factors with overall cancer cases and deaths during 2014 in the USA ranked modifiable risk factors, of which the top five are presented in Table 13.3.[14]

Table 13.3: Top five modifiable risk factors for cancer with the impact on cancer cases and mortality

Risk factor	Responsible for % of cancer	
	Diagnoses	Deaths
Cigarette smoking	19.0	29.0
Excess body weight	7.8	6.5
Alcohol consumption	5.6	4.0
UV radiation	5.0	1.5
Physical inactivity	2.9	2.2

The researchers found the combination of excess body weight, alcohol intake, poor diet, and physical inactivity accounted for the highest number of cancer cases in women (24%) and was second only to cigarette smoking in men (13.9% and 24% respectively). These findings highlight the importance of observing guidelines for reducing risk of cancer, discussed below.

The study also mapped the extent to which each risk factor contributed to specific cancer types (Table 13.4).[14,16] While this data concerns first primary cancers, these risk factors are potentially implicated in the formation of subsequent primary cancers. They highlight the importance of lifestyle behaviours for reducing risk of all cancers.

Table 13.4: Mapping risk factors to cancer types

Risk factor	Cancer type (% of cases)
Smoking	Lung (81.7), laryngeal (73.8), oesophageal (50), bladder (46.9)
Excess body weight	Uterine (60.3), liver (33.9), breast (11.3), colorectal (5.2)
Alcohol consumption	Oral cavity/pharyngeal (46.3 in males, 27.4 in females), liver (24.8 in males, 11.9 in females), colorectal (17.1 in males, 8.1 in females), female breast (6.4)
Low consumption of vegetables/fruit	Oral cavity/pharyngeal (17.6), laryngeal (17.4), lung (8.9)
Physical inactivity	Uterine (26.7), colorectal (16.3), female breast (3.9)
HPV infection	Cervical (100), anal (88.2), vaginal (64.6), penile (56.9)
Consumption of red/processed meats	Colorectal (5.4 red meat, 8.2 processed)
UV radiation	Melanomas (96 in males, 93.7 in women)
Low dietary fibre	Colorectal (10.3)
Low dietary calcium	Colorectal (4.9)

Guidelines for reducing risk of cancer (lifestyle advice)

Guidelines (Box 13.1) recommended by many cancer and health organisations are broadly similar throughout many countries, with minor variations or changes in emphasis.[12,17–19]

Box 13.1: Guidelines for reducing risk of cancer

- Avoid smoking or using any form of tobacco; make your home smoke free.
- Maintain a healthy body weight.
- Avoid overexposure to UV radiation, including sunshine and tanning beds.
- Limit alcohol intake.
- Eat a healthy diet.
- Be physically active.
- Avoid infections, such as HPV (human papillomavirus) or Hepatitis B and C.
- Reduce air pollution (indoor and outdoor).
- Take part in organised screening programmes.
- Limit exposure to carcinogens (substances that can cause cancer, e.g. asbestos).

Guidelines for diet

What does 'eat a healthy diet' mean? In an age where food and diet have become controversial subjects, this is not an easy question to answer. Numerous recommendations about what constitutes a good diet come from many sources, many of which have vested interests. These create confusion and often heated debate.

The World Cancer Research Fund (WCRF) Network is a global research organisation that focuses on how diet, weight, and physical activity affect the risk of developing and surviving cancer.[20] Its evidence-based recommendations (Box 13.2) offer guidance that is simple to use, aims to be realistic and achievable, and is formulated to be culturally relevant globally.[21]

The following notes apply to the WCRF recommendations:[22]

- These recommendations are applicable to people who are cancer free and may be followed by cancer survivors post treatment unless advised otherwise by a health professional.
- Individuals should aim to follow as many of the cancer prevention recommendations as possible. However, adopting any of the recommendations will go some way to reducing cancer risk.
- Following these guidelines is also likely to reduce risks of other diseases that are common with ageing as well as being common in people living beyond cancer (including diabetes and chronic respiratory disease).[21]

Box 13.2: World Cancer Research Fund Cancer Prevention Recommendations[21,22]

Be a healthy weight: Keep your weight within the healthy range and avoid weight gain in adult life.

Be physically active: Be physically active as part of everyday life – walk more and sit less.

Eat a diet rich in wholegrains, vegetables, fruit, and beans: Make wholegrains, vegetables, fruit, and pulses (legumes) such as beans and lentils a major part of your usual daily diet.

Limit consumption of 'fast foods' and other processed foods high in fat, starches, or sugars: Limiting these foods helps you control calorie intake and maintain a healthy weight.

Limit consumption of red and processed meat: Eat no more than moderate amounts of red meat, such as beef, pork, and lamb. Eat little, if any, processed meats.

Limit consumption of sugar-sweetened drinks: Drink mostly water and unsweetened drinks.

Limit alcohol consumption: For cancer prevention, it is best not to drink alcohol.

Do not use supplements for cancer prevention: Aim to meet nutritional needs through diet alone.

For mothers, breastfeed your baby if you can: Breastfeeding is good for both mother and baby.

After a cancer diagnosis, follow these recommendations if you can: Check with your health professional what is right for you. Not smoking and avoiding other exposure to tobacco and excess sun are also important in reducing cancer risk.

Following these recommendations is likely to reduce intake of salt, and saturated and trans fats, which together will help prevent other non-communicable diseases.

A note about healthy weight

Healthy weight is defined as a body mass index (BMI) in the range of 18.5–24.9. While BMI has shortcomings as a measurement, this is the currently accepted means of assessing healthy weight.

413

A note about physical activity

Physical activity is a key healthcare recommendation, implicated in reducing risk of certain cancers plus a range of other health conditions, including high blood pressure, stroke, type 2 diabetes, metabolic syndrome, and depression.[21] There is strong evidence that being physically active decreases risk of cancers of the colon, breast (post menopausal), and endometrium, while vigorous activity decreases the risk of pre- and post-menopausal breast cancer.[23]

TERMINOLOGY

Physical activity is 'any movement that uses skeletal muscles and requires more energy than resting'.[23] The term is carefully chosen to differentiate it from 'exercise', which is a subcategory of physical activity that is planned, structured, repetitive, and focused on improving or maintaining physical fitness.[24]

WCRF recommendations for being physically active are to:

- be at least moderately physically active and follow or exceed national guidelines
- limit sedentary habits.

In short, advice is to move more and sit less. The World Health Organization (WHO) details recommended levels of physical activity (Box 13.3).

Box 13.3: WHO recommendations for how much physical activity adults need[25]
Adults aged 18–64 years:

- should do at least 150–300 minutes of moderate-intensity aerobic physical activity; or at least 75–150 minutes of vigorous-intensity aerobic physical activity; or an equivalent combination of moderate- and vigorous-intensity activity throughout the week
- should also do muscle-strengthening activities at moderate or greater intensity that involve all major muscle groups on two or more days a week, as these provide additional health benefits
- may increase moderate-intensity aerobic physical activity to more than 300 minutes; or do more than 150 minutes of vigorous-intensity aerobic physical activity; or an equivalent combination of moderate- and vigorous-intensity activity throughout the week for additional health benefits.

Adults aged 65 years and above:

- should, in addition to the above, do varied multicomponent physical activity that emphasises functional balance and strength training at

---

moderate or greater intensity, on three or more days a week, to enhance functional capacity and to prevent falls.

All age groups should seek to limit sedentary activity, implicated in overweight and obesity, and indirectly implicated in cancer formation.

Clinical note

The WHO guidelines are complex and difficult to explain to patients. However, there are simple messages:

- **Any activity is better than none.**
- Physical activity is most effective and easier to maintain if it becomes part of everyday life. This can be done by adjusting daily habits, for example:
  - Walk or cycle instead of taking the car.
  - When using the car, park it in the furthest space away from the destination.
  - Get off public transport a stop early and walk the remainder of the journey.
  - Use stairs instead of a lift.
  - Take up an active hobby, such as gardening, dancing, sport, or going to the gym. The key criterion is that it should be enjoyable!
  - Activities such as housework and walking the dog count as physical activity.

The benefits of physical activity come from the total amount of activity during the week, and not how hard one pushes oneself. The benefits cannot be stored; physical activity needs to be regular to gain health benefits.

Cancer survivors who are elderly, frail, unaccustomed to physical activity, or who have physical limitation may need to increase their physical activity carefully and gradually. For these individuals, I recommend the traditional Chinese practice of 'walking 100 steps after a meal to live 100 years'. As well as amusing patients, this provides an achievable start towards what may seem a challenging goal.

Occasionally, patients need to be reminded not to do too much, or to avoid doing too much too soon. Rosa, whom we met in Chapters 4 and 5, exhausted herself doing too much physical activity too soon after major heart surgery.

Cancer screening

Screening is 'the use of simple tests across a healthy population to identify those individuals who have a disease, but do not yet have symptoms'.[26] Screening aims to:

- reduce mortality and morbidity through early detection and treatment (e.g. breast cancer)
- reduce the incidence of cancer by identifying and treating pre-cancerous disease, that is, abnormal cells that have the potential to develop into cancer over time (e.g. colorectal and cervical cancer).[27]

Screening programmes are only relevant for certain cancers; the WHO recommends programmes for cervical, colon, and breast cancers only.[27] There are known harms associated with screening, such as exposing healthy people to the potential harm of a screening intervention (such as mammography for breast cancer screening), false-positive diagnoses, and overtreating. Weighing the benefits of screening against the harms is a complex decision-making process for policy makers, and often for individuals.

CHAPTER SUMMARY

Acupuncturists:

- should be aware of the potential for recurrence and subsequent primary cancers in cancer survivors under their care
- should be aware of the signs and symptoms of cancer to monitor patients (cancer and non-cancer) and refer on for investigation, remembering that early diagnosis and treatment result in better outcomes
- can support all patients (cancer and non-cancer) to reduce risk of developing cancer or recurrence by helping them to adopt relevant lifestyle changes. These changes can also positively impact risk of other chronic diseases.

References

1. Morton LM, Onel K, Curtis RE, *et al.* The rising incidence of second cancers: patterns of occurrence and identification of risk factors for children and adults. Am. Soc. Clin. Oncol. Educ. Book 2014:e57–e67.
2. de Valois B, Glynne-Jones R Acupuncture in the supportive care of colorectal cancer survivors: four case studies, Part 2. Eur. J. Orient. Med. 2018;9(1):10–22.
3. Williams M, McConnell H, White R, *et al.* Beyond life and death: measuring recurrence, progression and functional outcomes in patients with cancer. Macmillan Cancer Support; 2016. Available from: www.macmillan.org.uk/_images/beyond-life-and-death_tcm9-298127.pdf
4. American Society of Clinical Oncology (ASCO) What is a second cancer? Alexandria, VA: ASCO; 2021. Available from: www.cancer.net/survivorship/what-second-cancer#:~:text=When%20a%20person%20who%20has,same%20as%20a%20cancer%20recurrence
5. American Cancer Society Cancer facts & figures 2009. Atlanta: American Cancer Society; 2009.
6. Utada M, Ohno Y, Hori M, *et al.* Incidence of multiple primary cancers and interval between first and second primary cancers. Cancer Sci 2014;105(7):890–806.
7. Rosso S, De Angelis R, Ciccolallo L, *et al.* Multiple tumours in survival estimates. Eur. J. Cancer 2009;45(6):1080–1094.
8. American Cancer Society Cancer treatment & survivorship facts & figures 2019–2021. Atlanta: American Cancer Society; 2019.
9. American Cancer Society Signs and symptoms of cancer. Atlanta: American Cancer Society; 2020. Available from: www.cancer.org/treatment/understanding-your-diagnosis/signs-and-symptoms-of-cancer.html
10. Cancer Research UK Signs and symptoms of cancer. London: Cancer Research UK; 2020. Available from: www.cancerresearchuk.org/about-cancer/cancer-symptoms
11. American Society of Clinical Oncology (ASCO) Understanding cancer risk. Alexandria, VA: ASCO; 2018. Available from: www.cancer.net/navigating-cancer-care/prevention-and-healthy-living/understanding-cancer-risk
12. World Health Organization Preventing cancer. WHO; no date. Available from: www.who.int/activities/preventing-cancer
13. Cancer Research UK Statistics on preventable cancers. London: Cancer Research UK; 2018. Available from: www.cancerresearchuk.org/health-professional/cancer-statistics/risk/preventable-cancers

---

14. Islami F, Goding Sauer A, Miller KD, *et al.* Proportion and number of cancer cases and deaths attributable to potentially modifiable risk factors in the United States. CA. Cancer J. Clin. 2018;68(1):31–54.

15. American Cancer Society Cancer facts & figures 2022. Atlanta: American Cancer Society; 2022.

16. Mendes E More than 4 in 10 cancers and cancer deaths linked to modifiable risk factors. American Cancer Society; 2017. Available from: www.cancer.org/latest-news/more-than-4-in-10-cancers-and-cancer-deaths-linked-to-modifiable-risk-factors.html

17. Australian Government Department of Health Preventing cancer. Canberra; 2021. Available from: www.health.gov.au/health-topics/cancer/about-cancer/preventing-and-diagnosing-cancer

18. PDQ° Screening and Prevention Editorial Board PDQ Cancer Prevention Overview. Bethesda, MD: National Cancer Institute; February 25, 2022. Available from: www.cancer.gov/about-cancer/causes-prevention/hp-prevention-overview-pdq

19. Cancer Research UK Can cancer be prevented? London: Cancer Research UK; 2022. Available from: www.cancerresearchuk.org/about-cancer/causes-of-cancer/can-cancer-be-prevented-0

20. World Cancer Research Fund Who we are. London: World Cancer Research Fund; no date. Available from: www.wcrf-uk.org/about-us/who-we-are

21. World Cancer Research Fund, American Institute for Cancer Research Continuous update project expert report 2018: Recommendations and public health and policy implications. 2018. Available from: www.wcrf.org/wp-content/uploads/2021/01/Recommendations.pdf

22. World Cancer Research Fund After a cancer diagnosis: follow our Recommendations, if you can. London: World Cancer Research Fund; no date. Available from: www.wcrf-uk.org/preventing-cancer/our-cancer-prevention-recommendations/after-cancer-diagnosis

23. World Cancer Research Fund, American Institute for Cancer Research Continuous update project expert report 2018. Physical activity and the risk of cancer; 2018. Available from: www.wcrf.org/wp-content/uploads/2021/02/Physical-activity.pdf

24. Dasso NA How is exercise different from physical activity? A concept analysis. Nurs. Forum. 2019;54(1):45–52.

25. World Health Organization Physical activity. Geneva: World Health Organization; 2020. Available from: www.who.int/news-room/fact-sheets/detail/physical-activity

26. World Health Organization Cancer – screening and early detection. World Health Organization; 2010. Available from: www.who.int/europe/news-room/fact-sheets/item/cancer-screening-and-early-detection-of-cancer

27. World Health Organization A short guide to cancer screening. Increase effectiveness, maximize benefits and minimize harm. Copenhagen: WHO Regional Office for Europe; 2022.

Part IV

ACUPUNCTURE FOR TRANSFORMATION AND RENEWAL

Chapter 14

Getting My Life Back:
A Detailed Case Study

Constant pain...lack of grip...makes you feel out of control...off balance. Some days I could cheerfully chop off my arm. It's ugly. It's a constant reminder of the cancer. (Ann, before her course of acupuncture)

I feel in control of my life. My arm is not so heavy. Pain is less and I have much better movement and control of my fingers...I feel more positive. I feel much calmer. (Ann, after 13 acupuncture treatments)

Introduction

This detailed case study of Ann brings together many of the aspects discussed in this book. It illustrates acupuncture's potential to help cancer survivors to thrive, not merely survive – to get their life back after cancer and its treatments.

A breast cancer survivor with lymphoedema, Ann experienced long-term and life-limiting consequences of cancer and its treatments. With her multiple comorbidities and a legacy of past and continuing traumatic life events, Ann's complex picture represents that of many cancer survivors. Her route through the Survivorship Pathway is marked by the shaded boxes in Figure 14.1.

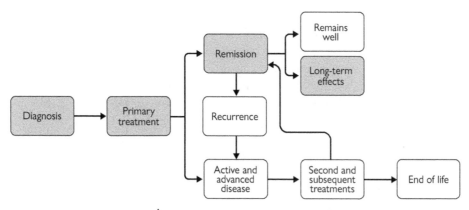

FIGURE 14.1: ANN'S ROUTE THROUGH THE SURVIVORSHIP PATHWAY

Ann was articulate about the damaging physical and emotional effects cancer and lymph-oedema had on her life. Coupled with her capacity to observe and communicate the benefits she experienced from acupuncture treatment, this provides a rich example that taught me a great deal about the challenges faced by survivors, and how acupuncture can help.

Her case is remarkable in that treatment was of short duration – 13 treatments over 16 weeks. It was also discrete – Ann had not had acupuncture prior to these sessions, nor did she have any for many years after. Yet she is clear about the short- and long-term effects, some of which have provided benefit for years.

In a world in which there is pressure to show that a specific acupuncture point or point protocol has a specific effect on a specific symptom, Ann's case demonstrates the breadth and depth of the effects of acupuncture. She reported a wide range of symptom improvements. While some of these may be categorised as specific (e.g. pain relief) and non-specific (e.g. improved energy and wellbeing) effects of acupuncture, her case demonstrates the systemic nature and resulting effects of acupuncture treatment.

We should expect a system based on a network of channels to have wide-ranging effects. To acupuncturists practising Chinese medicine, this comes as no surprise; for others, I hope this case is illuminating.

Ann's case also illustrates the importance of flexibility of approach. I changed the treatment principles and points as she changed through treatment.

Ann's story demonstrates how symptom relief combined with increased energy can improve motivation and lead to improved self-care, and build resilience and the ability to cope with life's continuing challenges (Figure 14.3 at the end of the chapter). These benefits are particularly important when people with chronic, incurable conditions must engage in the process of ongoing daily self-care to manage their condition.

Above all, Ann exemplifies how acupuncture can be a catalyst to change and transform the lives of cancer survivors.

Background to this case study

Ann participated in research into using acupuncture for people with cancer treatment-related lymphoedema.[1-3] This research focused on promoting wellbeing and improving quality of life for people with lymphoedema; acupuncture was an adjunct to usual care provided by the lymphoedema specialist clinic.

It was not an objective to use acupuncture to treat the lymphoedema itself; the aim was to treat the person, rather than the disease. For this reason, there are no objective measures (such as arm measurements) presented in this case study.

In the absence of clear evidence about the benefit or harm of applying acupuncture to an affected limb, the research protocol specified avoiding needling areas affected by lymph-oedema. In addition, for breast cancer participants, needling points in the torso quadrant on the affected side was also avoided. In consultation with the lymphoedema nurse specialist, it was agreed that points on the midline (Ren and Du channels) could be needled.

Participants were offered up to 13 acupuncture treatments. After completing a series of seven treatments, they could choose to have a further six treatments. They completed several questionnaires at intervals up to 12 weeks after the last treatment.

This case study can be read in conjunction with Chapter 9, Cancer Treatment-Related Lymphoedema, which is a full discussion of lymphoedema and acupuncture.

ANN'S STORY

Ann was involved in all stages of writing this case study and remains keen to share her experience of acupuncture.

Background

I met Ann when she participated in a preliminary focus group for the research. I was impressed by her clear articulation of the effects breast cancer treatment-related lymphoedema in her left arm had on her daily life, both practically and emotionally. Her descriptions were calm, clear, and powerful.

Although she knew little about acupuncture, she was eager to make changes in her life. She embraced the opportunity to participate in the research to facilitate significant personal change. I was pleased when some weeks after the focus group, the lymphoedema nurse specialist referred Ann to the treatment phase of the study.

Physical presentation

Ann was 60 years old when she joined the study. She dressed neatly and comfortably; her complexion was dull-pale. Although softly spoken, she had an air of quiet determination. Her left arm, encased in the flesh-coloured compression garment used in lymphoedema maintenance treatment, was considerably swollen, as were her fingers.

Cancer and lymphoedema history

Ann had been diagnosed eight years previously with Stage II oestrogen receptive-negative carcinoma of the left breast, with lymph node involvement. The breast cancer was treated with surgery (a wide local excision with axillary node clearance), chemotherapy, and radiotherapy.

Swelling of the left arm appeared during chemotherapy and was diagnosed as lymphoedema. Ann had been referred to the hospital's lymphoedema service and was now under maintenance treatment to control the swelling and manage her anxiety about it. Treatment was also aimed at preventing complications such as cellulitis; she had a history of idiopathic incidents of this secondary complication of lymphoedema.

Her prescribed self-management routine (Table 14.4) adhered to the four corner-stones of lymphoedema maintenance and included:

- daily self-massage
- exercise
- skin care (moisturising and protecting from injury)
- wearing a compression sleeve and glove.

In addition, Ann self-bandaged with kinesiology tape and wore a compression bra at night.

Main complaints

Ann presented with two main complaints, one physical and one emotional.

Physical complaint

Discomfort in her lymphoedema-affected arm was Ann's main physical complaint. Her arm felt 'heavy' and was affected by 'constant pain' extending across the front of her left shoulder and across the back to her spine.

Swelling affected her fingers, which were 'like sausages – I can't bend them'. A seamstress by profession, she was unable to sew. Attempting to do one hour of sewing caused increased pain and swelling 'for the next two or three days'. Her grip was so unreliable that taking a roast joint from the oven was dangerous as she risked losing her grip and burning herself with hot fat.

The condition profoundly affected her daily life, from 'silly little things' like not being able to wear a watch on her left arm to being unable to change her grandchildren's nappies. Ann was frustrated at the length of time even simple tasks took.

Furthermore, strangers noticed her hand and asked what the matter was. Finding clothes to fit was difficult. She felt her arm was 'ugly…it's a constant reminder of the cancer' and some days she felt she could 'cheerfully chop it off'. The discomfort and swelling fluctuated. She referred to these consequences as 'the monkey' and said that 'on a bad day the monkey jumps off your shoulder and slaps you in the face'.

Emotional complaint

This led to her emotional symptom. All this made Ann feel 'out of control' and she felt she had been 'emotionally off-balance since the cancer'. Prior to diagnosis, she was 'comfortable with myself', but now she felt 'lost somewhere'. Along with loss of confidence, she felt guilty about surviving cancer, a feeling intensified by the death of a young friend from cerebral palsy. Why had Ann survived, when this young woman had not?

Ann's treatment priorities

Ann was clear about the results she desired from acupuncture, which were:

- physical: relief of the pain in her arm and shoulder
- emotional: to 'get back in balance'
- active: to be able to resume sewing.

Questioning the systems

Diagnosis by interrogation, or 'questioning the systems', is part of diagnosis in Chinese medicine. It is a discussion between practitioner and patient to explore the condition, its history, and its context. This line of questioning explores the health of the physiological 'systems', such as digestion, gynaecological, and urinary, and is also the foundation for pattern diagnosis.[4,5]

Using a system called the 'Ten Questions' (Box 14.1), each of the main areas of questioning may have many more specific questions to explore that area of health.

This semi-structured format is used flexibly according to the patient, and in the discussion below, I present those pertinent to Ann's case.

Box 14.1: The Ten Questions

1. Sleep
2. Appetite, food, and taste
3. Thirst and drink
4. Bowels and urine
5. Sweating and temperature preference
6. Head and body
7. Eyes and ears
8. Thorax and abdomen
9. Pain
10. Climate and season

Two additional areas of questioning concern women (gynaecological) and children. Additional areas may be questioned, such as personal and family health histories, relationships, and present situation.[5]

Sleep: Ann's sleep pattern had been poor for 25 years, since the birth of her youngest child. At most, she slept four hours, and often stayed up all night reading. Frequent nightmares had started with her cancer diagnosis; she often woke up 'terrified' with her cries 'waking the entire household'. She described these later in a focus group:

> I've had terrible nightmares, to the point that I was frightened to go to sleep. I couldn't tell you what they were when I woke up, but I'd wake up screaming, crying, sweating. My husband, the whole house was up it was really…and it's been like that ever since [the diagnosis of cancer].

Appetite, food, and drink: Poor appetite, coupled with fear of further weight gain (Ann was 7 stone overweight (44.5kg or 98lb)) meant she ate little. She sometimes had an evening meal with the family, but often would 'go a couple of days without eating'. She lived on tea, consuming 10–12 cups daily. Ann suffered heartburn with acid reflux at night. Lying on her left side eased this discomfort but increased that in her arm. She felt exhausted!

Bowels and urine: Ann was constipated 'most of the time', managing a bowel movement 'every two or three days', a condition helped by eating peanuts. She had bladder repair surgery 15 years previously, and although she urinated frequently, she passed little urine.

Gynaecological history: Periods had stopped with a hysterectomy at the age of 38 (22 years previously), following three years of excessive bleeding after the birth of her fifth child. Ann's periods had always been heavy, frequent, and long, lasting eight to ten days in a short cycle of 21 days. Two of her five pregnancies were caesarean sections. Menopause commenced after the hysterectomy and was managed with hormone replacement therapy (HRT) until her cancer diagnosis.

Head and body: Ann experienced three to four headaches a week, which affected the back of her eyes. Controlled with Disprin (aspirin), they lasted about two hours. Dizziness affected her about once a month; mostly these incidents made her light-headed, but sometimes 'everything goes round' for a few seconds. Breathing was difficult when she went uphill; she rarely had colds.

Pain: As well as pain related to lymphoedema, she had arthritis in the knees (managed with Brufen® Retard (ibuprofen)), and back pain from a prolapsed disc between lumbars 4 and 5.

Sweating and temperature: Ann felt that her temperature was 'normal'; nightmares caused cold sweats.

Additional information: Ann's height was 167cm (5'7'). Her weight was 18 stone (252lb or 114kg). This is a BMI (body mass index) of 40.9 which falls into the range categorised as 'obese'. This is a significant comorbidity, as there are strong links between obesity and lymphoedema.[6,7]

Personal health history: In addition to the cancer and gynaecological histories, Ann had a shadow on her lung as a child. She also had a smoking history, starting at the age of 19 and smoking 20 cigarettes a day until the cancer diagnosis at the age of 52.

Prescription medications taken daily included doxazosin (1mg) and bendroflumethiazide (2.5mg) to manage blood pressure.

Relationships: Ann was almost three decades into her second marriage and enjoyed a supportive and loving relationship with her husband. Two of Ann's five adult children lived at home. Her youngest, with Down syndrome, required Ann's constant care. Although committed to caring for her child, this limited Ann's options in life. She was unable to work outside the home, finances were limited, and she knew that she would be her daughter's carer for the rest of her life.

Committed to family life, Ann put the needs of others before her own, describing herself as a 'doormat' to her large family. She was particularly anxious about her elder daughter's pregnancy as she had 'premonitions' that she 'would bury this child'. Also, Christmas (Ann commenced treatment in late October) was a particularly difficult time emotionally. The anniversary of her cancer diagnosis in December coincided with a pattern of deaths and bad news over the years, influencing her mood and increasing her anxiety levels during this season.

Physical examination: Tongue: Swollen, reddish purple, with a very red tip. A thin,

GETTING MY LIFE BACK: A DETAILED CASE STUDY

sticky, dirty-coloured coating extended from the back over the top, diminishing from the Spleen/Stomach area to the tip. Blue veins on the underside extended to the tip but were not distended. **Pulse:** Overall deep and weak on the left side; intensity and quality varying from almost impalpable on the left rear position to slippery on the dominant left middle position. Big across all three positions on the right. Even rhythm; normal rate.

Verbal and non-verbal behaviours: Softly spoken, Ann was candid and willing to share information about her circumstances. The clear verbal articulation that I noticed in the focus group was also present in the clinic. She was forthcoming, but never overwhelming.

Although her symptoms were burdensome and aspects of her life were clearly challenging, she appeared determined to regain control of her situation.

She was nervous about having acupuncture, describing her aversion to needles, especially after experiencing chemotherapy, in a focus group:

> I must admit, as I say, I was nervous, I don't like needles, I can't look at anyone on television having an injection! It says to me how desperate I was that I would even consider having needles put into me!

Over time, she grew to trust me, and became more confident about what she could divulge.

Diagnosis
Initial diagnosis
Figure 14.2 is a diagrammatic representation illustrating my initial diagnosis for Ann.

Non-cancer-related factors
Many symptoms were long-standing, such as the gynaecological history and insomnia. Diet was a long-standing aetiological factor contributing to much of her symptom picture.

Cancer and cancer treatment-related factors
Main complaints related to the cancer diagnosis and treatment, with two main aetiological factors:

- Trauma, a miscellaneous cause of disease in Chinese medicine, associated with surgical removal of lymph nodes, leading to the lymphoedema in her arm.
- Emotions, an internal cause of disease in Chinese medicine (see Chapter 3, Cancer Survivorship and the Emotions):
  - **Shock** of diagnosis scatters the qi, causing an imbalance in Heart and Kidney qi.
  - **Fear** about the progress of the disease and mortality is common for cancer patients and may contribute to weakening the Kidney qi.
  - **Worry** about cancer treatment as well as other practical issues is also a commonly experienced emotion and may contribute to weakening the Spleen.
  - **Anger**, in the form of Ann's continuous frustration about her incapacity to carry out her daily activities, may have affected the Liver qi.

Additional life events, such as the frequent deaths and associated grief, may also have impacted the Lungs and Large Intestine (not illustrated).

Blocks to treatment

I was also concerned about the presence of blocks to treatment, specifically, Aggressive Energy (AE) and Possession (see Chapter 5, Toolkit).

AE is indicated if a person has had serious or life-threatening physical illness and when there is a history of intensive drug therapy.[5] The combination of Ann's cancer diagnosis, chemotherapy treatment, and emotional history suggested it was appropriate to check for AE.

Possession is indicated when a person has underlying poor physical or psychological health and has experienced emotional shocks as well as physical shocks (such as surgery). Ann had these predisposing factors. In addition, she exhibited two key symptoms of possession: she felt out of control, and she experienced intense, terrifying nightmares.[5]

The constitutional factor

At this stage, I had not identified her constitutional factor.

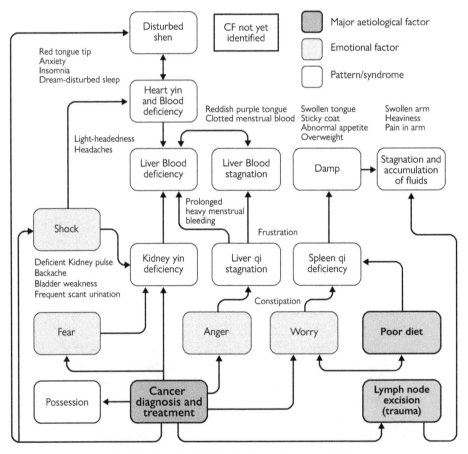

FIGURE 14.2: INITIAL DIAGNOSIS DIAGRAM FOR ANN

Initial treatment principles
Treatment strategy
My treatment plan was to use mixed methods, drawing on Chinese medicine approaches to influence the arm, and Five Element acupuncture to support the constitution and spirit.

Chinese medicine approaches
The interdiction to needling the affected area turned my focus away from attempting to treat the manifestation (*biao*, the swollen arm) to addressing the root (*Ben*, the underlying cause of the swelling).

With little in the literature to guide me, I was intrigued by Maciocia's discussion of activating the Triple Burner to move and transform qi and Fluids, which is fully discussed in Chapter 9, Cancer Treatment-Related Lymphoedema. Maciocia also recommends opening the Directing Vessel (*Ren Mai*) to promote transformation, transportation, and excretion of fluids, combining this with points on the Directing Vessel to stimulate the Triple Burner's capacity to metabolise Fluids.[8]

Five Element approaches
Clearing blocks to treatment: In view of the assessment (Figure 14.2), my initial treatment principles were to clear the blocks to treatment (Table 14.1), by:

- administering an AE Drain
- addressing Possession using Internal Dragons (IDs).

Identifying the CF: The ability to assess colour, sound, emotion, odour (CSEO) for a Five Element diagnosis is something that develops over time, and this was the case with Ann. It was not until well into the course of treatment that I began to identify these aspects and incorporate them into the treatment principles.

At this early stage, I suspected Ann might be an Earth CF, given her need to constantly look after others. However, I had no substantiation of this from her CSEO, so I continually observed and kept an open mind.

Treatment
Notes on treatment
Ann attended for acupuncture once a week and the treatments are detailed below. The techniques used in Ann's treatment are described fully in Chapter 5, Toolkit.

In general, I used an even needle technique and direct moxa.

- Needling was avoided in the left arm and associated torso quadrant, as this is the side of the arm affected by lymphoedema. Therefore, all arm and torso points were needled in the right side only.
- Other points were needled bilaterally, unless otherwise indicated.
- When using the extraordinary vessels, the Directing Vessel (*Ren Mai*) and Yang Stepping Vessel (*Yang Qiao Mai*):

- Maciocia's gender-based needling procedure – that is, needling the opening point on the right side (RS) and the coupled point on the left side (LS) for women – was possible when using the Directing Vessel, as Ann's affected arm was the on the left. It was not possible when using the Yang Stepping Vessel, and I needled the coupled point (SI-3) on the right.
- The extraordinary vessel points were needled first, followed by any additional points. Needles were retained for 20 minutes.
- When removing needles, all needles were removed, finishing with the coupled point of the extraordinary vessel as the penultimate needle removed, and the opening point removed last. These techniques are described in Chapter 5, Toolkit.

• When treating the CF, I needle without retention, removing the needles immediately after deqi.

Ann's first three treatments

I commenced by clearing blocks to treatment and using direct moxa unilaterally on Kidney chest points to support the spirit. At the third treatment, I began to focus on the arm pain and swelling.

Table 14.1: Ann's first three treatments

Abbreviations: Tx treatment; **RS** right side; **LS** left side; **(n)** shows number of direct moxa cones applied

Tx	Treatment principles	Points	Notes
1	Clear block to treatment: Aggressive Energy (AE) Drain	BL-13 *Feishu* BL-14 *Jueyinshu* BL-15 *Xinshu* BL-18 *Ganshu* BL- 20 *Pishu* BL-23 *Shenshu* Plus 3 check needles	Unilateral needling, RS only.
2	Clear block to treatment: Internal Dragons	Master point 0.25 cun below REN-15 *Jiuwei* ST-25 *Tianshu* ST-32 *Futu* ST-41 *Jiexi*	
	Help patient regain control (yuan source points of fire)	SI-4 *Wangu* HE-7 *Shenmen*	RS only.

3	Treat spirit	KID-25 *Shencang* KID-27 *Shufu*	Direct moxa (3) RS only, no needling.
	Promote transformation, transportation, and excretion of fluids[4]	Open *Ren Mai*: LU-7 *Lieque* (RS) KID-6 *Zhaohai* (LS)	
		REN-4 *Guanyuan*	Direct moxa (5), no needling.
	Treat arm pain and swelling[5]	TB-5 *Waiguan* LI-11 *Quchi*	On RS, contralateral to affected arm.

Ann's response to treatment

Ann responded strongly to treatment. She carefully observed and clearly expressed the changes she experienced. She overcame her fear of needles, and particularly enjoyed having moxa treatment; she loved the smell and found the warmth comforting and relaxing.

Tx 1: She reported that after the AE Drain she was 'extremely thirsty' for two days, better able to cope with the arm pain, was very 'laid back', and had slept for an 'unheard of' six hours on the night of treatment. Her husband had remarked that she was noticeably calmer.

Tx 2: After clearing IDs, Ann said she had much more energy, was very alert, and felt very positive. Her sleep improved, as did her emotional state. She felt less anxious about her daughter's pregnancy and less guilty about surviving cancer. Her relationship with her daughter with Down syndrome also began to change, and Ann began to treat her 'as she would treat her other children' rather than 'doing everything' for her.

Tx 3: Ann felt quite 'disoriented' after this treatment and slept almost continuously for nearly 18 hours. The next day she woke up 'feeling good' and she 'spent the day peeing!' The weekend marked the anniversary of the death of Ann's friend, and Ann noted that she felt sad but not guilty.

Changes to the arm

During this early stage of treatment, her arm responded as well:

- After IDs (treatment 2), it felt less heavy and she had not needed to bandage with kinesiology tape the following week.
- After treatment 3, the pain in her shoulder disappeared, and the usual 'screaming pain' around the lower forearm and wrist reduced to a 'constant nagging ache'.
- Although still swollen, the arm had softened, her grip began to improve, and she completed a small sewing project!

Progress: from looking after others to looking after herself

These responses were promising, but alas, progress was not straightforward. The improvements of the first three treatments seemed to be set back by a succession of acute episodes.

My treatment plan to consistently address Ann's priorities (the discomfort of her arm and balancing her emotions) was thwarted by the acute onset of sciatica on her right side, followed by severe lower back pain, followed by flu (during which Ann missed a week of treatment). I changed my treatment plan to address these acute conditions during treatments 4 to 6, while still managing to pay some attention to addressing the arm (Table 14.2).

Table 14.2: Ann's treatments 4–7

Abbreviations: Tx treatment; **RS** right side; **LS** left side; **(n)** shows number of direct moxa cones applied

Tx	Treatment principles	Points	Notes
4	Treat sciatic pain (RS): Open Yang Stepping Vessel (*Yang Qiao Mai*)*	BL-62 *Shenmai* SI-3 *Houxi*	All points on RS.
	Needle points on affected channel[3]	GB-32 *Zhongdu* GB-34 *Yanglingquan* GB-39 *Xuanzhong*	
		2 *ah shi* points in right buttock	
	Warm channel	Stick moxa along GB channel	
5	Treat spirit	KID-24 *Lingxu*	Direct moxa (3) RS only, no needling.
	Promote transformation, transportation, and excretion of fluids (PTTE)	Open *Ren Mai*: LU-7 *Lieque* (RS) KID-6 *Zhaohai* (LS) Plus REN-9 *Shuifen* REN-12 *Zhongwan*	
	Warm lower jiao (for back pain)**	Moxa stick along Ren channel from REN-2 *Qugu* to REN-8 *Shenque*[7]	
6	PTTE	As per Tx 5	
	Treat catarrh (after flu):		
	Resolve damp and phlegm***	ST-40 *Fenglong* (RS) SP-9 *Yinlingquan* (LS)	
	Clear sinuses***	LI-4 *Hegu* (RS) LI-20 *Yingxiang* M-HN-3 *Yintang*	

7	Treat spirit	KID-25 *Shencang* KID-27 *Shufu*	Direct moxa (3 cones on each point) RS only, no needling.
	PTTE	As per Tx 5 plus REN-5 *Shimen*	
		REN-4 *Guanyuan*	Direct moxa (5), no needling.

*Maciocia, pages 572–573.[8]

**Warming the Ren channel from REN-2 to REN-8 with stick moxa is a technique I discovered in clinical practice that is often effective for relieving spasm and pain associated with lower back pain.

***Deadman *et al.*, see relevant entries for functions of the points.[9]

Ann's response to treatment

These acute attacks were frustrating and disappointing for both practitioner and patient.

With hindsight, it appears they provided Ann with the opportunity to start putting her needs ahead of others. Taking to her bed, she realised her adult children could not only look after themselves, but they could also help her as well. She began to delegate; her adult son who was living at home took on household tasks and ironed his own shirts. She established boundaries and stopped pushing herself to keep going. She gave herself permission to look after herself.

Changes to the arm

During this period, her arm continued to improve. Although the pain increased because she was sleeping on her left side due to the sciatic and lower back pain, she reported that the arm continued to feel less heavy, movement was easier, and her grip continued to improve.

Overall changes

After treatment 6, flu-related sinusitis disappeared immediately after treatment, which she found 'so amazing…my family noticed the difference'. The arm pain also reduced, the 'heaviness (was) all but gone', and Ann could do the ironing without discomfort. She declared that she felt 'much better…back in balance'.

Progress: from symptom to self
Reviewing priorities

After completing seven treatments, Ann chose to continue having acupuncture, taking advantage of the six additional sessions offered as part of the research. In reviewing her priorities, Ann specified:

- physical: keep the arm discomfort under control
- emotional: focus on building confidence
- active: sewing remained the priority activity.

Adjusting the treatment strategy

I changed the treatment strategy during this phase. With the arm pain under control, and function restored to her hand, Ann could turn her attention from her physical symptoms to her overall wellbeing.

This change is described as a shift in orientation from symptom to self and is discussed in Chapter 4, Offering Complex Patients a Simple Piece of Heaven. It marks a patient's awareness that acupuncture can do more than deal with physical symptoms. Ann came for treatment intuitively aware that acupuncture could help restore her emotional balance; it was now time to focus on this. For this phase, I chose to utilise a more Five Element style.

Death, dreams, and dragons

This sequence of six treatments (Table 14.3) began in the new year. Ann returned from the break reporting it was 'the best Christmas in nine years'. However, death still haunted the festive season, with her uncle's death on Christmas morning. This brought up 'lots of memories' and her tummy 'felt knotted'.

She recounted a dream in which she was enclosed underwater in a clear box and could not get out. She was able to breathe, but unable to attract attention. We discussed the pattern of deaths at Christmas time, her anxieties about attending her uncle's funeral, and we noted that her dream might be related to her feelings about death.

Clearing blocks to treatment

I interpreted the reappearance of troubling dreams as the recurrence of a block, and administered IDs, supplementing this with moxa on KID-24 *Lingxu* and REN-17 *Shanzhong* to support the spirit and calm the shen. Ann subsequently reported that she was able to deal with the funeral and mourning without disturbance from nightmares or anxiety.

Addressing the CF – wood

For the remaining five treatments, I shifted the treatment principles to supporting the wood element.

Over the previous weeks, I became aware of a consistent and marked green hue in her face. Her gentle voice 'lacked shout',[5] and she spoke of how she had lost her assertiveness since the cancer diagnosis. In view of this, I suspected a Gall Bladder imbalance, indicated by '…timidity, a definite lack of self-assertion and a lack of balance, regulation, and good decision making'.[5]

I addressed this using GB-40 *Qiuxu* and other points on the Liver and Gall Bladder channels. In addition to addressing the wood element, I continued to support the spirit and calm the shen using moxa on Kidney chest points and on REN-17 *Shanzhong*. I continued to use the protocol for promoting transformation, transportation, and excretion of fluids to maintain and continue to improve her arm and hand.

Table 14.3: Ann's treatments 8–13

Abbreviations: Tx treatment; **RS** right side; **(n)** shows number of direct moxa cones applied

Tx	Treatment principles	Points	Notes
8	Treat spirit	KID-24 *Lingxu* (RS) REN-17 *Shanzhong*	Direct moxa (3 cones on each point) RS only, no needling.
	Clear block to treatment: Internal Dragons	Master point 0.25 cun below REN-15 *Jiuwei* ST-25 *Tianshu* ST-32 *Futu* ST-41 *Jiexi*	
	Help patient regain control (yuan source points of fire)	SI-4 *Wangu* HE-7 *Shenmen*	RS only.
9	Treat spirit	KID-20 *Futonggu* (RS) KID-21 *Youmen* (RS) REN-17 *Shanzhong*	Direct moxa (3 cones on each point) RS only, no needling.
	Treat CF – wood*	GB-40 *Qiuxu* LIV-3 *Taichong*	Bilateral needling.
10	Treat spirit	KID-25 *Shencang* KID-27 *Shufu* REN-17 *Shanzhong*	Direct moxa (3 cones on each point) RS only, no needling.
		REN-4 *Guanyuan*	Needled.
	Treat CF – wood	GB-37 *Guangming* LIV-5 *Ligou* GB-41 *Zulinqi*	Bilateral needling.
11	Promote transformation, transportation, and excretion of fluids (PTTE)	As per Tx 5, Table 14.2	
	Resolve damp	SP-9 *Yinlinquan* (RS)	
	Calm shen	REN-17 *Shanzhong*	Direct moxa (3), no needling.
		M-HN-3 *Yintang*	Needled.
	Treat CF – Wood	GB-40 *Qiuxu* LIV-3 *Taichong*	LS only.
12	Clear entry/exit block:** Spleen/Heart	SP-21 *Dabao* HE-1 *Jiquan*	RS only.
13	PTTE	As per Tx 7, Table 14.2	
	Treat spirit, calm shen	REN-17 *Shazhong*	Direct moxa (3), no needling.
	Treat CF – wood – spring seasonal treatment* (wood points of wood)	GB-41 *Zulinqi* LIV-1 *Dadun*	Bilateral needling.

*For theory and practice of treating the constitutional factor, see Hicks *et al.*, pages 321–326 for information about specific points.[5]

**Entry/exit blocks are another block to treatment used widely in Five Element acupuncture. See Hicks *et al.*, pages 250–253.[5]

Ann's response to treatment

As she progressed through these treatments, Ann's confidence increased. She reported that she 'had a go' at her chemist one morning, and she was assertive with troublesome builders doing renovations in her home. She was able to 'put (her) self first' and manage boundaries.

Her sleep patterns were consistently good; there were no more troublesome dreams. Her arm continued to improve, and although there were fluctuations in swelling and pain, recovery was more rapid than it had been prior to starting acupuncture.

Addressing lifestyle

Ann's poor eating habits were damaging to her health, and I encouraged her to eat regular meals. Initially she resisted this advice, convinced it would only exacerbate her weight problem.

Encountering resistance

During the first series of treatments, I persisted in my encouragement, explaining that by eating so little, she was pushing her body into starvation mode and making weight loss unlikely. I also explained that this was damaging her Spleen energy, which was in turn contributing to many of her symptoms.

Making changes

Ann remained deeply sceptical, and her efforts to eat breakfast every day were unsuccessful. Therefore, I was surprised at her New Year's decision to change her diet. She said she felt 'mentally able' to consider starting to manage her weight problem and she wanted to lose up to 7 stone (98lb or 44.5kg).

She made a conscious effort to eat three meals a day. Eating breakfast became less of a challenge; in fact, she began to want to eat in the morning. Lunch remained a struggle, but Ann attempted to eat then as well as to have dinner at 6.30pm.

Reaping rewards

Her persistence was rewarded and at her final treatment Ann reported:

> I am eating regularly, which I did not before, I have lost 10lb in weight and no long suffer with constipation.

The headaches decreased, and her energy improved.

End of treatment and follow-up

The end of treatment

After her 13th and final treatment, Ann summarised the physical and emotional benefits she experienced:

> The degree of heaviness and pain in my arm is much less than when I started and I am able to do the fine sewing I was finding impossible before. My fingers are not as swollen

and my grip has improved… Since having cancer I have been lacking in self-confidence and felt very vulnerable emotionally. The acupuncture/moxibustion has helped me regain control of my emotions and given me back self-confidence. I feel more positive and more like the person I was before the cancer. Family and friends have commented on these changes – particularly on the energy I now have compared to before…

Progress following the end of treatment
Continuous self-care is important, especially when managing chronic conditions such as lymphoedema.

An acute episode of cellulitis
Three weeks after the last acupuncture session, Ann had cellulitis, an acute infection associated with lymphoedema. This potentially life-threatening condition requires imme-diate medical attention and treatment with antibiotics.

In a research questionnaire sent out at this time, Ann wrote that although she experienced severe pain with this infection, her arm still felt lighter, and she was able to cope with the pain far better than in previous episodes of cellulitis. More importantly, she had sought immediate medical attention:

> Normally, I 'put off' going to the doctor until things are really bad; this time I had the confidence to request an urgent appointment and get prompt treatment. I feel this is due to the acupuncture/moxibustion treatment I received.

Long-term observations
Twelve weeks after treatment ended, Anne reflected on how acupuncture had changed her life. She was now eating three meals a day and continued to find time for herself. Her arm still felt lighter, and finger movement was better.

Although her arm could still become painful, she was coping with this better, saying 'I now rest it immediately and do not feel guilty.' This included not feeling guilty about asking family members to do her tasks! Ann later described this:

> And I think having the acupuncture helped me to find myself and actually say to the family 'I'm sorry, I'm tired, my arm hurts, either do it yourself or leave it 'til tomorrow!' And the funny thing was the roof didn't fall in, and people did still speak to me. But I'd lost that confidence and people keep saying that I'm like my old self now, I can't tell you what it means.[1]

The longer-term effects of treatment
Ann continued to support promoting acupuncture in the management of lymphoedema. She contributed to projects such as writing this chapter, which we did three years after treatment.

The cost of private treatment was a barrier to Ann having further acupuncture treatment; however, the benefits from her 13 treatments were remarkably long term. A bout of ill-health around the time of our writing raised concerns about cancer recurrence.

During this anxious time, Ann felt that she was still benefitting from the acupuncture sessions and was able to manage her anxieties while undergoing investigations for what was eventually diagnosed as chronic obstructive pulmonary disease (COPD).

In reviewing this text, Ann wrote:

> Reflecting back over what I was like before the treatment, I am amazed at how far acupuncture has enabled me to come and am so grateful that you did not 'give up' on me.
>
> I am able to cope with problems again – to keep things in perspective, deal with things and move on. More importantly, I enjoy life liked I used to – the monkey is still there but I now recognise that he always will be and he no longer frightens me, I am finally comfortable with him, and more importantly with myself!
>
> My lymphoedema is, of course, still there and sometimes is quite troublesome but it no longer rules my life because I am back in control.

In her letter containing this text, Ann included the changes in her self-management for lymphoedema (Table 14.4). The burden of self-care remained but had reduced considerably. This change raises a question of how much this might have improved if acupuncture treatment had continued.

Table 14.4: Ann's self-management of lymphoedema

Self-care activity	Before acupuncture series commenced	After acupuncture series ended
Arm and back massage	≥ 3x/day	2x/day
Arm exercises	≥ 3x/day	2x/day
Moisturising	2x/day	2x/day
Kinesiology taping	3x/week	Rarely (only if has a flare-up)
Wearing compression garments for arm and hand	Daily, for all activity	Only when doing heavy or repetitive work
Wearing compression bra	Every night	Rarely (only if has a flare-up)

What I learned from Ann

I am grateful to Ann for her openness during and after treatment, and for the rich learning experience that treating her afforded me.

Changes to the arm

Objective measures of any changes in the lymphoedema were not available to me. However, it was particularly illuminating to observe how Ann's perception of her condition changed, even when it was not possible to needle in the arm and torso quadrant on the lymphoedema-affected side. Furthermore, the arm responded early on, even when the focus was on clearing blocks to treatment.

The patient's process

Reflecting on Ann's journey through treatment was an important reminder that patients have their own process. My plan for the course of Ann's treatment needed to be responsive to her changes. While the series of acute conditions was disheartening at the time, it appears that these 'setbacks' were an integral part of her healing process. They provided her with an opportunity to make the changes she felt were necessary in her life, shifting her focus from caring for others to caring for herself.

The journey towards finding the CF

Reflecting on Ann's journey also made me reflect on the journey of the practitioner in identifying the CF. Students are often taught that the CF should be identified at the first treatment. I have rarely been able to do this and find that my ability to diagnose the CF emerges over time. Allied to the process of forming the deep therapeutic relationship is that of uncovering the deep constitutional areas of lifelong vulnerability, which we identify as the CF. This process of uncovering takes time, as deeper levels of contact and sharing develop between patient and practitioner. Hence, my journey from initially suspecting Earth to my diagnosis of wood.

Acupuncture as a catalyst for long-term healthcare and resilience

Ann's early progress through treatment illustrates the phenomenon of enabled coping, a person's capacity to manage both physical discomfort and emotional distress.[10,11] This is achieved through the combined actions of relieving symptoms and increasing the person's energy.

Reducing Ann's symptoms freed her energy so that she could take better care of herself. Less burdened by the continuous dragging discomfort of her arm, and by the exhaustion from poor sleep and poor diet, Ann was able to move from symptom to self. Her confidence was restored, and she took control of her life. She actively decided to make lifestyle changes to improve her health and was motivated to be more proactive in dealing with her lymphoedema. Overall, she was able to recover and develop resilience, and was better able to cope with life's challenges.

It was through observing this pattern demonstrated by Ann (as well as others in the lymphoedema research) that I was able to develop the diagram illustrating this process (Figure 14.3).

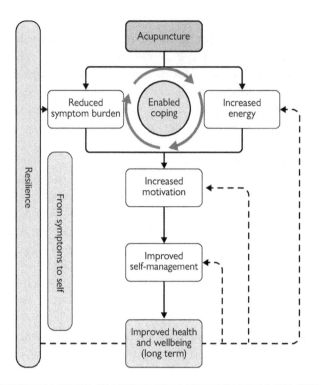

FIGURE 14.3: A MODEL OF ACUPUNCTURE FOR IMPROVING LONG-TERM
HEALTH AND WELLBEING AND DEVELOPING RESILIENCE

CHAPTER SUMMARY

That acupuncture can play a significant role in facilitating improved self-management of chronic conditions is an important message for acupuncturists, patients, and healthcare providers alike. As Ann expressed it:

> The biggest thing that it's done for me is to put me back in balance …it [lymph-oedema] doesn't let you forget the cancer I think, because it's a physical reminder of the fact that at one point in your life you were so very vulnerable. So it's a bit like a monkey sitting on your shoulder; most of the time he's on your shoulder but every now and then he comes and slaps you in the face. I just feel I can slap him back now, you know.[1]

Acknowledgements

Thank you to my colleagues and collaborators on the research team: Teresa Young, Rosemary Lucey, and Professor Jane Maher (Lynda Jackson Macmillan Centre), Professor Christine Moffatt (International Lymphoedema Framework), Anita Wallace (Lymph-oedema Support Network), Elaine Melsome (Mount Vernon Lymphoedema Service),

Dr Charlotte Paterson, and Anthea Asprey (University of Exeter), and Rachel Peckham BSc LicAc MBAcC.

Thank you also to Isobel Cosgrove for her insights into the process of finding the CF. I am especially grateful to Ann.

A brief version of Ann's story was first published in the *European Journal of Oriental Medicine*.[2]

This chapter presents an aspect of independent research commissioned by the National Institute for Health Research (NIHR) under its Research for Innovation, Speculation and Creativity (RISC) Programme (Grant Reference Number PB-PG-0407-10086). The views expressed are those of the author(s) and not necessarily those of the NHS, the NIHR, or the Department of Health.

References

1. de Valois B, Asprey A, Young T 'The monkey on your shoulder': a qualitative study of lymphoedema patients' attitudes to and experiences of acupuncture and moxibustion. Evid. Based Complement. Alternat. Med. 2016;Article ID 4298420.
2. de Valois B, Peckham R Treating the person and not the disease: acupuncture in the management of cancer treatment-related lymphoedema. Eur. J. Orient. Med. 2011;6(6):37–49.
3. de Valois B, Young T, Melsome E Assessing the feasibility of using acupuncture and moxibustion to improve quality of life for cancer survivors with upper body lymphoedema. Eur. J. Oncol. Nurs. 2012;16(3):301–309.
4. Maciocia G The foundations of Chinese medicine: a comprehensive text for acupuncturists and herbalists. Edinburgh: Churchill Livingstone; 1989.
5. Hicks A, Hicks J, Mole P Five element constitutional acupuncture. Edinburgh: Churchill Livingstone; 2004.
6. Lymphoedema Framework Best practice for the management of lymphoedema. International consensus. London: MEP Ltd; 2006.
7. Meeske KA, Sullivan-Halley J, Smith AW, *et al.* Risk factors for arm lymphedema following breast cancer diagnosis in Black women and White women. Breast Cancer Res. Treat. 2009;113(2):383–391.
8. Maciocia G The channels of acupuncture: clinical use of the secondary channels and eight extraordinary vessels. Edinburgh: Churchill Livingstone; 2006.
9. Deadman P, Al-Khafaji M, Baker K A manual of acupuncture. Hove: The Journal of Chinese Medicine; 2007.
10. Price S, Long A, Godfrey M What is traditional acupuncture – exploring goals and processes of treatment in the context of women with early breast cancer. BMC Complement. Altern. Med. 2014;14(1):201.
11. Price S, Long AF, Godfrey M Exploring the needs and concerns of women with early breast cancer during chemotherapy: valued outcomes during a course of traditional acupuncture. Evid. Based. Complement. Alternat. Med. 2013;2013:165891.

Conclusion

I think having cancer is the worst thing to have, but then having people around you who really want to care for you was very, very, very positive. I said it is the best thing that can happen from the worst thing that you have gone through. (A head and neck cancer survivor commenting on acupuncture treatment)

Recovery

Throughout this book, we have seen how acupuncture helps people with a cancer diagnosis recover after cancer treatment. Acupuncture has the capacity to address the physical consequences of treatment and the psychological trauma associated with having cancer. It can reduce the symptom burden, sometimes as much as or more effectively than biomedicine. The rich diversity of acupuncture, and its flexibility in practice, makes it an intervention that can address wide-ranging needs of the growing population of cancer survivors throughout the world.

Renewal

Acupuncture has the potential to do more than deal with symptoms. We can see through the patient stories how many survivors gain a sense of renewal though treatment. In experiencing an increase in energy levels and a greater ability to cope, they are empowered to take control of their health and self-care, facilitating improved wellbeing in the long term. Many can enjoy life again.

Transformation

Acupuncture transforms lives. This is a statement unlikely to be found in the medical or scientific literature! We are all thankful that biomedicine enables the survival of people with cancer. Acupuncture takes that process one step deeper, allowing people to thrive, as well as survive. This is demonstrated many times throughout this book, perhaps most extensively in Ann's case study. Acupuncture helps people live fully again; as so many survivors have said: 'I've got my life back'.

When teaching, I conclude my sessions about using acupuncture in cancer survivorship with the story of Coventry Cathedral:

In 1940, the medieval St Michael's Cathedral in Coventry, a city in the UK's West Midlands, was destroyed by bombing. In 1956, building commenced on a new cathedral as a sign of faith, trust, and hope for the future. Its radical modernist style was nothing like its ancient predecessor, whose ruined shell was preserved as an integral part of its overall design.

This parallels the cancer experience. Life, devastated by cancer diagnosis and treatments, continues, and is reshaped to the 'new normal'. This life, quite unlike the old life, carries with it the reminders of the devastating experience.

One of the glories of the new cathedral is John Piper's Baptistry Window, illustrated on the back cover of this book. This dazzlingly majestic masterpiece is said to represent renewal, while containing the reminder of destruction: 'Each viewer will find their own meaning.' For me, this represents what acupuncture can add to the cancer experience – transformation!

Subject Index

Subheadings in *italics* indicate tables and figures.

Author Index